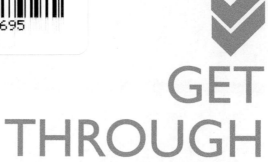

# GET
# THROUGH

**MRCPsych**
**Paper A2:** Mock
Examination Papers

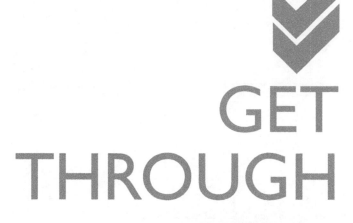

# GET
# THROUGH

## MRCPsych
## Paper A2: Mock
## Examination Papers

**Melvyn WB Zhang** MBBS, DCP, MRCPsych
National HealthCare Group, Singapore

**Cyrus SH Ho** MBBS, DCP, MRCPsych
National University of Singapore

**Roger Ho** MBBS, DPM, DCP, Gdip Psychotherapy,
MMed (Psych), MRCPsych, FRCPC
National University of Singapore

**Ian H Treasaden** MB, BS, LRCP, MRCS, FRCPsych, LLM
West London Mental Health NHS Trust,
Imperial College Healthcare NHS Trust, and
Bucks New University, UK

**Basant K Puri** MA, PhD, MB, BChir, BSc (Hons) MathSci,
DipStat, PG Dip Maths, MMath, FRCPsych, FSB
Hammersmith Hospital and Imperial College London, UK

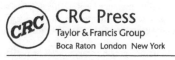

## CRC Press
Taylor & Francis Group
Boca Raton  London  New York

CRC Press is an imprint of the
Taylor & Francis Group, an **informa** business

CRC Press
Taylor & Francis Group
6000 Broken Sound Parkway NW, Suite 300
Boca Raton, FL 33487-2742

© 2016 by Taylor & Francis Group, LLC
CRC Press is an imprint of Taylor & Francis Group, an Informa business

No claim to original U.S. Government works

Printed in Great Britain by Ashford Colour Press Ltd, Gosport, Hants
Version Date: 20160513

International Standard Book Number-13: 978-1-4987-9668-2 (Paperback)

**Visit the Taylor & Francis Web site at**
**http://www.taylorandfrancis.com**

**and the CRC Press Web site at**
**http://www.crcpress.com**

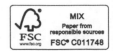

# TABLE OF CONTENTS

# INTRODUCTION

The two volumes that comprise this book consist of over 1800 questions. They correspond to the new format of Paper A of the Royal College of Psychiatrists' examinations, which has been revised recently. The questions (a mixture of both multiple choice questions [MCQs] as well as extended matching items [EMIs]) have been set so as to reflect the type and the current standard of the questions of the examinations, at the time of writing.

A good proportion of the questions featured in this book have been set so as to model against the core themes that have been commonly tested in the examinations in recent years. A good proportion of the questions are also being set based on the core domains of knowledge assessed in the examination. The authors have provided detailed explanation for each of the questions included in the mock examination paper. Readers are provided with references to which they could refer to, if they are in doubt with regards to any of the theoretical concepts. The format of the mock examination paper has been organized such that at least a third of the questions are EMIs, and the remaining two-thirds are MCQs.

We welcome any feedback from those of you who are using this book. Please also let us know further the type of questions you would like to see in the next edition of this book.

We wish to thank all the authors who have contributed to this revision guide-book and mock examination series.

*Melvyn WB Zhang*
*Cyrus SH Ho*
*Roger CM Ho*
*Ian H Treasaden*
*Basant K Puri*

# AUTHORS

**Dr Melvyn Zhang,** MBBS, DCP, MRCPsych, is a specialist registrar/senior resident at the National Healthcare Group, Singapore. He graduated from the National University of Singapore and received his postgraduate training with the Royal College of Psychiatrists (UK). He is currently working with the Institute of Mental Health, Singapore. He has a special interest in the application of web-based and smartphone technologies for education and research and has been published extensively in this field. He is a member of the Public Education and Engagement Board (PEEB), Royal College of Psychiatrists (UK), as well as a member of the editorial board of the *Journal of Internet Medical Research (Mental Health)*. He has published extensively in the *British Medical Journal (BMJ)*, *Lancet Psychiatry* and *BJPsych Advances*.

**Dr Cyrus SH Ho,** MBBS, DCP, MRCPsych, is an associate consultant psychiatrist and clinical lecturer from the National University Hospital, Singapore. He graduated from the National University of Singapore, Yong Loo Lin School of Medicine and subsequently obtained the Diploma of Clinical Psychiatry from Ireland and Membership of the Royal College of Psychiatrists from the United Kingdom. As a certified acupuncturist with the Graduate Diploma in Acupuncture conferred by the Singapore College of Traditional Chinese Medicine, he hopes to integrate both Western and Chinese medicine for holistic psychiatric care. He is actively involved in education and research work. His clinical and research interests include mood disorders, neuropsychiatry, pain studies and medical acupuncture.

**Dr Roger Ho,** MBBS, DPM, DCP, Gdip Psychotherapy, MMed (Psych), MRCPsych, FRCPC, is an assistant professor and consultant psychiatrist at the Department of Psychological Medicine, National University of Singapore. He graduated from the University of Hong Kong and received his training in psychiatry from the National University of Singapore. He is a general adult psychiatrist and in charge of the Mood Disorder Clinic, National University Hospital, Singapore. He is a member of the editorial board of *Advances of Psychiatric Treatment*, an academic journal published by the Royal College of Psychiatrists. His research focuses on mood disorders, psychoneuroimmunology and liaison psychiatry.

**Dr Ian H Treasaden,** MB, BS, LRCP, MRCS, FRCPsych, LLM, is currently an honorary consultant forensic psychiatrist at West London Mental Health NHS Trust and Imperial College Healthcare NHS Trust, as well as a visiting senior lecturer at Bucks New University.

Until 2014, he was a consultant forensic psychiatrist at Three Bridges Medium Secure Unit, West London Mental Health NHS Trust, where he was also the clinical director, College and Coordinating Clinical Tutor for the Charing Cross Rotational Training Scheme in Psychiatry, and tutor in law and ethics and honorary senior clinical lecturer at Imperial College London.

He has authored papers on forensic and general psychiatry, and he is co-author of the books *Textbook of Psychiatry* (3 editions), *Mental Health Law: A Practical Guide* (2 editions), *Emergencies in Psychiatry, Psychiatry: An Evidence-Based Text* and *Revision MCQs and EMIs for the MRCPsych* and the forthcoming *Forensic Psychiatry: Fundamentals and Clinical Practice*.

He qualified in medicine from the London Hospital Medical College, University of London, in 1975 where he was awarded the James Anderson Prize in Clinical Medicine. He undertook training in forensic psychiatry at the Maudsley & Bethlem Royal Hospitals in London and Broadmoor Special Hospital, Berkshire, England between 1982 and 1984.

**Basant K Puri,** MA, PhD, MB, BChir, BSc (Hons) MathSci, DipStat, PG Dip Maths, MMath, FRCPsych, FSB, is based at Hammersmith Hospital and Imperial College London, United Kingdom. He read medicine at St John's College, University of Cambridge. He also trained in molecular genetics at the MRC MNU, Laboratory of Molecular Biology, Cambridge. He has authored or co-authored more than 40 books, including the second edition of *Drugs in Psychiatry* (Oxford University Press, 2013), third edition of *Textbook of Psychiatry* with Dr Ian Treasaden (Churchill Livingston, 2011) and, with the publisher of the present volume, the third edition of *Textbook of Clinical Neuropsychiatry and Neuroscience Fundamentals* with Professor David Moore (2012).

# MRCPSYCH PAPER A2 MOCK EXAMINATION 1: QUESTIONS

## GET THROUGH MRCPSYCH PAPER A2: MOCK EXAMINATION

Total number of questions: 184 (124 MCQs, 60 EMIs)
Total time provided: 180 minutes

**Question 1**
A 30-year-old male, a patient with antisocial personality traits, has been admitted to the inpatient psychiatric ward. The nurses are now complaining much about the difficulties with managing him. They are angry with him and want him to be transferred. Which of the following psychological process is occurring?
 a. Transference
 b. Countertransference
 c. Displacement
 d. Reaction formation
 e. Sublimation

**Question 2**
Based on epidemiological studies in the United Kingdom, which of the following is known to be the most common methodology of committing suicide?
 a. Analgesic overdose
 b. Antidepressant overdose
 c. Antipsychotic overdose
 d. Hanging
 e. Drowning

**Question 3**
In which of the following inherited genetic conditions would dietary restriction and close monitoring of dietary habits be of use in terms of management?
 a. Down's syndrome
 b. Hunter's syndrome
 c. Lesch–Nyhan syndrome
 d. Prader–Willi syndrome
 e. Turner's syndrome

## Question 4

A 25-year-old male has tried two antipsychotic medications, but both of them did not help him with his symptoms. The team has recommended and started him on clozapine, with which he has not experienced much improvement still. He is currently on clozapine 400 mg ON. Based on the guidelines, which one of the following could be used to help him with his symptoms?

a. Continue clozapine treatment but titrate the medication to 1000 mg/day, as he is treatment resistant.
b. Continue clozapine treatment but titrate the medication to a maximum of 900 mg/day, as he is treatment resistant.
c. Consider commencement of intramuscular depot.
d. Consider adding lithium to augment the effects of the drug.
e. Consider adding omega-3 fatty acids to enhance the effectiveness of clozapine.

## Question 5

A 28-year-old male was admitted to the emergency department following a collapse at the shopping mall. A routine CT brain was performed, and the radiologist reported marked atrophy of the caudate nucleus. Which of the following clinical diagnoses would be the most appropriate?

a. Alzheimer's dementia
b. Frontotemporal dementia
c. Huntington's disease
d. Lewy body dementia
e. Parkinsonism-related dementia

## Question 6

Based on your understanding about psychotherapy, which of the following statements about interpersonal therapy is incorrect?

a. It is focused much on the earlier childhood events that the client has undergone.
b. It usually lasts for 16 sessions.
c. It involves dealing with grief.
d. It involves dealing with role transition.
e. It involves dealing with deficits in interpersonal relationships.

## Question 7

A medical student wonders which of the following anxiety disorders would have the earliest age of onset. The correct answer would be

a. Obsessive-compulsive disorder
b. Generalized anxiety disorder
c. Panic disorder
d. Specific phobia
e. Social phobia

## Question 8

Which of the following statements about the aetiology of autism is incorrect?

a. The heritability of autism is around 50%.
b. The male to female ratio is around 4:1.

c. Genetic causative factors might include a positive family history of schizophrenia like psychosis or affective disorder.
d. Maternal use of sodium valproate might cause autism.
e. Perinatal injuries and antenatal infections are aetiological factors that are responsible for the development of autism.

**Question 9**
It is known that some genetic disorders are caused by mutations that have occurred in the body cells and are inherited to the next generation. Which particular type of genetic mutation would not have an impact on the next generation?
a. Frameshift mutation
b. Missense mutation
c. Nonsense mutation
d. Polymorphic mutation
e. Somatic mutation

**Question 10**
In order for the transcribed RNA to be processed for translation, which of the following must happen first?
a. The introns must be separated first.
b. There must be methylation happening to the start end of the transcribed RNA.
c. There must be methylation happening to the tail end of the transcribed RNA.
d. There must be the splicing of the cap of the transcribed RNA.
e. There must be splicing and methylation of the cap of the transcribed RNA.

**Question 11**
Which of the following therapies would be the most effective for a patient with obsessive-compulsive disorder, whose main fears are that of contamination and compulsions are that of repeated washing?
a. Exposure and response prevention
b. Flooding
c. Cognitive analytical therapy
d. Rational emotive behavioural therapy
e. Interpersonal therapy

**Question 12**
A 28-year-old female just had a recent first episode of schizophrenia and she has been concordant with her medications since discharge. Her mother is worried about the long-term side effects of the medication and wanted to know for how long pharmacological treatment should be continued. The correct answer would be
a. For 3 months
b. For 6 months
c. For at least 1 year
d. For more than 2 years
e. For life

## Question 13

In which of the following conditions would there be the presence of eosinophilic inclusion with high amyloid content in the cingulated gyrus?

a. Alzheimer's disease
b. Frontotemporal dementia
c. Vascular dementia
d. Lewy body dementia
e. Parkinsonism dementia

## Question 14

A 22-year-old male would like to have some help with regards to his alcohol addiction issues. He has read about 'disulfiram' and is wondering how this medication can help him. What is the mechanism of action of the drug?

a. It is an aversive agent which inhibits aldehyde dehydrogenase 2 (ALDH2), thus leading to acetaldehyde accumulation after drinking alcohol.
b. It works as a GABA agonist and glutamate antagonist.
c. It inactivates the N-methyl-D-aspartate (NMDA) receptors and helps to prevent calcium influx.
d. It is an opioid antagonist.
e. It is a dopamine antagonist.

## Question 15

For a patient with OCD, whose main obsessions are that of fears of contamination and main compulsions are that of repeated washing, which of the following correctly describes how exposure and response prevention would help?

a. Therapist telling the patient to keep using deep breathing when she is anxious
b. Therapist challenging the automatic thoughts of the patient
c. Therapist telling the patient to intentionally touch something contaminated, but preventing her from doing her usual compulsion
d. Therapist gradually limiting the number of times the patient is allowed to perform the compulsion
e. Therapist advising the patient to consider other forms of distractions when she is compelled to perform her compulsions

## Question 16

Genetic studies have identified that trinucleotide repeat expansions are responsible for the following genetic disorder:

a. Down's syndrome
b. Fragile X syndrome
c. Lewy body dementia
d. Rett syndrome
e. Turner syndrome

## Question 17

A 27-year-old female has bipolar disorder and is currently on treatment. She presented to the emergency department with the following symptoms: nausea, diarrhoea and coarse tremors. She claimed that she has just seen her GP last week

and has just been started on some painkillers for her lower back pain. Which of the following is the likely cause of her current symptoms?
  a. Extrapyramidal side effect
  b. Electrolytes disturbances
  c. Neuroleptic malignant syndrome
  d. Lithium toxicity
  e. Serotonin syndrome

## Question 18
A 55-year-old male suffered from a stroke around a year ago. His wife has noticed that his memory has been deteriorating and he is currently no longer able to manage himself. An MMSE was conducted during the out-patient visit, but he was also referred to a psychologist for an evaluation of his cognitive abilities prior to the onset of the stroke. Which toolkit would be the most helpful in this case?
  a. Luria Test
  b. National Adult Reading Test
  c. Tower of London Test
  d. Verbal fluency test
  e. WAIS-IIII

## Question 19
A 60-year-old female has been referred to the mental health service, as she has been increasingly paranoid. After ruling out medical conditions, she has been diagnosed with late-onset schizophrenia. Which of the following statements about late-onset schizophrenia is true?
  a. Most of those with late-onset schizophrenia are females.
  b. Most of those with late onset schizophrenia are males.
  c. The treatment for late-onset schizophrenia is different from the treatment of early-onset schizophrenia.
  d. Late-onset schizophrenia is not mediated by genetic factors.
  e. Sensory impairment has not been associated with the development of paraphrenia.

## Question 20
Which of the following chromosomal types is characterized by the central location of a centromere?
  a. Acrocentric
  b. Holocentric
  c. Metacentric
  d. Submetacentric
  e. Telocentric

## Question 21
During a routine outpatient review, the core trainee noted that the patient whom he is seeing has tardive dyskinesia. Which of the following treatments would help with the symptoms?
  a. Addition of lithium
  b. Addition of an anticholinergic

c. Increasing the dose of the antipsychotics
d. Reducing the dose of the antipsychotics
e. Stopping all medications

## Question 22
Following a cerebrovascular accident, a 35-year-old male finds that he is unable to read, but when words are spelt out by his wife, he is able to recognize the words immediately. This is most commonly due to a lesion involving which one of the following arteries?
a. Anterior cerebral artery
b. Anterior communicating artery
c. Middle cerebral artery
d. Posterior communicating artery
e. Posterior cerebral artery

## Question 23
As compared to normal individuals, patients who are diagnosed with schizophrenia are more likely to have an increased mortality rate. This rate has been established to be around
a. 1–2 times increased in incidence
b. 2–3 times increased in incidence
c. 4–6 times increased in incidence
d. 6–8 times increased in incidence
e. 10 times increased in incidence

## Question 24
The dermatologist has referred a patient with schizophrenia to see the psychiatrist, as the patient has been having long-standing paranoid delusions and auditory hallucinations. Which of the following antipsychotics would be contraindicated if the patient has a dermatological condition that is photosensitive?
a. Chlorpromazine
b. Clozapine
c. Olanzapine
d. Quetiapine
e. Risperidone

## Question 25
Which of the following is one of the metabolites of serotonin?
a. 5-Hydroxytryptamine
b. 5-Hydroxytrytophan
c. 5-Hydroxyindoleacetic acid
d. 5-Aminoglycine
e. 5-Aminophosphate

## Question 26
Based on previous genetic studies, which of the following statements about autosomal recessive transmission is true?
a. Individuals who marry their siblings are at a high risk.
b. High female-to-female transmission risk.

c. High male-to-male transmission risk.
d. Paternal transmission is implicated.
e. Maternal transmission is implicated.

## Question 27
Studies have shown that there has been an association between deficits in smooth eye pursuit tracking and which of the following psychiatric disorders?
a. Anxiety disorder
b. Bipolar disorder
c. Dementia
d. Depressive disorder
e. Schizophrenia

## Question 28
Which of the following is the main artery that supplies Broca's area?
a. Anterior cerebral artery
b. Basilar artery
c. Middle cerebral artery
d. Posterior cerebral artery
e. Vertebral artery

## Question 29
A 32-year-old female has been diagnosed with bipolar disorder since she was 20. She is now planning to start a family. She is concerned about the risk of foetal malformations as she has been on sodium valproate. The risk associated with the use of sodium valproate in pregnancy has been estimated to be
a. 1 in 100
b. 3 in 100
c. 5 in 100
d. 7 in 100
e. 10 in 100

## Question 30
A neurologist is seeing a patient who has presented to his clinic with sudden onset of coarse and hoarse voice. In addition, he has been having swallowing difficulties. Injury to which of the following cranial nerves should be suspected?
a. Facial
b. Hypoglossal
c. Olfactory
d. Trigeminal
e. Vagus nerve

## Question 31
Based on epidemiology studies, which of the following is the second most common cause of dementia?
a. Alzheimer's dementia
b. Frontotemporal dementia
c. Mixed dementia

d. Lewy body dementia

e. Vascular dementia

**Question 32**

Antipsychotics have been known to have an effect on the corrected QT (QTC) interval. Which of the following antidepressants would also have an effect on the QTC interval?

a. Agomelatine

b. Fluoxetine

c. Paroxetine

d. Sertraline

e. Trazodone

**Question 33**

Based on previous research, the estimated incidence of a child developing schizophrenia if one parent has been affected has been estimated to be

a. 3%

b. 6%

c. 10%

d. 13%

e. 15%

**Question 34**

The tract that connects the Wernicke's and the Broca's area is commonly referred to as the arcuate fasciculus. Lesions involving this particular tract would lead to which one of the following?

a. Broca's aphasia

b. Conduction aphasia

c. Global aphasia

d. Nominal aphasia

e. Wernicke's aphasia

**Question 35**

A forensic psychiatrist was giving a lecture to medical students and asked them to guess the estimated prevalence of antisocial personality disorder amongst the general population in the United Kingdom. The correct answer should be

a. 3%

b. 4%

c. 5%

d. 6%

e. 7%

**Question 36**

An 18-year-old male was involved in a road traffic accident nearly 3 months ago. Currently, he has symptoms of avoidance, hyper-arousal and emotional numbing. Which of the following psychotherapies would be suitable to help him with his condition?

a. Trauma-focused cognitive behavioural therapy

b. Cognitive analytical therapy

c. Brief psychodynamic therapy
d. Supportive therapy
e. Cognitive behavioural therapy

## Question 37
It is not uncommon for adolescents to have suicidal ideations. What has been the estimated proportion of them having suicidal ideations over the past 1 year?
a. 1%
b. 2%
c. 5%
d. 10%
e. 15%

## Question 38
Post-mortem examination of the brains of those who have died from Wernicke's encephalopathy revealed that there have been petechial haemorrhages in all of the following structures expect?
a. Mammillary bodies
b. Periaqueductal grey matter
c. Inferior colliculi
d. Walls of the third ventricle
e. Walls of the lateral ventricle

## Question 39
Roughly what percentage of patients with Wernicke's encephalopathy would have the classical triad of ataxia, ophthalmoplegia and memory disturbances?
a. 2%
b. 4%
c. 6%
d. 8%
e. 10%

## Question 40
Chlorpromazine is known to be one of the first antipsychotics discovered. It is known to be an effective antiemetic as well. This is mainly due to its action on which of the following receptors?
a. Serotonin receptors
b. Noradrenaline receptors
c. Acetylcholine receptors
d. Histamine receptors
e. Dopamine receptors

## Question 41
It is known that the stimulation of the opioid receptors would produce all of the following effects, with the exception of?
a. Analgesia
b. Euphoria

c. Miosis
d. Hypotension
e. Hypertension

## Question 42
Which of the following opiate receptors is responsible for the development of opioid dependence?
a. Mu-receptor
b. Kappa-receptor
c. Delta-receptor
d. Alpha-receptor
e. Beta-receptor

## Question 43
Which of the following structures is part of the brain's reward pathway that has been implicated in addictive behaviours?
a. Basal ganglia
b. Cerebellum
c. Lateral geniculate nucleus
d. Suprachiasmatic nucleus
e. Ventral tegmental area

## Question 44
A 65-year-old male, Simon, has been referred by his nursing home doctor to the old-age psychiatrist for restlessness during sleep. The psychiatrist feels that Simon has signs and symptoms of REM sleep disorder. Which of the following medications would help in his signs and symptoms?
a. Clonazepam
b. Fluoxetine
c. Haloperidol
d. Mirtazapine
e. Lithium

## Question 45
A core trainee is new to forensic psychiatry. He understands from his consultant that a patient was scheduled for a personality testing. He wonders which one of the following psychometric instruments would be able to assess the patient across at least nine different psychopathological domains. The correct answer would be
a. Minnesota Multiphasic Personality Inventory
b. NEO Personality Inventory
c. Wechsler Adult Intelligence Scale (WAIS)-III
d. Eysenck's Personality Questionnaire
e. None of the aforementioned

## Question 46
With regards to the epidemiology of substance misuse in the United Kingdom, which of the following statements in incorrect?
a. The peak age of substance misuse is 15 years old.
b. The male-to-female ratio for substance misuse has been estimated to be 3:1.

c. Fifty percent of the adolescents and young adults in the United Kingdom have taken illicit drugs at some point in time.
d. Twenty percent of them have used illicit substances in the previous month.
e. Five percent of them have used at least a minimum of two substances in the past one month.

## Question 47

Astrocytes are present in the central nervous system (CNS). They are known to be multipolar and their functions involve all the following except:
a. Contributing to the blood–brain barrier
b. Formation of the CNS neuroglial scar tissue
c. Neuromodulation
d. Phagocytosis
e. Structural support of neurons

## Question 48

Which of the following is the main pathological change in patients who have multiple sclerosis?
a. Presence of neuritic plaques
b. Presence of Lewy bodies
c. Presence of demyelination of neurons
d. Presence of gliosis
e. Presence of amyloid plaques

## Question 49

A 38-year-old female has been diagnosed with moderate depression and the consultant psychiatrist is recommending to her antidepressant treatment. She is not keen about antidepressants, as she feels that they would lead to weight gain. Which of the following antidepressants is likely to cause the maximum weight gain?
a. Doxepin
b. Duloxetine
c. Fluoxetine
d. Phenelzine
e. Venlafaxine

## Question 50

A 22-year-old was involved in a road traffic accident around 3 hours ago. He did not sustain any obvious injuries, but now he is complaining that he is having the worst headache of his life. Which of the following would be the most appropriate immediate investigation?
a. CT brain scan
b. MRI brain scan
c. Positron emission tomography (PET)-CT scan
d. Ultrasound carotids
e. X-ray of skull

## Question 51

A core trainee was taking his MRCPsych CASC examination. He noted that on examination, the patient was not able to perform the Luria's hand sequence and also the Go–No–Go Test. Which area of the cerebral cortex is most likely to be implicated given the changes observed?

a. Cerebellum
b. Frontal lobe
c. Parietal lobe
d. Temporal lobe
e. Occipital lobe

### Question 52
Zolpidem is one of the hypnotics that have a relatively short half-life. Its main mechanism of action is on which of the following receptors?

a. Alpha subunit of the GABA receptor
b. Beta subunit of the GABA receptor
c. Gamma subunit of the GABA receptor
d. Omega 1 subunit of the GABA receptor
e. Omega 2 subunit of the GABA receptor

### Question 53
There are various neuronal mechanisms regulating the intake of food. Which of the following is a gut hormone that is released to help in the regulation of intake?

a. Cholecystokinin
b. Corticotrophin
c. Somatostatin
d. Thyrotropin
e. Vasoactive intestinal peptide

### Question 54
Corticotropin release factor (CRF) regulates the release of adrenocorticotropic hormone from the anterior pituitary. Which of the following statements about the clinical relevance of this neuropeptide is incorrect?

a. CRF concentration is elevated in patients who are depressed.
b. With antidepressant treatment, there would be an expected reduction in the CRF level in the cerebrospinal fluid (CSF) of depressed patients.
c. There would be an increase in the ACTH release in depressed patients who are being challenged with CRF.
d. CRH overactivity has a correlation with panic attacks.
e. CRH overactivity has a correlation with alcohol withdrawal.

### Question 55
Alcohol is metabolized by which of the following?

a. Alcohol dehydrogenase
b. Alcohol oxidase
c. Alcohol dihydrogenase
d. Alcohol reductase
e. Microsomal ethanol reduction system

## Question 56

At which of the following ages would an infant display or show the characteristic stranger anxiety syndrome?
a. 3 months
b. 6 months
c. 9 months
d. 12 months
e. 15 months

## Question 57

This refers to the proportion of a defined population that has or has had a given disease (at any time during each individual's lifetime thus far) at a given point in time. Which terminology is correct?
a. Birth defect rate
b. Disease rate at post-mortem
c. Lifetime prevalence
d. Point prevalence
e. Period prevalence

## Question 58

Which of the following is known to be the smallest brain peptide?
a. Cholecystokinin
b. CRF
c. Somatostatin
d. Thyrotropin-releasing factor
e. Vasoactive intestinal peptide

## Question 59

Which of the following medications acts as a partial agonist at a receptor site?
a. Acamprosate
b. Buprenorphine
c. Disulfiram
d. Naltrexone
e. Naloxone

## Question 60

Which of the following is the correct terminology describing a structure whose ultrastructure consists of protein neurofilaments, granular materials, dense core vesicles, microtubule assembly protein, ubiquitin and tau protein?
a. Creutzfeldt–Jakob disease (CJD) plaques
b. Lewy bodies
c. Pick bodies
d. Neuritic plaques
e. None of the aforementioned

### Question 61
These are cells that are present in the nervous system, which aid in the flow of the CSF. Which of the following is correct?
a. Astrocytes
b. Ependyma
c. Microglia
d. Oligodendrocytes
e. Schwann cells

### Question 62
Juvenile delinquency is defined as a law-breaking behaviour engaged by those who are between 10 and 21 years old. The factors associated with juvenile delinquency include all of the following, with the exception of
a. Conduct disorder
b. Parental criminality
c. Low intelligence quotient
d. Inappropriate child rearing
e. Small family size

### Question 63
Based on the social class classification system, a 17-year-old female, Alice, and her family belong to the lower social class. As compared to the upper social class, which one of the following psychiatric conditions would Alice be less susceptible to acquire?
a. Anorexia
b. Anxiety disorder
c. Alcohol dependence
d. Cocaine dependence
e. Depression

### Question 64
It has been known that clozapine has the highest affinity for which of the following dopamine receptors?
a. Dopamine D1
b. Dopamine D2
c. Dopamine D3
d. Dopamine D4
e. Dopamine D5

### Question 65
Somatostatin is a neuropeptide that has an inhibitory effect on growth hormone release. A decrease in its concentration in the CSF is expected for patients with which one of the following conditions?
a. Alzheimer's disease
b. Bipolar disorder – manic phase
c. Generalized anxiety disorder
d. Panic disorder
e. Schizophrenia

## Question 66

Based on epidemiology studies, what percentage of dementia in the general population is due to vascular causes?

a. 5%
b. 10%
c. 15%
d. 25%
e. 30%

## Question 67

Based on the World Health Organization classification system, which one of the following terminologies correctly describes the number of stillbirths and deaths in the first week of life per 1000 live births?

a. Absolute mortality rate
b. Case mortality rate
c. Crude mortality rate
d. Perinatal mortality rate
e. Neonatal mortality rate

## Question 68

Who was responsible for proposing a dimensional rather than a categorical approach to the description of personality?

a. Prichard
b. Schneider
c. Kernberg
d. Eysenck
e. Skinner

## Question 69

Which of the following medications would be the most appropriate for patients who need minimal night sedation, without hangover effects the next day?

a. Clonazepam
b. Lorazepam
c. Diazepam
d. Zolpidem
e. Zopiclone

## Question 70

Which of the following is not one of the structures of the peripheral nervous system?

a. Arachnoid mater
b. Cranial nerves
c. Cell bodies lying outside the CNS
d. Neuronal process
e. Spinal nerve

## Question 71

Which of the following defence mechanisms is considered to be a mature defence mechanism?

a. Sublimation
b. Regression

c. Displacement
d. Repression
e. Denial

## Question 72

All of the following medications would have an interaction with the mood
stabilizer lithium, with the exception of
a. Fluoxetine
b. Diclofenac
c. Ibuprofen
d. Frusemide
e. Thiazides

## Question 73

A 22-year-old female has always been afraid of heights. She is increasingly finding
it difficult to get to work, as her new workplace is on the twentieth floor in central
London. Which of the following psychological therapies would be best indicated
for her?
a. Exposure and response prevention
b. Brief psychodynamic psychotherapy
c. Interpersonal therapy
d. Desensitization therapy
e. Cognitive analytical therapy

## Question 74

Which of the following statements with regards to mortality statistics is
incorrect?
a. The mortality rate refers to the number of deaths in a defined population
during a given period of time divided by the population size during that
period.
b. The mortality rate is sometimes also referred to as the crude mortality rate.
c. The standardized mortality rate is the mortality rate that has been adjusted to
compensate for a potential confounder.
d. The age-standardized mortality rate is the mortality rate that has been adjusted
to compensate for the confounding effect of age.
e. The standardized mortality ratio is obtained from the standardized mortality
rate multiplied by 100.

## Question 75

Thomas and Chess previously described several different kinds of temperaments.
Which of the following is not described by them?
a. Easy
b. Difficult
c. Slow to warm up
d. Avoidant
e. None of the aforementioned

## Question 76

Amongst the following options, which is the commonest defence mechanism used by patients with borderline personality disorder?
a. Splitting
b. Reaction formation
c. Sublimation
d. Displacement
e. Denial

## Question 77

A medical student is curious as to which of the following antipsychotics has the same structure and belongs to the same family as paliperidone. The correct answer would be
a. Clozapine
b. Haloperidol
c. Quetiapine
d. Olanzapine
e. Risperidone

## Question 78

A medical student attached to the Child and Adolescent Mental Health Service (CAMHS) service was keen to know the estimated prevalence of psychiatric disorders in adolescence. The correct answer would be
a. 1%–5%
b. 6%–10%
c. 11%–20%
d. 21%–30%
e. More than 30%

## Question 79

This refers to the proportion of a defined population that has a given disease during a given interval of time. Which terminology is correct?
a. Birth defect rate
b. Disease rate at post-mortem
c. Lifetime prevalence
d. Point prevalence
e. Period prevalence

## Question 80

Which of the following statements with regards to the measures of incidence is incorrect?
a. The alternative name for incidence is that of incidence rate.
b. The alternative name for cumulative incidence is that of risk.
c. Incidence refers to the number of new events during a specified period.
d. Cumulative incidence refers to the proportion of a population who develops the disease of interest in a defined period.
e. Incidence is affected by the disease survival.

## Question 81
The interaction between lamotrigine and which of the following medications would cause a marked increase in the serum levels of lamotrigine?
a. Carbamazepine
b. Lithium
c. Olanzapine
d. Risperidone
e. Sodium valproate

## Question 82
As compared to the normal population, what is the increase in the risk of acquiring schizophrenia for a monozygotic twin?
a. 5 times higher
b. 10 times higher
c. 15 times higher
d. 20 times higher
e. 50 times higher

## Question 83
Based on epidemiological studies, what has been estimated to be the 1-year prevalence of schizophrenia?
a. 0.5%
b. 1%
c. 2%
d. 3%
e. 4%

## Question 84
The lifetime risk of adults in the general population suffering from bipolar disorder has been estimated to be around
a. 1%
b. 3%
c. 6%
d. 8%
e. 10%

## Question 85
Which of the following statements about the epidemiology of depressive disorder is incorrect?
a. The prevalence in the general population has been estimated to be around 2%–5%.
b. The female-to-male ratio is around 1:2.
c. The peak age of onset of the first episode of depression has been estimated to be around 30 years old.
d. Social factors that contribute to depressive disorder include unemployment, separation and divorce.
e. The first major depressive episode in old people is often associated with an undiagnosed neurological disorder.

## Question 86
A 35-year-old male has been advised by his colleagues to seek help from his local GP. His colleagues have noted that he has been more irritable at work recently. He shares that he is having some marital relationship issues with his wife. Which of the following defence mechanisms is in play?
a. Displacement
b. Reaction formation
c. Sublimation
d. Projection
e. Projective identification

## Question 87
Which of the following statements about polyploidy is correct?
a. It refers to the presence of $3n$ number of chromosomes.
b. It refers to the presence of $4n$ number of chromosomes.
c. It refers to the presence of multiple sets of chromosomes.
d. It refers to the replicated nuclear material prior to cellular replication and duplication.
e. It refers to the presence of multiple mutations within a set of chromosomes.

## Question 88
The cerebellum is derived from which of the following primitive brain structures?
a. Telencephalon
b. Diencephalon
c. Mesencephalon
d. Metencephalon
e. None of the aforementioned

## Question 89
Which of the following statements about the epidemiology of schizophrenia is incorrect?
a. The lifetime prevalence of the disorder has been estimated to be around 1.4%.
b. There is an unequal gender ratio, with males being more affected than females.
c. The mean age of onset for men is between 15 and 25 years.
d. The mean age of onset for women is between 25 and 35 years.
e. The association between schizophrenia and low social class is seen as a consequence rather than an aetiology of schizophrenia.

## Question 90
Which of the following chromosomal types is characterized by the presence of a centromere at the tail?
a. Metacentric
b. Acrocentric
c. Holocentric
d. Submetacentric
e. Telocentric

## Question 91
A medical student attending the neurology class has been having difficulties with understanding and comprehending the concepts in neurology. He wonders which of the following is not considered a type of neuroglia in the CNS. The correct answer would be
a. Astrocytes
b. Oligodendrocytes
c. Microglia
d. Ependyma
e. Satellite cells

## Question 92
The main functions of astrocytes include all of the following, with the exception of
a. They help in the support of neurons.
b. They are actively involved in phagocytosis.
c. They are responsible for forming the CNS neuroglial scar tissue.
d. They are responsible for immune control.
e. They help to contribute to the blood–brain barrier.

## Question 93
What are the chances of children acquiring an autosomal recessive disorder, in situations in which both parents carry one abnormal copy of the gene?
a. 10% chance
b. 25% chance
c. 50% chance
d. 75% chance
e. 100% chance

## Question 94
A 22-year-old female is about to enter university. She has come for an assessment at the university health centre, as she is concerned about her chances of acquiring bipolar disorder, given that her sister has it. The chances of her acquiring the disorder would be
a. 1%–2%
b. 4%–6%
c. 5%–15%
d. 20%–25%
e. More than 50%

## Question 95
A lesion involving which of the following would lead to expressive motor aphasia?
a. Frontal operculum on the dominant side
b. Frontal operculum on the non-dominant side
c. Superior mesial region
d. Inferior mesial region
e. Orbital cortex

## Question 96
Prior research has demonstrated that a lesion involving this area could potentially lead to a form of acquired sociopathy. Which of the following is correct?
a. Frontal operculum on the dominant side
b. Frontal operculum on the non-dominant side
c. Superior mesial region
d. Inferior mesial region
e. Orbital cortex

## Question 97
A psychiatrist started a patient on a new antidepressant and he presented back to the clinic with swollen eyes and lips. Which type of adverse drug reaction would this be classified as?
a. Type I
b. Type II
c. Type III
d. Type IV
e. Type V

## Question 98
A lesion involving which of the following structures would lead to akinetic mutism?
a. Frontal operculum on the dominant side
b. Frontal operculum on the non-dominant side
c. Superior mesial region
d. Inferior mesial region
e. Orbital cortex

## Question 99
What is the prevalence of dysthymia in the general population based on epidemiological studies?
a. 2%
b. 4%
c. 5%
d. 8%
e. 10%

## Question 100
A 30-year-old male who has been an inpatient for the past 3 months has been recently commenced on clozapine for his treatment-resistant schizophrenia. The consultant psychiatrist in charge of his case was alerted by the lab, as he has developed neutropenia. Which type of adverse drug reaction would neutropenia be classified under?
a. Type I
b. Type II
c. Type III
d. Type IV
e. Type V

## Question 101
Haloperidol is classified as a typical antipsychotic. Based on the structure of haloperidol, which family or class of antipsychotics would it belong to?
a. Butyrophenes
b. Dibenzodiazepines
c. Benzoxazoles
d. Dibenzothiazepines
e. Substituted benzamides

## Question 102
Studies have shown that there is less than the normal number of chromosomes in some genetic disorders. Which of the following is correct?
a. Down syndrome
b. Fragile X syndrome
c. Huntington disease
d. Turner's syndrome
e. Rett syndrome

## Question 103
Which of the following techniques can be used to detect trinucleotide repeat expansion?
a. ELISA
b. Polymerase chain reaction
c. Southern blot
d. Western blot
e. None of the aforementioned

## Question 104
Which of the following antipsychotics and its related antipsychotic class is correctly matched?
a. Dibenzodiazepines – Clozapine
b. Dibenzothiazepines – Olanzapine
c. Thienobenzodiazepines – Quetiapine
d. Benzoxazoles – Haloperidol
e. Substituted benzamides – Chlorpromazine

## Question 105
A core trainee has been asked to review one of the patients in the gastroenterology ward. The patient was noted to have alcohol withdrawal syndrome. The most recent investigation showed that his liver function test was abnormal. Which one of the following medications would be the most appropriate?
a. Lorazepam
b. Midazolam
c. Diazepam
d. Zopiclone
e. Oxazepam

## Question 106

Chlorpromazine has been known to be the one of the first antipsychotics discovered. It belongs to the class of phenothiazines, but differs from the rest of the members of the same class as it has

a. An aliphatic side chain
b. A piperidine side chain
c. A piperazine side chain
d. A benzamide side chain
e. A quinolone side chain

## Question 107

Which of the following statements regarding discontinuation of antidepressants is incorrect?

a. It would be wise to gradually reduce the dose of antidepressants over a period of 4 weeks.
b. For antidepressants that have a shorter half-life, a shorter period is required for discontinuation.
c. For antidepressants that have a longer half-life, a shorter period is required for discontinuation.
d. If the patient experiences unpleasant discontinuation symptoms, it would be wise to consider reintroduction of the original antidepressant at the dose that was effective.
e. Fluoxetine is a medication with a long half-life, whereas paroxetine is a medication with a short half-life.

## Question 108

A medical student wonders which one of the following would not be caused by a lesion involving the dorsolateral prefrontal cortex. The correct answer would be

a. Impairments in cognitive executive functions
b. Impairments in verbal functioning
c. Impairments in non-verbal functioning
d. Impairments affecting judgements
e. Sociopathy

## Question 109

Which of the following statements pertaining to epidemiological findings with regards to schizoaffective disorder is incorrect?

a. The incidence is not known, but it is known to be relatively less common than schizophrenia.
b. The prevalence is usually less than 1%.
c. It affects women more than men.
d. The age of onset is earlier for women compared with men.
e. The depressive subtype of schizoaffective disorder is more common in elders than in young persons.

## Question 110
Which of the following theorists suggested the 'split mind' of schizophrenia and influenced Bleuler to develop a theory of fragmentation of mental activities in schizophrenia?
a. Kahlbaum
b. Kraepelin
c. Hecker
d. Freud
e. Griesinger

## Question 111
Which of the following statements with regards to the gender differences in people with schizophrenia is false?
a. Men have bimodal peak of incidence.
b. Men have an earlier onset.
c. Men have a higher incidence.
d. Men have a higher mortality.
e. Men have more structural abnormalities.

## Question 112
A 30-year-old motorcyclist suffers from head injuries after a road traffic accident. His partner comments that his memory has become very poor. Which of the following is not a standardized test to assess his memory?
a. Auditory–Verbal Learning Test (AVLT)
b. California Verbal Learning Test (CVLT)
c. Recognition Memory Test (RMT)
d. Wechsler Memory Test (WMT)
e. Weigl Colour–Form Sorting Test (WCFST)

## Question 113
Which of the following symptoms of schizophrenia is not a first-rank symptom?
a. Audible thoughts
b. Delusional perception
c. Formal thought disorder
d. Thought insertion
e. Voices discussing or arguing

## Question 114
A 50-year-old woman was admitted to the ward and the nurses are having difficulty with her. She appears to be arrogant, refuses to follow ward rules and insists to drink alcohol in the ward. She believes that she is a 'special' patient and requests first-class treatment. Her husband mentions that she tends to exploit others and most people try to avoid her. Which defence mechanism is most often used by people with such disorder?
a. Acting out
b. Denial
c. Projection

d. Rationalization
e. Splitting

## Question 115
You are the specialist trainee on the inpatient psychiatric ward. A patient with schizophrenia is admitted to the ward. He complains of having tremor and rigidity after taking haloperidol. The specialist trainee has consulted you on the appropriate scale to assess the potential side effects of antipsychotics. Which of the following scale would you recommend?
a. Abnormal Involuntary Movement Scale
b. Acute Dystonia Rating Scale
c. Barnes Akathisia Scale
d. Extrapyramidal Side-Effect Scale
e. Simpson–Angus Scale

## Question 116
Which of the following movement disorders is not typically associated with schizophrenia?
a. Ambitendency
b. Mannerism
c. Mitgehen and Mitmachen
d. Negativism
e. Stupor

## Question 117
The copying of a genetic message from mRNA to protein via tRNA is known as
a. Coding
b. Degradation
c. Polyadenylation
d. Translation
e. Transcription

## Question 118
Which of the following statements regarding molecular genetics is false?
a. Polymerase chain reaction (PCR) can detect small changes caused by mutations.
b. PCR requires large amounts of DNA.
c. Southern blotting can detect large triplet repeat expansions better than PCR can.
d. Northern blotting involves the analysis of RNA.
e. In expression microarray, mRNA from the tissue is converted into cDNA using reverse transcriptase and the cDNA is then labelled using different-coloured fluorochromes.

## Question 119
What is the increased risk for developing Alzheimer's disease in an individual with ε2/ε4 alleles for the ApoE4 gene compared with the general population?
a. 4 times higher
b. 10 times higher

c. 15 times higher
d. 20 times higher
e. 25 times higher

## Question 120
Which of the following diseases has an autosomal dominant form in a proportion of cases?
a. Hunter syndrome
b. Niemann–Pick disease
c. Hurler's syndrome
d. Parkinson's disease
e. Rett syndrome

## Question 121
Mutations in all of the following genes are associated with the development of schizophrenia, with the exception of
a. Dopamine D3 receptor gene
b. 5-HT2A receptor gene
c. Dysbindin gene
d. Neuregulin gene
e. EPN2

## Question 122
Genetic knockout mice lacking the gene for which of the following neuropeptides have been reported to exhibit narcolepsy?
a. Cholecystokinin
b. Orexin
c. Neuropeptide Y
d. Substance P
e. Vasoactive intestinal peptide

## Question 123
Which of the following statements regarding trisomy and non-disjunction of chromosome 21 is false?
a. Non-disjunction involves failure of a pair of chromosomes to separate normally during one of the meiotic divisions.
b. In 50% of Down syndrome cases, the non-disjunction event occurs during anaphase in maternal meiosis.
c. If non-disjunction occurs during anaphase in maternal meiosis, the result is two maternal copies of chromosome 21 plus one paternal copy.
d. If non-disjunction occurs during maternal meiosis, then the foetus inherits two copies of one of its mother's number 21 chromosomes.
e. Non-disjunction occurs more frequently in maternal meiosis owing to its longer duration compared with paternal meiosis.

**Question 124**
Which of the following statements regarding Klinefelter's syndrome is false?
  a. The incidence is approximately 1 in 1000 newborn boys.
  b. Eighty percent of males with Klinefelter's syndrome have a 47,XXY karyotype with the additional X chromosome being derived equally from meiotic errors in each parent.
  c. Newborn boys with Klinefelter's syndrome are clinically normal.
  d. Fertility in Klinefelter's syndrome is severely impaired, and risks to offspring are usually irrelevant.
  e. Patients with Klinefelter's syndrome usually have affected siblings.

# Extended Matching Items (EMIs)

## Theme: Psychoanalytic concepts
**Lead in:** Please identify the correct answer for each one of the following questions.

**Options:**
  a. Oral phase
  b. Anal phase
  c. Phallic phase
  d. Latency phase
  e. Genital phase

**Question 125**
This usually occurs around 15–30 months of age.

**Question 126**
This is the stage in which pleasure is derived mainly from sucking.

**Question 127**
This is the stage that occurs from around age 5–6 years to the onset of puberty.

**Question 128**
This is the stage in life is which there is a strong resurgence in the sexual drive.

## Theme: Genetics
**Lead in:** Please identify the correct answer for each one of the following questions.

**Options:**
  a. Trisomy 21
  b. Trinucleotide CAG repeats
  c. Trinucleotide CGG repeats
  d. 45X or 46XX
  e. 47XXY
  f. XYY

**Question 129**
Males with this particular karyotype will show an increased rate of petty crime.

**Question 130**
A 22-year-old male has been referred to your service. He has some degree of learning disability and has come to seek help for fertility-related problems. Physical examination shows small testes.

**Question 131**
Fetuses with this particular syndrome tend to develop hydrops fetalis due to delayed maturation of the lymphatic drainage system.

**Question 132**
This is an X-linked dominant disorder with low penetrance. Verbal intelligence quotient (IQ) is usually better than performance IQ.

**Question 133**
This is the most common cytogenetic cause of learning disability.

## Theme: Inheritance of diseases
**Lead in:** Please identify the correct answer for each one of the following questions.
**Options:**
   a. X-linked dominant with trinucleotide repeats
   b. Maternal or paternal non-disjunction
   c. Spontaneous mutation
   d. Non-disjunction of the parental XY
   e. Autosomal dominant
   f. Autosomal recessive

**Question 134**
Patients with this disorder usually have a short stature, seizure (20% of patients), strabismus, mitral valve prolapse and single transverse palmar crease

**Question 135**
Patients with this disorder have a short stature, a low hairline, shield-shaped thorax, widely spaced nipples and coarctation of the aorta.

**Question 136**
Newborn boys with this syndrome are clinically normal. Sexual orientation is usually normal and results in heterosexual marriage. They might be passive and compliant in childhood and aggressive and antisocial past puberty.

**Question 137**
Patients with this syndrome usually have recurrent respiratory infections and death before the age of 10 years.

## Theme: Genetics

**Lead in:** Please identify the correct answer for each one of the following questions.

**Options:**
  a. DISC1
  b. DISC2
  c. Presenilin 1
  d. Presenilin 2
  e. Chromosome 2q
  f. Chromosome 5p
  g. Chromosome 7q
  h. Chromosome 11p
  i. Chromosome 19
  j. Chromosome 20

### Question 138
This gene is associated with the development of schizophrenia and bipolar disorder.

### Question 139
Which of the following pairs of chromosomes are responsible for the development of autism?

### Question 140
This chromosome is involved in the regulation of the amount of brain-derived neurotrophic factor and is also one of the chromosomes responsible for the development of bipolar affective disorder.

### Question 141
Which of the following chromosomes and genes are responsible for the development of Alzheimer's disease?

### Question 142
Which of the following is a chromosome that is implicated in CJD?

## Theme: Neurology and neurological examination

**Options:**
  a. Holmes–Adie pupil
  b. Hutchison's pupil
  c. Argyll Robertson pupil
  d. Horner's syndrome
  e. Papilloedema
  f. Nystagmus

**Question 143**
This particular pathology of the pupil is associated with diminished and absent knee jerk.

**Question 144**
This particular pathology of the eye is associated with rapidly raising unilateral intracranial pressure.

**Question 145**
This particular pathology of the eye is due to an underlying neurosyphilis and diabetes mellitus.

**Question 146**
This particular pathology of the eye is due to an underlying brain stem stroke, pancoast tumour at the lung apex or carotid dissection.

## Theme: Neurology and neurological examination
**Options:**
a. Central cord lesions
b. Anterior cord syndrome
c. Dorsal column loss
d. Brown-Sequard syndrome
e. Total spinal transection

**Question 147**
The common clinical features include preservation of the dorsal column function, but the loss of all other functions. Which spinal cord lesion is this?

**Question 148**
The common clinical features include early sphincter disturbances, spinothalamic loss and loss of pain and temperature sensation. There is noted to be spasticity below the level of the lesions. Which spinal cord lesion is this?

**Question 149**
The common clinical features include ipsilateral spasticity and pyramidal signs. There might also be posterior column sensory loss and contralateral spinothalamic loss. Which spinal cord lesion is this?

**Question 150**
In this condition, there is loss of all functions below the level of the lesion. Which spinal cord lesion is this?

## Theme: Neuroanatomy
**Options:**
a. Anterior corticospinal tract
b. Reticulospinal tract

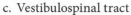

c. Vestibulospinal tract
d. Tectospinal tract
e. Lateral corticospinal tract
f. Rubrospinal tract
g. Lateral reticulospinal tract
h. Descending autonomic fibres
i. Olivospinal tract

**Question 151**
This is a descending anterior tract that is involved in motor functioning.

**Question 152**
This is a descending anterior tract that is involved in voluntary movement.

**Question 153**
This is a descending anterior tract that is involved in muscle tone control.

**Question 154**
This is a descending lateral tract involved in visceral function control.

## Theme: Psychopathology of memory
**Options:**
a. Anterograde amnesia
b. Retrograde amnesia
c. Post-traumatic amnesia
d. Psychogenic amnesia
e. False memory
f. Transient global amnesia
g. Amnestic syndrome
h. Amnesia involving episodic memory

**Lead in:** Select the most appropriate answer for each of the following. Each option may be used once, more than once or not at all.

**Question 155**
The individual usually presents with an abrupt onset of disorientation, loss of ability to encode recent memories and retrograde amnesia for variable duration. The patient, however, still has a remarkable degree of alertness and responsiveness. The episode usually lasts for a few hours and is never repeated.

**Question 156**
This involves confabulation, report of false events and false confessions.

**Question 157**
This is defined as the memory loss from the time of accident to the time that the patient can give a clear account of the recent events.

**Question 158**
This refers to the inability to form new memories.

**Question 159**
This refers to the loss of memory for events that occurred prior to an event or condition.

## Theme: Neuropathology
**Options:**
  a. Alzheimer's disease
  b. Pick's disease
  c. Lewy body dementia
  d. CJD
  e. Punch-drunk syndrome

**Lead in:** Select the most appropriate answer for each of the following. Each option may be used once, more than once or not at all.

**Question 160**
The typical macroscopic changes for this particular condition include cerebral atrophy, ventricular enlargement, perforation of the cavum septum pellucidum and thinning of the corpus callosum. Which condition is this?

**Question 161**
The typical macroscopic changes for this particular condition include selective cerebellar atrophy, generalized cerebral atrophy and also ventricular enlargement. Which condition is this?

**Question 162**
The typical macroscopic changes for this particular condition include selective symmetrical atrophy of the anterior temporal lobes and the frontal lobes, knife-blade gyri and ventricular enlargement. Which condition is this?

**Question 163**
The typical macroscopic changes for this particular condition include global brain atrophy and low brain mass, ventricular enlargement and sulcal widening. Which condition is this?

## Theme: Neuroimaging
**Options:**
  a. X-ray
  b. CT scan
  c. PET scan
  d. Single-photon emission tomography scan
  e. MRI

**Lead in:** Select the most appropriate answer for each of the following. Each option may be used once, more than once or not at all.

**Question 164**
The main use of this form of imaging is for trauma assessment.

**Question 165**
One of the main uses of this form of imaging is for neuropsychiatric research. It is able to pick up shifts of intracranial pressure and cerebral infarction.

**Question 166**
This particular form of imaging can give information about metabolic changes.

**Question 167**
This particular form of imaging is of use in conditions in which the onset of symptoms is being studied.

**Question 168**
This is the preferred form of neuroanatomical imaging for clinical and research studies that require high-resolution neuroanatomical imaging.

## Theme: Psychiatric epidemiology – concepts
**Options:**
   a. Incidence
   b. Prevalence
   c. Chronicity
   d. Point prevalence
   e. Incidence rate
   f. Cumulative incidence
   g. Risk

**Lead in:** Select the most appropriate answer for each of the following. Each option may be used once, more than once or not at all.

**Question 169**
This term is also known as risk.

**Question 170**
This term is also known as incidence rate.

**Question 171**
This term takes into account both the incidence and the chronicity.

**Question 172**
This refers to the average duration of an illness condition.

**Question 173**
This terminology refers to the rate of occurrence of new cases of the disease in a defined population over a given period of time.

**Question 174**
This terminology refers to the proportion of a defined population that has disease at a given time.

## Theme: Psychiatric epidemiology

**Options:**
  a. Standardized mortality rate
  b. Age-standardized mortality rate
  c. Standardized mortality ratio
  d. Life expectancy
  e. Standardized morbidity rate
  f. Age-standardized morbidity rate
  g. Standardized morbidity ratio
  h. Relative risk
  i. Attributable risk
  j. Absolute risk reduction
  k. Relative risk reduction
  l. Number needed to treat
 m. Odd ratio

**Lead in:** Select the most appropriate answer for each of the following. Each option may be used once, more than once or not at all.

**Question 175**
This terminology is also otherwise known as the risk difference of absolute excess risk.

**Question 176**
This refers to the ratio of the odds that subjects in the disease group were exposed to the factor to the odds that subjects in the control group were exposed to the factor.

**Question 177**
This refers to the ratio of the incidence of the disease in people exposed to that risk factor to the incidence of the disease in people not exposed to the same risk factor.

**Question 178**
This refers to the mortality rate that is adjusted to compensate for a confounder.

**Question 179**
This terminology refers to the ratio of the observed standardized mortality rate derived from the population being studied to the expected standardized mortality rate derived from a comparable standard population.

### Question 180
This terminology refers to the mean length of time that an individual can be expected to live based on the assumption that the mortality rates used remain constant.

## Theme: Psychotherapy

**Options:**
   a. Acting out
   b. Denial
   c. Displacement
   d. Intellectualization
   e. Projection
   f. Rationalization
   g. Repression
   h. Sublimation

**Lead in:** A 55-year-old man who was working in a multinational company as a manager, with a background of poorly controlled diabetes, underwent a right below-knee amputation 3 months ago because of complications of his diabetes. Since then, he has been feeling depressed with passive thoughts of suicide. Select the most appropriate defence mechanism for each of the following situations. Each option may be used once, more than once or not at all.

### Question 181
He denies being depressed and says that everything is fine. When the psychiatrist asks him how he feels about the amputation, he always evades the question and talks about something else.

### Question 182
He becomes angry with the psychiatrist for asking him questions about his work and family situation. He says that the psychiatrist deliberately makes his mood worse and there is nothing that can be done to help him.

### Question 183
He is made to resign from work, as he cannot keep up to the demands of his job. He overhears colleagues saying sarcastic remarks about him. When he is at home, he scolds his wife badly for a trivial matter.

### Question 184
Two months later, after adequate pharmacological and psychotherapy treatment, he appears to be coping well and tells his psychiatrist that he has decided to help out in a volunteer social service catering to support the disabled.

## GET THROUGH MRCPSYCH PAPER A2: MOCK EXAMINATION

**Question 1 Answer: b, Countertransference**
*Explanation*: This is commonly referred to as the therapist's own feelings, emotions and attitudes towards his or her patient.

*Reference*: Puri BK, Hall A, Ho R (2014). *Revision Notes in Psychiatry*. London: CRC Press, p. 132.

**Question 2 Answer: d, Hanging**
*Explanation*: It is essential to note that psychiatric patients tend to use violent methods such as hanging, shooting and jumping from heights. For the general population, two thirds of the British men and one third of the British women commit suicide by hanging or via inhalation of vehicular exhaust fumes. Drowning is the most common amongst older people.

*Reference*: Puri BK, Hall A, Ho R (2014). *Revision Notes in Psychiatry*. London: CRC Press, p. 269.

**Question 3 Answer: d, Prader–Willi syndrome**
*Explanation*: The commonest presentation for the disorder would be that of irresistible hunger drive and also excessive skin picking with associated compulsion and anxiety. Given that insatiable appetite is a core diagnostic feature, dietary restriction should be used as it would help to reduce obesity.

*Reference*: Puri BK, Hall A, Ho R (2014). *Revision Notes in Psychiatry*. London: CRC Press, p. 675.

**Question 4 Answer: b, Continue clozapine treatment, but titrate the medication to a maximum of 900 mg/day as he is treatment resistant.**
*Explanation*: Clozapine is indicated usually for patients with schizophrenia that is not well controlled despite the sequential usage of two or more of the antipsychotics, of which one should be atypical, and the medication should have

been used for the past 6–8 weeks. The average dose in the UK is around 450 mg/day. Response could be seen in the range 150–900 mg/day. Commencement of an intramuscular depot, addition of lithium and addition of Omega 3 Fatty acids are unlikely to be helpful in his condition.

*Reference*: Puri BK, Hall A, Ho R (2014). *Revision Notes in Psychiatry*. London: CRC Press, p. 366.

### Question 5 Answer: c, Huntington's disease
*Explanation*: This is defined as a genetic disorder that has the following features: continuous involuntary movements and a slowly progressive dementia. CT scan might show a reduction in the volume of the caudate nucleus.

*Reference*: Puri BK, Hall A, Ho R (2014). *Revision Notes in Psychiatry*. London: CRC Press, p. 760.

### Question 6 Answer: a, It is focused much on earlier childhood events that the client has undergone.
*Explanation*: Interpersonal therapy deals with the following areas: grief, interpersonal disputes, role transitions and interpersonal role deficits. The main objective is to create a therapeutic environment with meaningful therapeutic relationship and the ability to recognize the client's underlying attachment needs.

*Reference*: Puri BK, Hall A, Ho R (2014). *Revision Notes in Psychiatry*. London: CRC Press, p. 341.

### Question 7 Answer: e, Social phobia
*Explanation*: Social phobia would have the earliest age of onset. Based on epidemiological studies, generalized anxiety disorder would first occur in the 20s; panic disorder at the age of 15–24 years and social phobia usually at the ages of 11–15 years.

*Reference*: Puri BK, Hall A, Ho R (2014). *Revision Notes in Psychiatry*. London: CRC Press, p. 291.

### Question 8 Answer: a, The heritability of autism is around 50%.
*Explanation*: The heritability of autism is around 90% instead of 50%. The male-to-female ratio is estimated to be 4:1. Autism accounts for around 25%–60% of all autistic disorders. There have not been studies demonstrating an association between autistic disorder and any socioeconomic status. The recurrent rate in siblings is roughly 3% for narrowly defined autism but is about 10%–20% for milder variants. Perinatal injuries (such as maternal bleeding after the first trimester or meconium in the amniotic fluid) or antenatal infections or the use of sodium valproate in pregnancy might result in the development of autism.

*Reference*: Puri BK, Hall A, Ho R (2014). *Revision Notes in Psychiatry*. London: CRC Press, p. 623.

**Question 9 Answer: e, Somatic mutation**
*Explanation*: A mutation is a change in the DNA sequence that can be transmitted from the parent cell to its daughter cells. There are two main types of mutations: germline mutation and somatic mutation. A somatic mutation occurs after fertilization and is only present in a subpopulation of somatic cells. This differs from a germline mutation, which refers to a mutation that originates from a gamete that is then fused with another gamete during fertilization, thus leading to conception of an individual who has mutation in every cell.

*Reference*: Puri BK, Hall A, Ho R (2014). *Revision Notes in Psychiatry*. London: CRC Press, p. 263.

**Question 10 Answer: a, The introns must be separated first.**
*Explanation*: Once transcription has taken place, it is followed by splicing and nuclear transport, so that the information (minus that from the introns) then exists in the cytoplasm of the cell on messenger RNA. The splicing out of the introns is guided by the recognition of the GT and AG dinucleotides that mark the beginning and the end of the intron.

*Reference*: Puri BK, Hall A, Ho R (2014). *Revision Notes in Psychiatry*. London: CRC Press, p. 262.

**Question 11 Answer: a, Exposure and response prevention**
*Explanation*: Based on the NICE guidelines, for the initial treatment of OCD, exposure and response prevention (up to 10 therapist hours per client) should be offered. For adults with mild-to-moderate functional impairment, more intensive CBT (including ERP) (more than 10 therapist hours per client) would be recommended.

*Reference*: Puri BK, Hall A, Ho R (2014). *Revision Notes in Psychiatry*. London: CRC Press, p. 418.

**Question 12 Answer: c, For at least one year**
*Explanation*: In the maintenance phase of schizophrenia, antipsychotic drugs should be continued for at least 1 or 2 years after the last acute episode. It is still important to continue to monitor for adverse effects related to the treatment. Withdrawal of antipsychotic medication should be gradual and monitored. Following the withdrawal of drugs, patients should be monitored for the signs of relapse for at least 2 years after the last acute episode.

*Reference*: Puri BK, Hall A, Ho R (2014). *Revision Notes in Psychiatry*. London: CRC Press, p. 364.

**Question 13 Answer: d, Lewy body dementia**
*Explanation*: Lewy bodies are commonly located in the cingulated gyrus, the cortex and the substantial nigra. They contain eosinophilic inclusion with

high amyloid content, but with the absence of tau pathology. Lewy bodies are alpha-synuclein and ubiquitin positive. Alpha-synuclein is an aggregated and insoluble protein, which is pathognomonic of Lewy body dementia and idiopathic Parkinson's disease.

*Reference*: Puri BK, Hall A, Ho R (2014). *Revision Notes in Psychiatry*. London: CRC Press, p. 702.

### Question 14 Answer: a, It is an aversive agent which inhibits ALDH2, thus leading to acetaldehyde accumulation after drinking alcohol

*Explanation*: The medication works as an aversive agent, and the doctor who prescribes has to make sure that the patient has not consumed alcohol over the past 1 day prior to commencement. It would inhibit ALDH2 and this would lead to an accumulation of acetaldehyde, which would result in unpleasant side effects on consumption of alcohol. Aversive effects include flushing, headache, palpitations, tachycardia, nausea and vomiting with ingestion of small amounts of alcohol, and air hunger, arrhythmias and severe hypotension with large amounts of alcohol. These effects occur 10–30 minutes after drinking and are dose dependent. The reaction to alcohol discourages the person from drinking and reduces the number of days spent on drinking.

*Reference*: Puri BK, Hall A, Ho R (2014). *Revision Notes in Psychiatry*. London: CRC Press, p. 524.

### Question 15 Answer: c, Therapist telling the patient to intentionally touch something contaminated, but preventing her from doing her usual compulsion

*Explanation*: In this example, in order to prevent the response of excessive washing, the therapist should tell the patient to intentionally touch something contaminated, but prevent her from doing her usual compulsions.

*Reference*: Puri BK, Hall A, Ho R (2014). *Revision Notes in Psychiatry*. London: CRC Press, p. 422.

### Question 16 Answer: b, Fragile X syndrome

*Explanation*: The clinical features of the fragile X syndrome are due to the failure of the FMR1 gene transcription due to hyper-methylation, thus resulting in the absence of the FMR1 gene protein. Normal number of repeats is 30, and the repeats for carriers range from 55 to 2000. Full mutation with more than 200 repeats leads to hyper-methylation at the gene.

*Reference*: Puri BK, Hall A, Ho R (2014). *Revision Notes in Psychiatry*. London: CRC Press, p. 666.

### Question 17 Answer: d, Lithium toxicity

*Explanation*: The presentation is very likely lithium toxicity. It is important to note that the therapeutic index of lithium is low, and therefore regular lithium level monitoring would be required. At a toxic dose of above 2 mM, the following effects could occur: hyper-reflexia, hyperextension of all the limbs, toxic psychosis, convulsions, syncope, oliguria, circulatory failure, coma and death.

*Reference*: Puri BK, Hall A, Ho R (2014). *Revision Notes in Psychiatry*. London: CRC Press, p. 254.

### Question 18 Answer: b, National Adult Reading Test
*Explanation*: The National Adult Reading Test is a reading test consisting of phonetically irregular words that have to be read aloud by the subject. If a patient suffers deterioration in intellectual abilities, their premorbid vocabulary may remain less affected or even unaffected. The NART thus could be used to estimate the premorbid IQ.

*Reference*: Puri BK, Hall A, Ho R (2014). *Revision Notes in Psychiatry*. London: CRC Press, p. 96.

### Question 19 Answer: a, Most of those with late-onset schizophrenia are females.
*Explanation*: It has been established that late-onset schizophrenia is actually more prevalent in females. Individuals with late-onset psychosis are likely to be unmarried and have a lower reproductive rate as compared to controls. Late-onset schizophrenia is partly genetically determined, but the part played by inheritance requires further investigation and research. In a subset of patients, there is a history of those who have long-standing paranoid personalities, which are thought to predispose to the development of the disorder in the old age. Hearing impairment and sensory impairment have been associated with the development of paranoid symptoms.

*Reference*: Puri BK, Hall A, Ho R (2014). *Revision Notes in Psychiatry*. London: CRC Press, p. 712.

### Question 20 Answer: a, Metacentric
*Explanation*: Metacentric chromosome refers to a chromosome with a centrally or almost centrally positioned centromere. This should be distinguished from acrocentric chromosome, in which the centromere is very near to one end.

*Reference*: Puri BK, Hall A, Ho R (2014). *Revision Notes in Psychiatry*. London: CRC Press, p. 259.

### Question 21 Answer: d, Reducing the dose of the antipsychotics
*Explanation*: Tardive dyskinesia refers to a wide variety of movements that can occur, such lip smacking or chewing, tongue protrusion, choreiform hand movements (pill rolling or piano playing) and pelvic thrusting. The severe movements involving the facial muscles might lead to much difficulty with speaking, eating or breathing. Movements are usually worst when under stressful situations. These movements tend to be more common in elderly women and those with affective illness. In order to reduce the side effects, anti-cholinergic (if prescribed) should be stopped. The existing dose of the antipsychotics could

be reduced. If a typical antipsychotic is used, it might be better to change to an atypical drug. Previous research has shown that clozapine is the antipsychotic most likely to be associated with resolution of these symptoms.

*Reference*: Taylor D, Paton C, Kapur S (2009). *The Maudsley Prescribing Guidelines* (10th edition). London: Informa Healthcare, p. 97.

**Question 22 Answer: e, Posterior cerebral artery**
*Explanation*: Posterior cerebral artery causes cortical blindness and denial of disability and sometimes alexia without agraphia. It is noted that the occlusion of the left posterior cerebral artery leads to infarction of the medial aspect of the left occipital lobe and the splenium of the corpus callosum. Thus, after the stroke, the lesion in the splenium prevents the transfer of information from the right to the left side. The primary language area is thus disconnected from the incoming visual information. Hence, as a consequence, he is unable to comprehend any written material even though he is able to write.

*Reference*: Puri BK, Hall A, Ho R (2014). *Revision Notes in Psychiatry*. London: CRC Press, p. 493.

**Question 23 Answer: b, 2–3 times increase in incidence**
*Explanation*: Based on the epidemiological studies of schizophrenia and schizoaffective disorder, it has been demonstrated that the mortality rates are at least two times higher than the general population as a result of suicide or metabolic diseases. The life expectancy is 10 years less than that of the general population. Approximately 10% do commit suicide. Risk factors include male gender, age younger than 30 years, university education, paranoia, depression and substance abuse.

*Reference*: Puri BK, Hall A, Ho R (2014). *Revision Notes in Psychiatry*. London: CRC Press, p. 284.

**Question 24 Answer: a, Chlorpromazine**
*Explanation*: Chlorpromazine would be contraindicated as it would lead to the side effects such as photosensitization, hypothermia or pyrexia, allergic reactions and even neuroleptic malignant syndrome. The adverse reactions have been believed to be caused by the antagonistic action on the neurotransmitters, including dopamine, acetylcholine, adrenaline and noradrenaline and histamine.

*Reference*: Puri BK, Hall A, Ho R (2014). *Revision Notes in Psychiatry*. London: CRC Press, p. 252.

**Question 25 Answer: c, 5-hydrooxyindoleacetic acid**
*Explanation*: 5-HIAA is one of the metabolites of serotonin and it is transferred out of the brain via the CSF or blood. The concentration of 5-HIAA in the CSF correlates with the concentration in the brain tissue. CSF 5-HIAA is a useful index

of the central 5-HIAA turnover. Low CSF 5-HIAA is found in patients with violent behaviours and untreated depression.

*Reference*: Puri BK, Hall A, Ho R (2014). *Revision Notes in Psychiatry*. London: CRC Press, p. 228.

**Question 26 Answer: a, Individuals who marry their siblings are at high risk**
*Explanation*: It has been noted that the rarer the disorder, the more likely it is that the parents are related for an autosomal recessive condition. Heterozygous individuals are generally carriers who do not manifest the abnormal phenotypic trait. The disorder tends to miss generations but the affected individual in a family tends to be found amongst siblings – horizontal transmission takes place. When both parents carry one abnormal copy of the gene, there is a 25% chance of a child inheriting both mutations, hence expressing the disease.

*Reference*: Puri BK, Hall A, Ho R (2014). *Revision Notes in Psychiatry*. London: CRC Press, p. 269.

**Question 27 Answer: e, Schizophrenia**
*Explanation*: Previous research has shown that there is a reduction in rapid visual processing for psychotic disorder. There has been noted to be other cognitive impairments in individuals diagnosed with schizophrenia, including deficits involving learning and memory, working memory, executive functioning, attentional deficits and functional deficits.

*Reference*: Puri BK, Hall A, Ho R (2014). *Revision Notes in Psychiatry*. London: CRC Press, p. 363.

**Question 28 Answer: c, Middle cerebral artery**
*Explanation*: Broca's area is the core of the frontal operculum on the dominant (usually left) side and consists of areas 44 and 45. A lesion in this region could lead to expressive (motor) aphasia. The blood supply is derived from the middle cerebral artery.

*Reference*: Puri BK, Hall A, Ho R (2014). *Revision Notes in Psychiatry*. London: CRC Press, p. 177.

**Question 29 Answer: a, 1 in 100**
*Explanation*: Valproate has been known to be one of the most teratogenic mood stabilizers and the NICE guidelines has not recommended it for pregnancy, as the incidence of foetal death has been estimated to be around 1 in 100. The current guidelines state that for women who are trying to conceive and require valproate, folate should be prescribed.

*References*: Puri BK, Hall A, Ho R (2014). *Revision Notes in Psychiatry*. London: CRC Press, p. 561; Taylor D, Paton C, Kapur S (2009). *The Maudsley Prescribing Guidelines* (10th edition). London: Informa Healthcare, p. 143.

### Question 30 Answer: e, Vagus nerve

*Explanation*: The clinical significance of the vagus nerve is that it aids in swallowing and speech. The motor component of the nerve supplies the soft palate, pharynx, larynx and the upper oesophagus. The sensory component of the nerve supplies the pharynx, larynx, oesophagus and external ear. It has also an autonomic component, which is parasympathetic in nature and supplies the thoracic and abdominal vessels.

*Reference*: Puri BK, Hall A, Ho R (2014). *Revision Notes in Psychiatry*. London: CRC Press, p. 165.

### Question 31 Answer: b, Vascular dementia

*Explanation*: Based on epidemiology studies, vascular dementia has been shown to be the second most common type of dementia. The prevalence of AD has been estimated to be around 50%, whereas the prevalence of vascular dementia is around 20%.

*Reference*: Puri BK, Hall A, Ho R (2014). *Revision Notes in Psychiatry*. London: CRC Press, p. 300.

### Question 32 Answer: e, Trazodone

*Explanation*: Trazodone does have an effect on QTC and it might cause prolongation of the QTC interval. It might cause a decrease in the heart rate more commonly, although an increase can also occur. It could result in significant postural hypotension. Fluoxetine, paroxetine and sertraline do not affect the QTC interval.

*Reference*: Taylor D, Paton C, Kapur S (2009). *The Maudsley Prescribing Guidelines* (10th edition). London: Informa Healthcare, p. 221.

### Question 33 Answer: d, 13%

*Explanation*: The approximate risk is 13%. If both parents are affected, then the approximate risk will be 46%.

*Reference*: Puri BK, Hall A, Ho R (2014). *Revision Notes in Psychiatry*. London: CRC Press, p. 358.

### Question 34 Answer: b, Conduction aphasia

*Explanation*: Damage to the arcuate fasciculus results in a conduction dysphasia in which the person cannot repeat what is said by another. Comprehension and verbal fluency remain intact. In contrast, global dysphasia usually results from a global left hemispheric dysfunction. For receptive dysphasia, the damage incurred to the Wernicke's area disrupts the ability to comprehend language, either written or spoken. In addition to the loss of comprehension, the person also is unaware that his or her dysphasic speech is difficult for others to follow.

For expressive dysphasia, damage to the Broca's area results in the loss of rhythm, intonation and grammatical aspects of speech. Comprehension is normal, and the person is aware that his or her speech is difficult for others to follow, resulting in marked distress and frustration. Speech is slow and hesitant, and often lacks connecting words.

*Reference*: Puri BK, Hall A, Ho R (2014). *Revision Notes in Psychiatry*. London: CRC Press, p. 105.

### Question 35 Answer: a, 3%
*Explanation*: The prevalence of antisocial personality disorder amongst individuals in the community has been estimated to be around 0.6%–3.0%. There are more males affected with this particular personality disorder as compared to females, with a gender ratio of 6:1.

*Reference*: Puri BK, Hall A, Ho R (2014). *Revision Notes in Psychiatry*. London: CRC Press, p. 295.

### Question 36 Answer: a, Trauma-focused cognitive behaviour therapy
*Explanation*: The NICE guidelines recommends that trauma-focused CBT should be offered to people with severe PTSD within 3 months of the trauma with fewer sessions in the first month after the trauma. The duration of the therapy will be 8–12 sessions, with at least 1 session per week.

*Reference*: Puri BK, Hall A, Ho R (2014). *Revision Notes in Psychiatry*. London: CRC Press, p. 428.

### Question 37 Answer: d, 10%
*Explanation*: Based on epidemiology studies, it has been estimated that around 10% of adolescents would have had suicidal ideations over the past 1 year.

*Reference*: Puri BK, Hall A, Ho R (2014). *Revision Notes in Psychiatry*. London: CRC Press, p. 286.

### Question 38 Answer: e, Walls of the lateral ventricle
*Explanation*: Wernicke's encephalopathy is considered to be a medical emergency and it should be treated with intravenous thiamine and other B vitamins. Post-mortem examination has revealed that all of the aforementioned areas are affected, including the floor of the fourth ventricle. It is important to note that Wernicke's encephalopathy and Korsakov's psychosis have overlapping pathology; 80% of untreated Wernicke's encephalopathy would convert.

*Reference*: Puri BK, Hall A, Ho R (2014). *Revision Notes in Psychiatry*. London: CRC Press, p. 517.

**Question 39 Answer: e, 10%**
*Explanation*: The important clinical features would include ophthalmoplegia, nystagmus, ataxia and clouding of consciousness. Peripheral neuropathy may also be present at times. Around 10% of patients would have the classical triad. Wernicke's encephalopathy is caused by severe deficiency of thiamine (Vitamin B1), which is usually caused by alcohol abuse in Western countries. Other causes would include lesions of the stomach causing mal-absorption, lesions of the duodenum causing mal-absorption, lesions of the jejunum causing mal-absorption, hyperemesis and starvation.

*Reference*: Puri BK, Hall A, Ho R (2014). *Revision Notes in Psychiatry*. London: CRC Press, p. 517.

**Question 40 Answer: e, Dopamine receptors**
*Explanation*: Chlorpromazine was one of the first antipsychotic medications discovered in the 1950s. It has its action mainly on the dopamine receptors. It is important to note that all clinically effective antipsychotic drugs occupy a substantial proportion of the D2 receptors in the brain (70%–80%).

*Reference*: Puri BK, Hall A, Ho R (2014). *Revision Notes in Psychiatry*. London: CRC Press, p. 361.

**Question 41 Answer: e, Hypertension**
*Explanation*: Stimulation of the opiate receptors would usually produce analgesia, euphoria, miosis, hypotension, bradycardia and respiratory depression. The binding of the morphine to the mu receptors inhibits the release of GABA from the nerve terminal, reducing the inhibitory effect of GABA on the dopaminergic neurons. The increased activation of the dopaminergic neurons in the nucleus accumbens and the ventral tegmental areas that are part of the brain's reward pathway, and the release of the dopamine into the synapse result in sustained activation of postsynaptic membrane. Continued activation of the dopaminergic reward pathway leads to feelings of euphoria.

*Reference*: Puri BK, Hall A, Ho R (2014). *Revision Notes in Psychiatry*. London: CRC Press, p. 531.

**Question 42 Answer: a, Mu-receptor**
*Explanation*: The main types of opioid receptors are mu, kappa and delta receptors. The mu receptor is believed to be essential for the development of opioid dependence. It is potassium channel linked and inhibits adenylate cyclase. When opiate binds to the mu receptors, it inhibits the release of GABA from the nerve terminals, reducing the inhibitory effect of GABA on the dopaminergic neurons. The increased activation of the dopaminergic neurons in the nucleus accumbens and the ventral tegmental areas that are part of the brain's reward pathway, and the release of the dopamine into the synapse result in sustained activation of postsynaptic membrane. Continued activation of the dopaminergic reward pathway leads to feelings of euphoria.

*Reference*: Puri BK, Hall A, Ho R (2014). *Revision Notes in Psychiatry*. London: CRC Press, p. 531.

### Question 43 Answer: e, Ventral tegmental area

*Explanation*: It has been shown that the increased activation of dopaminergic neurons in the nucleus accumbens and also the ventral tegmental area, which are part of the brain's intrinsic reward pathway, is responsible for the addictive behaviour. Activation would cause the release of increased amount of dopamine into the synapse, resulting in sustained activation of the postsynaptic membrane. The continued activation of the dopaminergic reward pathway leads to feelings of euphoria.

*Reference*: Puri BK, Hall A, Ho R (2014). *Revision Notes in Psychiatry*. London: CRC Press, p. 531.

### Question 44 Answer: a, Clonazepam

*Explanation*: For this condition, psychopharmacological treatment would be indicated if symptoms impairing sleep have lasted for more than two nights per week. Benzodiazepines such as clonazepam, anticonvulsants such as gabapentin and dopamine agonists such as levodopa might be of help. It is always essential to identify any organic causes and the organic causes should be treated first prior to the consideration of psychotropic medications.

*Reference*: Puri BK, Hall A, Ho R (2014). *Revision Notes in Psychiatry*. London: CRC Press, p. 619.

### Question 45 Answer: a, Minnesota Multiphasic Personality Inventory

*Explanation*: The final version of the MMPI contains over 550 questions related to attitudes, emotional reactions, physical symptoms and psychological symptoms. Scores are derived from several scales, which include the lie/social desirability, frequency, correction/defensiveness, hypochondriasis, depression, hysteria, psychopathic deviance, paranoia, schizophrenia, hypomania, social introversion–extraversion and masculinity–femininity.

*Reference*: Puri BK, Hall A, Ho R (2014). *Revision Notes in Psychiatry*. London: CRC Press, pp. 48–49.

### Question 46 Answer: a, The peak age of substance misuse is 15 years

*Explanation*: Based on nation-wide epidemiological studies, the peak age of substance misuse is 20 years.

*Reference*: Puri BK, Hall A, Ho R (2014). *Revision Notes in Psychiatry*. London: CRC Press, p. 296.

### Question 47 Answer: c, Neuromodulation

*Explanation*: Astrocytes are known to be multipolar and they serve all the aforementioned functions, with the exception of neuromodulation. There are two types of astrocytes or astroglia: fibrous astrocytes and protoplasmic astrocytes.

*Reference*: Puri BK, Hall A, Ho R (2014). *Revision Notes in Psychiatry*. London: CRC Press, p. 176.

### Question 48 Answer: c, Presence of demyelination of neurons
*Explanation*: In multiple sclerosis, there is demyelination of the neurons. Schwann cells are usually part of myelinated peripheral nerves and they do encircle some unmyelinated peripheral nerve axons as well.

*Reference*: Puri BK, Hall A, Ho R (2014). *Revision Notes in Psychiatry*. London: CRC Press, p. 177.

### Question 49 Answer: a, Doxepin
*Explanation*: Doxepin, via the blockage of the histamine H1 receptors, would cause marked weight gain as well as increased drowsiness and sedation.

*Reference*: Puri BK, Hall A, Ho R (2014). *Revision Notes in Psychiatry*. London: CRC Press, p. 254.

### Question 50 Answer: a, CT Brain scan
*Explanation*: CT Brain scan would be the most indicated first-line investigation. CT brain scan would be able to pick up any shifts on intracranial structures, intracranial expanding lesions, cerebral infarction, cerebral oedema, cerebral atrophy and ventricular dilation, atrophy of other structures and demyelination changes and other causes of radio-density change. CT is x-ray computerized tomography or computed tomography. The basis of CT is as follows. X-ray beams are passed through a given tissue plane in different directions. Scintillation counters record the emerging x-rays. There is computer reconstruction of emerging x-ray data and radio-density maps.

*Reference*: Puri BK, Hall A, Ho R (2014). *Revision Notes in Psychiatry*. London: CRC Press, p. 205.

### Question 51 Answer: b, Frontal lobe
*Explanation*: An impaired performance on the Luria's hand performance test implies a lesion involving most likely the frontal lobe. The left frontal lobe is involved in controlling language-related movement (Broca's area), and the right frontal lobe is involved in the non-verbal abilities. Left frontal lobe damage leads to non-fluent speech (excessive dysphasia) and depression.

*Reference*: Puri BK, Hall A, Ho R (2014). *Revision Notes in Psychiatry*. London: CRC Press, p. 110.

**Question 52 Answer: d, Omega 1 subunit of the GABA receptor**
*Explanation*: The proposed mechanism of action of benzodiazepine is binding to the GABA(A) receptors, and in particular, the omega 1 subunit of the GABA receptor.

*Reference*: Puri BK, Hall A, Ho R (2014). *Revision Notes in Psychiatry*. London: CRC Press, p. 247.

**Question 53 Answer: a, Cholecystokinin**
*Explanation*: This is a neuropeptide that is released from the small intestine and helps in the regulation of the postprandial release of bile locally in the gut itself and to control the appetite in the central nervous system. CCKa receptors are involved in appetite and feeding, whereas CCKb receptors are involved in emotional behaviour.

*Reference*: Puri BK, Hall A, Ho R (2014). *Revision Notes in Psychiatry*. London: CRC Press, p. 234.

**Question 54 Answer: c, There would be an increase in the ACTH release in depressed patients who are being challenged with CRF.**
*Explanation*: It has been noted that injections of CRH would lead to depressive symptoms such as reduction in appetite, sex drive, weight loss and altered circadian rhythms. A blunted ACTH response is noted to CRF challenge in depressed patients.

*Reference*: Puri BK, Hall A, Ho R (2014). *Revision Notes in Psychiatry*. London: CRC Press, p. 234.

**Question 55 Answer: a, Alcohol dehydrogenase**
*Explanation*: Ethanol is acted upon by alcohol dehydrogenase, whose gene is on chromosome 4, and is converted into acetaldehyde, which is then further acted upon by aldehyde dehydrogenase and converted into acetate. The gene that codes for the enzyme alcohol dehydrogenase is located on chromosome 4, whilst the gene for aldehyde dehydrogenase is located on chromosome 12.

*Reference*: Puri BK, Hall A, Ho R (2014). *Revision Notes in Psychiatry*. London: CRC Press, p. 524.

**Question 56 Answer: d, 12 months**
*Explanation*: This refers to what is commonly known as stranger anxiety. Fear of strangers is usually shown by infants between the age of 8 months and 1 year. It is not necessarily part of the attachment behaviour and may occur independent of separation anxiety.

*Reference*: Puri BK, Hall A, Ho R (2014). *Revision Notes in Psychiatry*. London: CRC Press, p. 64.

### Question 57 Answer: c, Lifetime prevalence
*Explanation*: The lifetime prevalence refers to the proportion of a defined population that has or has had a given disease (at any time during each individual's lifetime thus far) at a given point in time.

*Reference*: Puri BK, Hall A, Ho R (2014). *Revision Notes in Psychiatry*. London: CRC Press, p. 275.

### Question 58 Answer: d, Thyrotropin-releasing factor
*Explanation*: Thyrotropin-releasing factor is known to be the smallest brain peptide and has the ability to also reverse sedation caused by drugs due to the release of dopamine and acetylcholine in the brain.

*Reference*: Puri BK, Hall A, Ho R (2014). *Revision Notes in Psychiatry*. London: CRC Press, p. 234.

### Question 59 Answer: b, Buprenorphine
*Explanation*: The aforementioned drug is considered to be a partial mu-opioid agonist and a partial k-opioid antagonist. The peak plasma concentration of the drug is observed approximately 3 hours after dose administration. It has a terminal half-life of about 3–5 hours. The primary side effects of the medication include nausea, vomiting and constipation. The side effects may be less intense than those produced by the full opioid agonist opioids.

*Reference*: Puri BK, Hall A, Ho R (2014). *Revision Notes in Psychiatry*. London: CRC Press, p. 536.

### Question 60 Answer: b, Lewy bodies
*Explanation*: The aforementioned description correlates to the ultra-structural pathology of Lewy bodies.

*Reference*: Puri BK, Hall A, Ho R (2014). *Revision Notes in Psychiatry*. London: CRC Press, p. 196.

### Question 61 Answer: b, Ependyma
*Explanation*: These are cells that line the cavities of the CNS and their function is to aid in the flow of the CSF through cilial beating.

*Reference*: Puri BK, Hall A, Ho R (2014). *Revision Notes in Psychiatry*. London: CRC Press, p. 177.

### Question 62 Answer: e, Small family size
*Explanation*: All of the aforementioned are associated factors, with the exception of small family size. A large family size has been implicated.

*Reference*: Puri BK, Hall A, Ho R (2014). *Revision Notes in Psychiatry*. London: CRC Press, p. 723.

### Question 63 Answer: a, Anorexia

*Explanation*: Eating disorders such as anorexia have a higher prevalence in higher socioeconomic classes and Western Caucasians and a significant association with greater parental education.

*Reference*: Puri BK, Hall A, Ho R (2014). *Revision Notes in Psychiatry*. London: CRC Press, p. 575.

### Question 64 Answer: d, Dopamine D4

*Explanation*: Clozapine is almost 20–25 times more potent at the D4 receptors than the D2 receptors.

*References*: Puri BK, Hall A, Ho R (2014). *Revision Notes in Psychiatry*. London: CRC Press, p. 224; Taylor D, Paton C, Kapur S (2009). *The Maudsley Prescribing Guidelines* (10th edition). London: Informa Healthcare, p. 149.

### Question 65 Answer: a, Alzheimer's disease

*Explanation*: The CSF concentration is decreased in unipolar and bipolar depression as well as in Alzheimer's disease.

*Reference*: Puri BK, Hall A, Ho R (2014). *Revision Notes in Psychiatry*. London: CRC Press, p. 234.

### Question 66 Answer: c, 15%

*Explanation*: The estimated percentage of vascular dementia amongst the general population has been estimated to be around 15%.

*Reference*: Puri BK, Hall A, Ho R (2014). *Revision Notes in Psychiatry*. London: CRC Press, p. 300.

### Question 67
### Answer: d, Perinatal mortality rate

*Explanation*: Perinatal mortality rate refers to the number of deaths in infants aged 4–52 weeks divided by the number of live births in 1 year.

*Reference*: Puri BK, Hall A, Ho R (2014). *Revision Notes in Psychiatry*. London: CRC Press, p. 278.

### Question 68
### Answer: c, Kernberg

*Explanation*: In 1978, Eysenck proposed a dimensional rather than a categorical approach to the description of personality.

*Reference*: Puri BK, Hall A, Ho R (2014). *Revision Notes in Psychiatry*. London: CRC Press, p. 437.

## Question 69
**Answer: d, Zolpidem**
*Explanation*: Zolpidem has the shortest half-life when administered. It is believed to achieve a central hypnotic effect by acting on the same receptors as do benzodiazepines.

*References*: Puri BK, Hall A, Ho R (2014). *Revision Notes in Psychiatry*. London: CRC Press, p. 247; Taylor D, Paton C, Kapur S (2009). *The Maudsley Prescribing Guidelines* (10th edition). London: Informa Healthcare, p. 266.

## Question 70
**Answer: a, Arachnoid matter**
*Explanation*: All of the aforementioned are part of the structural components of the peripheral nervous system. The dura, arachnoid and pia mater are part of the meninges and not part of the peripheral nervous system.

*Reference*: Puri BK, Hall A, Ho R (2014). *Revision Notes in Psychiatry*. London: CRC Press, p. 175.

## Question 71
**Answer: a, Sublimation**
*Explanation*: Sublimation is a mature defence mechanism and it involves a process that utilizes the force of a sexual instinct in drives, affects and memories in order to motivate creative activities having no apparent connection to the sexual instincts.

*Reference*: Puri BK, Hall A, Ho R (2014). *Revision Notes in Psychiatry*. London: CRC Press, p. 137.

## Question 72 Answer: a, Fluoxetine
*Explanation*: Lithium would interact with all of the aforementioned with the exception of the antidepressant fluoxetine. It is important to note that oedema should not be treated with diuretics as both the thiazide and the loop diuretics can interact and lead to lithium toxicity.

*References*: Puri BK, Hall A, Ho R (2014). *Revision Notes in Psychiatry*. London: CRC Press, p. 254; Taylor D, Paton C, Kapur S (2009). *The Maudsley Prescribing Guidelines* (10th edition). London: Informa Healthcare, p. 149.

## Question 73 Answer: d, Desensitization therapy
*Explanation*: This is a form of behavioural technique. It was introduced by Wolpe, who combined relaxation with graded exposure.

*Reference*: Puri BK, Hall A, Ho R (2014). *Revision Notes in Psychiatry*. London: CRC Press, p. 407.

**Question 74 Answer: e, The standardized morality ratio is obtained from the standardized mortality rate multiplied by 100.**

*Explanation*: The standardized mortality ratio is actually the ratio of the observed standardized mortality rate, derived from the population being studied, to the expected standardized mortality rate, derived from a comparable standard population.

*Reference*: Puri BK, Hall A, Ho R (2014). *Revision Notes in Psychiatry*. London: CRC Press, p. 277.

**Question 75 Answer: d, Avoidant**

*Explanation*: (d) Avoidant is incorrect. They have proposed the following attachment types: easy child pattern (characterized by regularity, positive approach responses to new stimuli, high adaptability to change and expressions of mood that are mild/moderate in intensity and predominantly positive); difficult child pattern (characterized by irregularity in biological functions, negative withdrawal responses to new situations, nonadaptability or slow adaptability to change and intense, frequently negative expressions of mood); and slow to warm up the child (characterized by a combination of negative responses of mid intensity to new situations with slow adaptability after repeated contact).

*Reference*: Puri BK, Hall A, Ho R (2014). *Revision Notes in Psychiatry*. London: CRC Press, p. 67.

**Question 76 Answer: a, Splitting**

*Explanation*: (a) is the correct option. This refers to segregating good objects, affects and memories from bad ones.

*Reference*: Puri BK, Hall A, Ho R (2014). *Revision Notes in Psychiatry*. London: CRC Press, p. 137.

**Question 77 Answer: e, Risperidone**

*Explanation*: Paliperidone is a derivative of risperidone. For risperidone, it has a higher risk for extra-pyramidal side effects (EPSE) and galactorrhoea as compared to other second-generation antipsychotics. For paliperidone, the side effects include EPSE, QTC prolongation and hyperprolactinaemia.

*Reference*: Puri BK, Hall A, Ho R (2014). *Revision Notes in Psychiatry*. London: CRC Press, p. 367.

**Question 78 Answer: c, 11%–20%**

*Explanation*: Based on epidemiology studies, the estimated prevalence of psychiatric disorders in adolescence has been estimated to be around 10%–20%. A male-to-female ratio of approximately 1:1.5 has been observed.

*Reference*: Puri BK, Hall A, Ho R (2014). *Revision Notes in Psychiatry*. London: CRC Press, p. 619.

**Question 79 Answer: e, Period prevalence**
*Explanation*: Period prevalence refers to the proportion of a defined population that has a given disease during a given interval of time.

*Reference*: Puri BK, Hall A, Ho R (2014). *Revision Notes in Psychiatry*. London: CRC Press, p. 275.

**Question 80 Answer: e, Incidence is affected by the disease survival.**
*Explanation*: Incidence is not affected by the disease survival. The dominator usually includes those who are at risk.

*Reference*: Puri BK, Hall A, Ho R (2014). *Revision Notes in Psychiatry*. London: CRC Press, p. 276.

**Question 81 Answer: e, Sodium valproate**
*Explanation*: Sodium valproate works by increasing the amount of GABA, decreasing the GABA breakdown, increasing the GABA release and decreasing the turnover of GABA. Lamotrigine works by the inhibition of glutamate release. Interaction between lamotrigine and sodium valproate causes a marked increase in the levels of lamotrigine.

*Reference*: Puri BK, Hall A, Ho R (2014). *Revision Notes in Psychiatry*. London: CRC Press, p. 247.

**Question 82 Answer: e, 50 times higher**
*Explanation*: Based on prior studies, the concordance rate for monozygotic twin has been approximately 45%, whereas that for dizygotic twin has been approximately 10%.

*Reference*: Puri BK, Hall A, Ho R (2014). *Revision Notes in Psychiatry*. London: CRC Press, p. 358.

**Question 83 Answer: b, 1%**
*Explanation*: The estimated 1-year prevalence of schizophrenia has been estimated to be around 1%.

*Reference*: Puri BK, Hall A, Ho R (2014). *Revision Notes in Psychiatry*. London: CRC Press, p. 281.

**Question 84 Answer: a, 1%**
*Explanation*: The lifetime risk for adults in the general population that has bipolar disorder has been estimated to be around 1%.

*Reference*: Puri BK, Hall A, Ho R (2014). *Revision Notes in Psychiatry*. London: CRC Press, p. 283.

**Question 85 Answer: b, The female-to-male ratio is around 1:2.**
*Explanation*: Based on existing studies, the female-to-male ratio has been estimated to be around 2:1.

*Reference*: Puri BK, Hall A, Ho R (2014). *Revision Notes in Psychiatry*. London: CRC Press, p. 284.

**Question 86 Answer: a, Displacement**
*Explanation*: The defence mechanism in play is displacement. In displacement, emotions, ideas or wishes are transferred from their original objects to a more acceptable substitute.

*Reference*: Puri BK, Hall A, Ho R (2014). *Revision Notes in Psychiatry*. London: CRC Press, p. 137.

**Question 87 Answer: c, It refers to the presence of multiple sets of chromosomes.**
*Explanation*: Option (c) is the correct, as it refers to the presence of multiple sets of chromosomes.

*Reference*: Puri BK, Hall A, Ho R (2014). *Revision Notes in Psychiatry*. London: CRC Press, p. 271.

**Question 88 Answer: d, Metencephalon**
*Explanation*: The cerebellum is derived from the metencephalon. Other derivatives include the pons and also part of the medulla oblongata.

*Reference*: Puri BK, Hall A, Ho R (2014). *Revision Notes in Psychiatry*. London: CRC Press, p. 176.

**Question 89 Answer: b, There is an unequal gender ratio, with males being more affected than females.**
*Explanation*: Studies have shown that there is an equal gender ratio between males and females.

*Reference*: Puri BK, Hall A, Ho R (2014). *Revision Notes in Psychiatry*. London: CRC Press, p. 281.

**Question 90 Answer: b, Acrocentric**
*Explanation*: Acrocentric refers to a chromosome in which the centromere is very near to one end.

*Reference*: Puri BK, Hall A, Ho R (2014). *Revision Notes in Psychiatry*. London: CRC Press, p. 259.

### Question 91 Answer: e, Satellite cells
*Explanation*: Neuroglia, or interstitial cells, usually outnumber neurons by around 5–10 times. The main types of neuroglia in the central nervous system are astrocytes, oligodendrocytes, microglia and also ependymal cells. Satellite cells and also the Schwann cells are part of the peripheral nervous system.

*Reference*: Puri BK, Hall A, Ho R (2014). *Revision Notes in Psychiatry*. London: CRC Press, p. 176.

### Question 92 Answer: d, They are responsible for immune control.
*Explanation*: There are typically two main types of astrocytes: the fibrous and the protoplasmic astrocytes. They are responsible for all of the aforementioned, with the exception of immune mediation. Astrocytes are considered to be multi-polar.

*Reference*: Puri BK, Hall A, Ho R (2014). *Revision Notes in Psychiatry*. London: CRC Press, p. 176.

### Question 93 Answer: b, 25% Chance
*Explanation*: It has been noted that when both parents carry one abnormal copy of the gene, there is a 25% chance of a child inheriting both mutations, and hence expressing the disorder.

*Reference*: Puri BK, Hall A, Ho R (2014). *Revision Notes in Psychiatry*. London: CRC Press, p. 269.

### Question 94 Answer: c, 5%–15%
*Explanation*: The lifetime risk for first-degree relatives has been estimated to be around 4%–18%.

*Reference*: Puri BK, Hall A, Ho R (2014). *Revision Notes in Psychiatry*. London: CRC Press, p. 285.

### Question 95 Answer: a, Frontal operculum on the dominant side
*Explanation*: This usually involves a lesion of the frontal operculum on the dominant (and usually left) side, and areas 44 and 45.

*Reference*: Puri BK, Hall A, Ho R (2014). *Revision Notes in Psychiatry*. London: CRC Press, p. 177.

### Question 96 Answer: e, Orbital cortex
*Explanation*: Lesions involving the orbital cortex on either side have been shown to lead to a form of acquired sociopathy.

*Reference*: Puri BK, Hall A, Ho R (2014). *Revision Notes in Psychiatry*. London: CRC Press, p. 177.

### Question 97 Answer: Type I
*Explanation*: This is a type I adverse reaction as it is IgE-mediated.

*Reference*: Puri BK, Hall A, Ho R (2014). *Revision Notes in Psychiatry*. London: CRC Press, p. 252.

### Question 98 Answer: c, Superior mesial region
*Explanation*: The superior mesial region consists of the supplementary motor area as well as the anterior cingulate cortex. Lesions involving either the left or the right superior mesial region can lead to akinetic mutism.

*Reference*: Puri BK, Hall A, Ho R (2014). *Revision Notes in Psychiatry*. London: CRC Press, p. 177.

### Question 99 Answer: c, 5%
*Explanation*: The average prevalence of dysthymia in the general population has been estimated to be around 5%. Dysthymia is more common than severe depressive episode in the chronically medically ill patients.

*Reference*: Puri BK, Hall A, Ho R (2014). *Revision Notes in Psychiatry*. London: CRC Press, p. 283.

### Question 100 Answer: b, Type II
*Explanation*: A type II reaction is largely a cytotoxic reaction.

*Reference*: Puri BK, Hall A, Ho R (2014). *Revision Notes in Psychiatry*. London: CRC Press, p. 252.

### Question 101 Answer: a, Butyrophenes
*Explanation*: Haloperidol has been classified in the family of butyrophenes.

*Reference*: Puri BK, Hall A, Ho R (2014). *Revision Notes in Psychiatry*. London: CRC Press, p. 238.

### Question 102 Answer: d, Turner's syndrome
*Explanation*: In Turner's syndrome, there is less than the normal number of chromosomes. Non-disjunction of the paternal XY thus results in sex chromosomal monosomy. Fifty per cent of the patients have a karyotype consisting of 45X or 46XX mosaicism. Fifty per cent of the patients have 46 chromosomes with one normal X chromosome and the other X chromosome, which is abnormal in the form of a ring, a long arm isochromosome or a partially deleted X chromosome.

*Reference*: Puri BK, Hall A, Ho R (2014). *Revision Notes in Psychiatry*. London: CRC Press, p. 666.

### Question 103 Answer: c, Southern blot

*Explanation*: Southern blotting is a technique that allows for the transfer of DNA fragments from gel, where electrophoresis and DNA denaturation have taken place, to a nylon or nitro-cellular filter. It involves over-laying the gel with the filter and in turn overlaying the filter with paper towels. A solution is then blotted through the gel to the paper towels. Autoradiography can then be used to identify the fragments of interest on the filter. Northern blotting enables the detection of RNA, whereas Western blotting allows for the detection of proteins.

*Reference*: Puri BK, Hall A, Ho R (2014). *Revision Notes in Psychiatry*. London: CRC Press, p. 265.

### Question 104 Answer: a, Dibenzodiazepines – Clozapine

*Explanation*: (a) is correct.

*Reference*: Puri BK, Hall A, Ho R (2014). *Revision Notes in Psychiatry*. London: CRC Press, p. 238.

### Question 105 Answer: e, Oxazepam

*Explanation*: In this case, the patient has hepatic impairment due to the chronic use of alcohol. There is a reduced ability of the liver to metabolize and synthesize plasma proteins. Shorter-acting benzodiazepines are recommended for patients with alcohol withdrawal.

*Reference*: Puri BK, Hall A, Ho R (2014). *Revision Notes in Psychiatry*. London: CRC Press, p. 513.

### Question 106 Answer: a, An aliphatic side chain

*Explanation*: The difference between chlorpromazine and the rest of the members of the same family is that it contains an aliphatic side chain.

*Reference*: Puri BK, Hall A, Ho R (2014). *Revision Notes in Psychiatry*. London: CRC Press, p. 422.

### Question 107 Answer: b, For antidepressants that have a short half-life, a shorter period is required for discontinuation.

*Explanation*: Longer period is usually required, instead of a shorter period for drugs with a relatively short half-life, such as paroxetine and venlafaxine. There should be a gradual reduction of the dose of the antidepressant over a period of 4 weeks. In case the patient experiences unpleasant discontinuation symptoms, it would be wise to consider re-introduction of the original antidepressant at the previous dose that was effective.

*Reference*: Puri BK, Hall A, Ho R (2014). *Revision Notes in Psychiatry*. London: CRC Press, p. 391.

## Question 108 Answer: e, Sociopathy
*Explanation*: All of the aforementioned, with the exception of sociopathy, are changes related to lesions involving the dorsolateral prefrontal cortex. In addition, there would be other changes such as poor organization, poor planning, poor abstraction and disturbances in motor programming.

*Reference*: Puri BK, Hall A, Ho R (2014). *Revision Notes in Psychiatry*. London: CRC Press, p. 178.

## Question 109 Answer: d, The age of onset is earlier for women as compared to men.
*Explanation*: The age of onset has been found to be much later for women than for men.

*Reference*: Puri BK, Hall A, Ho R (2014). *Revision Notes in Psychiatry*. London: CRC Press, p. 281.

## Question 110 Answer: d, Freud
*Explanation*: Both Freud and Bleuler believed in the 'split mind' or 'fragmentation of mental activities'.

*Reference*: Puri BK, Treasaden I (eds) (2010). *Psychiatry: An Evidence-Based Text*. London: Hodder Arnold, pp. 12–13, 106, 215, 613, 615.

## Question 111 Answer: a, Men have bimodal peak of incidence.
*Explanation*: The incidence of schizophrenia is between 15 and 30 new cases per 100,000 of the population per year. The point prevalence is approximately 1%. The lifetime risk is approximately 1%. The age of onset is usually between 15 and 45 years, much earlier in men than in women. It is equally common in males and females. There is a higher incidence in those who are not married. For women, there is a bimodal peak of incidence in their late 20s and 50s.

*Reference*: Puri BK, Hall A, Ho R (2014). *Revision Notes in Psychiatry*. London: CRC Press, p. 283.

## Question 112 Answer: e, Weigl Colour–Form Sorting Test (WCFST)
*Explanation*: WCFST is a test mainly for executive function. AVLT is a 15-item five-trial test, from which recall (immediate and delayed) and recognition memory can be assessed. CVLT involves a list of 16 words. The list is repeated five times. Then, a second list is given, serving to interfere with the first list, after which recall of the first list is requested. RMT involves recognition of non-verbal material with interference from distracters after the first initial image is presented. The WMT assesses several memory components including concentration and summary

indices that can be derived with a mean of 100. Tasks under WMT include assessment of logical memory (subjects are asked to recall the content of two stores read to them with a 30-minute delay) and a verbal paired associates test (learning word pairs, e.g. baby cries, and recalling the second word when the first word is given).

*Reference*: Trimble M (2004). *Somatoform Disorders – A Medico-legal Guide*. Cambridge, UK: Cambridge University Press.

### Question 113 Answer: c, Formal thought disorder
*Explanation*: The following are first-rank symptoms: auditory hallucinations, delusions of passivity, somatic passivity and delusional perception. Second-rank symptoms include perplexity, emotional blunting, hallucinations and other delusions. First-rank symptoms can occur in other psychoses and, although highly suggestive of schizophrenia, are not pathognomic.

*Reference*: Puri BK, Hall A, Ho R (2014). *Revision Notes in Psychiatry*. London: CRC Press, p. 351.

### Question 114 Answer: d, Rationalization
*Explanation*: This person suffers from narcissistic personality disorder. Rationalization is the defence mechanism most commonly used by people with narcissistic personality disorder.

*Reference*: Gabbard GO, Beck JS, Holmes J (2005). *Oxford Textbook of Psychotherapy*. Oxford, UK: Oxford University Press.

### Question 115 Answer: e, Simpson Angus Scale
*Explanation*: The questionnaires listed under options B and D do not exist.

*Reference*: Puri BK, Hall A, Ho R (2014). *Revision Notes in Psychiatry*. London: CRC Press, p. 281.

### Question 116 Answer: b, Mannerism
*Explanation*: Mannerism involves repeated involuntary movements that appear to be goal directed, for example a person repeatedly moving his or her hand when he or she talks and tries to convey his or her message to the examiner.

*Reference*: Puri BK, Hall A, Ho R (2014). *Revision Notes in Psychiatry*. London: CRC Press, p. 2.

### Question 117 Answer: d, Translation
*Explanation*: Following transcription, splicing and nuclear transport, translation is the process in gene expression whereby mRNA acts as a template allowing

the genetic code to be deciphered to allow the formation of a peptide chain. This process involves tRNA molecules.

*Reference*: Puri BK, Hall A, Ho R (2014). *Revision Notes in Psychiatry*. London: CRC Press, p. 263.

**Question 118 Answer: b, PCR requires large amounts of DNA.**
*Explanation*: Polymerase chain reaction (PCR) is the most versatile technique for cloning or making copies of DNA. PCR starts with a mixture in a buffer solution comprising the template, Taq polymerase, the four deoxyribonucleotide triphosphates and DNA primers. PCR requires a small amount of DNA and can detect small mutations. It can be completed in less than 1–2 hours.

*Reference and Further Reading*: Puri BK, Treasaden I (eds) (2010). *Psychiatry: An Evidence-Based Text*. London: Hodder Arnold, pp. 466–467; Puri BK, Hall A, Ho R (2014). *Revision Notes in Psychiatry*. London: CRC Press, p. 264.

**Question 119 Answer: a, 4 times higher**
*Explanation*: It is three to four times higher. If the individual is homozygous for ε4/ε4 alleles for the ApoE4 gene, the risk of developing Alzheimer's disease is 10 times higher.

*Further Reading*: Puri BK, Treasaden I (eds) (2010). *Psychiatry: An Evidence-Based Text*. London: Hodder Arnold, pp. 1103–1104.

**Question 120 Answer: d, Parkinson's disease**
*Explanation*: Parkinson's disease with mutation in alpha synuclein gene, which is involved in neuronal plasticity, follows an autosomal dominant pattern of inheritance.

*Further Reading*: Puri BK, Treasaden I (eds) (2010). *Psychiatry: An Evidence-Based Text*. London: Hodder Arnold, pp. 541–543.

**Question 121 Answer: e, EPN2**
*Explanation*: All of the aforementioned genes are associated with the development of schizophrenia with the exception of EPN2. The EPN4 gene located on chromosome 5q33 has been implicated instead.

*Reference*: Puri BK, Hall A, Ho R (2014). *Revision Notes in Psychiatry*. London: CRC Press, p. 359.

**Question 122 Answer: b, Orexin**
*Explanation*: The genotype HLA-DQB1*0602 is present in nearly 99% of patients suffering from narcolepsy with cataplexy and 40% of patients suffering from

narcolepsy without cataplexy. Loss of hypocretin cells in the hypothalamus has been implicated. Orexin promotes wakefulness.

*References*: Chemelli RM, Willie JT, et al. (1999). Narcolepsy in orexin knockout mice: Molecular genetics of sleep regulation. *Cell*, 98: 437–451; Puri BK, Hall A, Ho R (2014). *Revision Notes in Psychiatry*. London: CRC Press, p. 616.

**Question 123 Answer: b, In 50% of Down syndrome cases, the non-disjunction event occurs during anaphase in maternal meiosis.**
*Explanation*: In 95% of Down syndrome cases, the non-disjunction event occurs in anaphase of maternal meiosis.

*Further Reading*: Puri BK, Treasaden I (eds) (2010). *Psychiatry: An Evidence-Based Text*. London: Hodder Arnold, pp. 467, 1082, 1087–1088.

**Question 124 Answer: e, Patients with Klinefelter's syndrome usually have affected siblings.**
*Explanation*: Option E is false, as Klinefelter's syndrome usually occurs as sporadic familial cases.

   Option C is correct as the diagnosis is usually first suspected in childhood because of mild learning disabilities or in adulthood because of infertility.

*Further Reading*: Puri BK, Treasaden I (eds) (2010). *Psychiatry: An Evidence-Based Text*. London: Hodder Arnold, pp. 467, 754, 763.

# Extended Matching Items (EMIs)

## Theme: Psychoanalytic concepts

### Question 125 Answer: b, Anal phase
*Explanation*: This happens from around 15–18 months to 30–36 months of age. Erotogenic pleasure is derived from stimulation of the anal mucosa, initially through faecal excretion and later also through faecal retention.

### Question 126 Answer: a, Oral phase
*Explanation*: The oral phase occurs from birth to around 15–18 months of age, Pleasure is derived from sucking. In addition to the mother's breast, the infant also has a desire to place other objects into his or her mouth.

### Question 127 Answer: d, Latency phase
*Explanation*: This happens from 5–6 years to the onset of puberty. The sexual drive remains relatively latent during this period.

### Question 128 Answer: e, Genital phase
*Explanation*: This occurs from the onset of puberty to young adulthood. Successful resolution of conflict from this and previous psychosexual stages leads to a mature well-integrated adult identity.

*Reference*: Puri BK, Hall A, Ho R (2014). *Revision Notes in Psychiatry*. London: CRC Press, p. 133.

## Theme: Genetics

**Question 129 Answer: f, XYY**

*Explanation*: Men with this particular karyotype show an increased rate of petty crime (an average of three times more common than in the general population). This is a result of underlying impulsiveness, and there is no propensity towards severe aggressive or violent crime.

**Question 130 Answer: e, 47XXY**

*Explanation*: Eighty per cent of individuals with this condition have this karyotype. They tend to have fertility-related problems that could be treated using haploid spermatocytes obtained by testicular biopsy.

**Question 131 Answer: d, 45X or 46XX**

*Explanation*: The syndrome being tested here is Turner's syndrome. Apart from the complications to note prior to delivery, at birth, the neonate always has a normal female feature with a residue of intrauterine oedema in the form of neck webbing and puffy extremities. Short stature would become apparent in early childhood.

**Question 132 Answer: c, Trinucleotide CGG repeats**

*Explanation*: Women with fragile X syndrome suffer from mild learning disability, whereas men with fragile X syndrome suffer from moderate-to-severe learning disability. Verbal IQ is usually more than performance IQ. The length of the tri-nucleotide repeat is usually inversely related to IQ.

**Question 133 Answer: a, Trisomy 21**

*Explanation*: Down's syndrome is the most common cytogenetic cause of learning disability. It accounts for 30% of all children with mental retardation. The prevalence is usually 1 in 800 live births.

*Reference*: Puri BK, Hall A, Ho R (2014). *Revision Notes in Psychiatry*. London: CRC Press, p. 664.

## Theme: Inheritance of diseases

**Question 134 Answer: a, X-linked dominance with tri-nucleotide repeats**

*Explanation*: These are the characteristics clinical features of patients with fragile X syndrome. The tri-nucleotide repeats are found on the long arm of X chromosome.

**Question 135 Answer: d, Non-disjunction of the parental XY**

*Explanation*: These are the characteristic clinical features of Turner's syndrome. It is due to non-disjunction of the paternal XY that results in sex chromosomal abnormality.

**Question 136 Answer: b, Maternal or paternal non-disjunction**
*Explanation*: The clinical features described refer Klinefelter's syndrome. Fifty per cent are due to maternal and another 50% are due to paternal non-disjunction.

**Question 137 Answer: f, Autosomal recessive**
*Explanation*: The condition referred to here is Hurler's syndrome, which is an autosomal recessive condition. Patients with this condition usually have short stature, hepato-splenomegaly and hirsutism.

*Reference*: Puri BK, Hall A, Ho R (2014). *Revision Notes in Psychiatry*. London: CRC Press, p. 669.

## Theme: Genetics

**Question 138 Answer: a, DISC-1**
*Explanation*: DISC-1 has been implicated in both schizophrenia and bipolar disorder, whereas DISC-2 has largely been implicated only in schizophrenia.

**Question 139 Answer: e and g, Chromosome 2q and Chromosome 7q**
*Explanation*: Chromosome 2q is implicated in the development of autistic spectrum disorder, whereas chromosome 7q is implicated in the development of autism.

**Question 140 Answer: h, Chromosome 11p**
*Explanation*: Chromosome 11p has been implicated in the regulation of the amount of brain-derived neuro-trophic factor and is also one of the chromosomes responsible for the development of bipolar affective disorder.

**Question 141 Answer: c, Presenilin 1, d, Presenilin 2, i, Chromosome 19**
*Explanation*: Presenilin 1 and 2 and APOE gene present on chromosome 19 are responsible for the development of Alzheimer's disease.

**Question 142 Answer: j, Chromosome 20**
*Explanation*: This chromosome is responsible for the PrP in inherited CJD.

*Reference*: Puri BK, Hall A, Ho R (2014). *Revision Notes in Psychiatry*. London: CRC Press, p. 260.

## Theme: Neurology and neurological examination

**Question 143 Answer: a, Holmes–Adie pupil**
*Explanation*: The clinical features include it being unilateral in 80% of the cases, moderately dilated, with poor reaction to light and slow reaction to accommodation. It is associated with diminished and absent knee jerk.

**Question 144 Answer: b, Hutchison's pupil**
*Explanation*: This is caused by rapidly rising unilateral intracranial pressure. The clinical features include the pupil being dilated and unreactive on the side of an

intracranial mass lesion as a result of compression of the oculomotor nerve on the same side.

**Question 145 Answer: c, Argyll Robertson pupil**
*Explanation*: The clinical features include constricted pupils, being unreactive to light but reactive to accommodation.

**Question 146 Answer: d, Horner's syndrome**
*Explanation*: Aetiology includes brain stem stroke, tumour at the lung apex or carotid dissection. A lesion to the sympathetic supply to the eye at the central brain stem, cervical spine, cervical ganglion and carotid body would result in this.

*Reference*: Puri BK, Hall A, Ho R (2014). *Revision Notes in Psychiatry*. London: CRC Press, pp. 161–162.

## Theme: Neurology and neurological examination
**Question 147 Answer: b, Anterior cord syndrome**
*Explanation*: For anterior cord syndrome, there is preservation of dorsal column functions such as joint position sense and discriminative touch. However, there is associated loss of all other functions.

**Question 148 Answer: a, Central cord syndrome**
*Explanation*: In central cord syndrome, there are early sphincter disturbances. There might be either unilateral or bilateral spino-thalamic loss. There is associated loss of pain and temperature sensation. Weakness, wasting and areflexia are noted in the affected segment, but there is spasticity below the level of the lesion.

**Question 149 Answer: d, Brown-Sequard syndrome**
*Explanation*: The aforementioned clinical features are typical of this syndrome.

**Question 150 Answer: e, Total spinal cord transection**
*Explanation*: For total spinal cord transection, there is loss of all functions below the level of the lesions. This is associated with urinary retention and constipation.

*Reference*: Puri BK, Hall A, Ho R (2014). *Revision Notes in Psychiatry*. London: CRC Press, p. 166.

## Theme: Neuroanatomy
**Question 151 Answer: b, Reticulospinal fibres**

**Question 152 Answer: a, Anterior corticospinal tract**

**Question 153 Answer: c, Vestibulospinal tract**

**Question 154 Answer: h, Descending autonomic fibres**

*Reference*: Puri BK, Hall A, Ho R (2014). *Revision Notes in Psychiatry*. London: CRC Press, p. 189.

## Theme: Psychopathology of memory

### Question 155 Answer: f, Transient global amnesia
*Explanation*: This is usually a result of transient ischaemia of the hippocampus–fornix–hypothalamic system. Functional neuroimaging may show transient reduction in metabolic and functional activities in the mesial temporal lobes.

### Question 156 Answer: e, False memory
*Explanation*: The false memory syndrome is a condition in which a person's identity and interpersonal relationship are centred around a memory of a traumatic experience, which is objectively false, but the person strongly believes that such experience did take place.

### Question 157 Answer: c, Post-traumatic amnesia
*Explanation*: Post-traumatic amnesia is defined as the memory loss from the time of the accident to the time the patient can give a clear account of the recent events.

### Question 158 Answer: a, Anterograde amnesia
*Explanation*: This is due either to the failure to consolidate what is perceived into permanent memory storage or because of inability to retrieve memory from the storage.

### Question 159 Answer: b, Retrograde amnesia
*Explanation*: Retrograde amnesia refers to the loss of memory for events that occurred prior to an event or condition. Such event is presumed to have caused the memory disturbance in the first place. Retrograde memory related to public events is more likely to be subjected to greater memory loss than personal events.

## Theme: Neuropathology

### Question 160 Answer: e, Punch-drunk syndrome
*Explanation*: This is also known as post-traumatic dementia or boxing encephalopathy. In addition to occurring in boxers who have received repeated punches to the head, other contact sports involving repeated head injury, such as rugby union, may also put participants at increased risk.

### Question 161 Answer: d, CJD
*Explanation*: This is a condition that is transmitted by infection with a prion. In addition to the brain changes, it is also associated with degeneration of spinal cord long descending tracts. It has an incubation period of many years. There may be little or no gross atrophy of the cerebral cortex evident in rapidly developing cases. In those surviving the longest, the common changes may

include selective cerebellar atrophy, generalized cerebral atrophy and ventricular enlargement.

**Question 162 Answer: b, Pick's disease**
*Explanation*: Pick's disease is one histological type of fronto-temporal dementia. Macroscopic changes include the aforementioned.

**Question 163 Answer: a, Alzheimer's dementia**
*Explanation*: These are the characteristic macroscopic pathological changes for Alzheimer's dementia. The atrophy is usually more marked in the frontal, medial, temporal and also the parietal lobes.

*Reference*: Puri BK, Hall A, Ho R (2014). *Revision Notes in Psychiatry*. London: CRC Press, pp. 195–197.

## Theme: Neuroimaging

**Question 164 Answer: a, X-ray**
*Explanation*: X-ray radio-imaging is a form of structural imaging. The main use currently is largely for the assessment of trauma. It is also useful for the detection of intracranial expanding lesions.

**Question 165 Answer: b, CT Scan**
*Explanation*: CT and MRI have largely replaced skull radiography these days. Its clinical use includes the detection of shifts of intracranial pressure, intracranial expanding lesions, cerebral infarction, cerebral oedema, cerebral atrophy and ventricular dilatation and atrophy of other structures

**Question 166 Answer: c, PET Scan**
*Explanation*: PET neuro-imaging can give information about metabolic changes, regional cerebral blood flow and ligand binding. Clinical application includes assessment of cerebrovascular disease, Alzheimer's disease, epilepsy (prior to neurosurgery) and head injury.

**Question 167 Answer: d, SPECT**
*Explanation*: SPECT is also of use in conditions in which the onset of the symptomatology being studied may occur at a time when the patient is not in or near any scanner; a suitable radio-ligand could be administered at around the material time and the patient be scanned afterward. Clinical applications of SPECT include assessment of Alzheimer's disease.

**Question 168 Answer: e, MRI**
*Explanation*: MRI is useful in most clinical and research studies requiring high-resolution neuroanatomical imaging.

*Reference*: Puri BK, Hall A, Ho R (2014). *Revision Notes in Psychiatry*. London: CRC Press, pp. 205–208.

## Theme: Psychiatric epidemiology – concepts

**Question 169 Answer: g, Cumulative incidence**
*Explanation*: Cumulative incidence refers to the proportion of a population who develops the disease of interest in a defined time period.

**Question 170 Answer: a, Incidence**
*Explanation*: Incidence or incidence rate refers to the number of new events during a specified time period.

**Question 171 Answer: d, Point prevalence**
*Explanation*: In the steady state, in which the incidence of a disease is constant over a given time period and the time between the case onset and ending is constant, the following relationship holds true: P (point prevalence) = I (incidence) × D (chronicity).

**Question 172 Answer: c, Chronicity**
*Explanation*: The chronicity of a disease is its average duration. It has the units of time.

**Question 173 Answer: a, Incidence**
*Explanation*: The incidence of a disease is the rate of occurrence of new cases of the disease in a defined population over a period of time. It is equal to the number of new cases over a given period of time divided by the total population at risk during the same period of time.

**Question 174 Answer: b, Prevalence**
*Explanation*: The prevalence of a disease is the proportion of a defined population that has the disease at a given time. The point prevalence is the proportion of a defined population that has a given disease at a given point in time. The period prevalence is the proportion of a defined population that has a given disease during a given interval of time.

*Reference*: Puri BK, Hall A, Ho R (2014). *Revision Notes in Psychiatry*. London: CRC Press, pp. 277–279.

## Theme: Psychiatric epidemiology

**Question 175 Answer: i, Attributable risk**
*Explanation*: This is the incidence of the disease in the group exposed to the risk factor of interest minus the incidence in the group not exposed to the risk factor. The attributable risk is also known as risk difference or the absolute excess risk.

**Question 176 Answer: m, Odd ratio**
*Explanation*: The odds ratio is the ratio of the odds that subjects in the disease group were exposed to the factor to the odds that subjects in the control group were exposed to the factor.

### Question 177 Answer: h, Relative risk

*Explanation*: In terms of analytical epidemiological studies, the relative risk of a disease with respect to a given risk factor is the ratio of the incidence of the disease in people exposed to that risk factor to the incidence of the disease in people not exposed to the same risk factor. The relative risk does not have any units, being the ratio of two numbers, and it can take on nonnegative real value, that is, relative risk more than zero.

### Question 178 Answer: a, Standardized mortality rate

*Explanation*: The standardized mortality rate is the mortality rate adjusted to compensate for a confounder.

### Question 179 Answer: c, Standardized mortality ratio

*Explanation*: Standardized mortality ratio refers to the ratio of the observed standardized mortality rate derived from the population being studied to the expected standardized mortality rate derived from a comparable standard population.

### Question 180 Answer: d, Life expectancy

*Explanation*: This is a measure of the mean length of time that an individual can be expected to live based on the assumption that the mortality rate used remains constant. It is calculated from the ratio of the total time a hypothetical group of people is expected to live to the size of that group.

*Reference*: Puri BK, Hall A, Ho R (2014). *Revision Notes in Psychiatry*. London: CRC Press, pp. 278–281.

## Theme: Psychotherapy

### Question 181 Answer: b, Denial

*Explanation*: Denial is the avoidance of awareness of an external reality that is difficult to face. In this case, the issue of amputation is difficult for the patient to face and he decides to avoid it by saying that everything is fine.

### Question 182 Answer: e, Projection

*Explanation*: In projection, unacceptable qualities, feelings, thoughts or wishes are projected onto another person or thing. This is often seen in paranoid patients. In this case, the patient gets defensive and blames the psychiatrist for probing too much about his situation and deliberately making his mood worse.

### Question 183 Answer: c, Displacement

*Explanation*: In displacement, emotions, ideas or wishes are transferred from their original object to a more acceptable substitute. In this case, the patient only vents his frustration to his wife instead of his colleagues, as it is safer and more acceptable for the patient.

**Question 184 Answer: h, Sublimation**

*Explanation*: Sublimation refers to channelling socially objectionable or internally unacceptable motives into socially acceptable ones. In this case, the patient copes by devoting his energy into doing volunteering work, which is socially acceptable and this helps his mood get better.

*References*: Puri BK, Hall A, Ho R (2014). *Revision Notes in Psychiatry*. London: CRC Press, pp. 136–137; Puri BK, Treasaden I, (eds) (2010). *Psychiatry: An Evidence-Based Text*. London: Hodder Arnold, pp. 717, 809, 1034–1035.

# MRCPSYCH PAPER A2 MOCK EXAMINATION 2: QUESTIONS

## GET THROUGH MRCPSYCH PAPER A2: MOCK EXAMINATION

Total number of questions: 174 (110 MCQs, 64 EMIs)
Total time provided: 180 minutes

**Question 1**
Which of the following is true with regards to the differences between a lesion involving the left side of the dorsolateral prefrontal cortex and a lesion involving the right sided dorsolateral prefrontal cortex?
 a. Left-sided lesions are associated with significant impairment in judgement.
 b. Left-sided lesions are associated with more impaired verbal fluency.
 c. Left-sided lesions are associated with poorer organization.
 d. Left-sided lesions are associated with more memory impairments.
 e. Left sided lesions are associated with more impaired nonverbal fluency.

**Question 2**
The mesial temporal region consists of all of the following with the exception of
 a. Para-hippocampal gyrus
 b. Amygdala
 c. Entorhinal cortex
 d. Hippocampus
 e. Hypothalamus

**Question 3**
A 25-year-old male came to the outpatient clinic for his routine review. He has a lot of concerns with regards to the antipsychotics that he is on. He is keen to consider an antipsychotic that has the least amount of side effects. Which one of the following has the least number of side effects?
 a. Clozapine
 b. Risperidone
 c. Haloperidol
 d. Olanzapine
 e. Aripiprazole

## Question 4

A 30-year-old female had a relapse of bipolar affective disorder and has since been started on lithium. She has recently seen her GP, who has noted that she has hypertension (BP measured was 150/90). He is keen to start her on treatment for her hypertension. Which of the following is the most suitable drug he could consider for treatment of her hypertension?
a. Enalapril
b. Captopril
c. Thiazide diuretics
d. Furosemide
e. All are contraindicated; better to watch closely

## Question 5

Which of the following statements regarding the inferior parietal lobule is incorrect?
a. It consists of both the angular gyrus and also the supramarginal gyrus.
b. Lesions on the right side lead to conduction aphasia.
c. Lesions on the left side lead to tactile agnosia.
d. Lesions on the right side lead to anosognosia, neglect and tactile agnosia.
e. Lesions on the right side lead to anosodiaphoria.

## Question 6

Patients who have been on antipsychotics for some time are likely to develop metabolic syndrome. Based on the CATIE study, which of the following antipsychotics has been proven to be greatly associated with metabolic syndrome?
a. Olanzapine
b. Quetiapine
c. Risperidone
d. Ziprasidone
e. Perphenazine

## Question 7

Autosomal dominant disorders result from the presence of an abnormal dominant allele, which would cause individuals to manifest the abnormal phenotype. Which of the following statements about autosomal dominant transmission is incorrect?
a. The phenotype is usually present in all individuals carrying the dominant allele.
b. The phenotype does not skip generations, and vertical transmission takes place.
c. Only males are affected.
d. Male-to-male transmission could take place.
e. If one parent is homozygous for the abnormal dominant allele, all the members will manifest the abnormal phenotype trait.

**Question 8**

All of the following are autosomal dominant disorders, with the exception of
a. Huntington's disease
b. Phacomatosis
c. Early-onset Alzheimer's disease
d. Hurler's syndrome
e. Early-onset Parkinson's disease

**Question 9**

Balint's syndrome occurs due to a lesion involving the occipital lobe. In this syndrome, it consists of all of the following clinical signs and symptoms, with the exception of
a. Simultanagnosia
b. Ocular apraxia
c. Psychic gaze paralysis
d. Optic ataxia
e. Nystagmus

**Question 10**

Which of the following statements about autosomal recessive disorders is correct?
a. Heterozygous individuals are usually carriers who do not manifest the abnormal phenotype trait.
b. The more uncommon the disorder, the more unlikely that the parents are consanguineous.
c. Horizontal transmission of the disorder tends to take place.
d. In the event that both parents carry one abnormal copy of the gene, there is a 25% chance that a child would inherit both mutations, hence expressing the disease.
e. When both parents are affected, all the children would be affected.

**Question 11**

Which of the following statements about the methods of suicide used, based on previous epidemiological studies, is incorrect?
a. It has been found that psychiatric patients tend to use violent methods such as hanging, shooting and jumping from heights.
b. It has been estimated that two thirds of British men would commit suicide by hanging or via the usage of vehicle exhaust fumes.
c. Approximately one third of British women commit suicide by jumping.
d. It has been shown that drowning is more frequent in older people.
e. It has been shown that jumping from height is more frequent in young people who commit suicide.

**Question 12**

Which of the following statements about deliberate self-harm (DSH) is incorrect?
a. Within the United Kingdom, the rate of DSH is rising among the Asian women.
b. The Goth subculture in the UK is not strongly associated with self-harm.

c. It is known that adverse life events do tend to have occurred just prior to the act of self-harm.
d. A known history of DSH has been shown to be a long-term predictor of suicide, and the risk of suicide is 100 times greater than that of the general population.
e. Fifteen percent of people who have attempted self-harm are likely to attempt another episode within the next 1 year.

## Question 13
Which of the following statements about the hippocampus is incorrect?
a. It lies mainly in the floor of the inferior horn of the lateral ventricle.
b. Anteriorly, it forms what is known as the pes hippocampus.
c. Posteriorly, it ends inferior to the splenium of the corpus callosum.
d. It is histologically made up of four different layers.
e. Axons from each alveus converge medially to form the fimbria and the crus of the fornix.

## Question 14
All of the following statements about X-linked recessive inheritance are correct, with the exception of which of the following?
a. Male-to-male transmission usually does not take place.
b. Female heterozygotes are usually carriers.
c. A heterozygote carrier women would pass the allele to half of her son (who would have features of the disease) and half of her daughters (who do not have features of the disease).
d. Males are more likely to be affected with the X-linked recessive disorders.
e. Females are equally likely to be affected with the X-linked recessive disorders.

## Question 15
The age of onset of bipolar disorder has been known to be much earlier than for that of unipolar disorder. What is the average mean age of onset?
a. 15
b. 20
c. 25
d. 30
e. 35

## Question 16
Which of the following syndromes does not involve chromosomal deletion?
a. Angelman syndrome
b. Cri-du-chat syndrome
c. Di George syndrome (velocardiofacial syndrome)
d. Fragile X syndrome
e. William syndrome

**Question 17**

Which of the following is not considered as autosomal recessive disorders?
a. Phenylketonuria
b. Niemann–Pick disease
c. Hurler's syndrome
d. Laurence–Moon–Biedl syndrome
e. Fragile X syndrome

**Question 18**

Which of the following statements about the epidemiology of bipolar disorder is incorrect?
a. Women are as likely to have the disorder as men.
b. Rapid cycling is much more common in women than in men.
c. The first onset is usually that of a manic episode.
d. Bipolar disorder is usually found in occupations that require marked creativity, such as artists, writers and pop stars.
e. Genetic factors do play a significant role in the transmission of bipolar disorder.

**Question 19**

A 25-year-old woman has come to consult you for the management of her insomnia. She has never managed to sleep before 3 AM since adolescence. She does not much of a problem in the university as she used to skip morning lecture. She has recently taken a job which requires her to wake up at 6:00 AM. Which of the following is the most likely diagnosis?
a. Circadian rhythm sleep disorder
b. Delayed sleep phase syndrome
c. Poor sleep hygiene
d. Restless leg syndrome
e. Sleep disorder related to chaotic lifestyle in university

**Question 20**

The Papez circuit was a concept introduced in 1937, which proposed that there is a circuit mediating the neuronal mechanism of emotions. All of the following are part of this circuit, with the exception of
a. Hippocampus
b. Hypothalamus
c. Anterior nucleus of the thalamus
d. Posterior nucleus of the thalamus
e. Cingulate gyrus

**Question 21**

Which of the following is considered to be the largest of all the cranial nerves?
a. Optic nerve
b. Oculomotor nerve

c. Trochlear nerve
d. Trigeminal nerve
e. Facial nerve

## Question 22

The consultant psychiatrist decides to start a 22-year-old male Jonathan on olanzapine for his first-episode psychosis. He was noted to be unwell after the commencement of the antipsychotics and the consultant has made the decision to immediately transfer him to the medical unit. He explained to Jonathan's parents that Jonathan might be having a rare side effect to the medication, which is known as neuroleptic malignant syndrome. All of the following are clinical signs and symptoms observed in the syndrome, with the exception of
a. Rapidly varying and fluctuating changes in blood pressure
b. Elevated bodily temperatures
c. Rigidity of muscles
d. Elevated creatine kinase levels
e. Myoclonus

## Question 23

Which of the following terminology describes best the following concept: 'the disorder tends to occur at earlier ages of onset or with greater severity in the succeeding generations?'
a. Anticipation
b. Mosaicism
c. Uniparental disomy
d. Genomic imprinting
e. Mitochondrial inheritance

## Question 24

Age-specific mortality rate is correctly described as
a. The number of deaths over the midyear population in 1 year
b. The number of deaths of a specific age over the mid-year population of a specific age in 1 year
c. The mortality due to a condition over the population of people with the condition within a specified time period
d. The number of deaths over the midyear population over 10 years
e. The number of deaths of a specific age over the midyear population of a specific age over a course of 5 years

## Question 25

A 65-year-old man had a stroke 4 months ago. He subsequently developed low mood, irritability, poor sleep and anhedonia. He was diagnosed by the psychiatrist to have post-stroke depression. The stroke is most likely to affect which part of the brain in this case?
a. Left frontal cortex
b. Left cerebellum

c. Right cerebellum
d. Right temporal
e. Right occipital

## Question 26

This usually refers to the phenomenon in which an individual inherits both homologues of a chromosome pair from the same parent. Which terminology is correct?
a. Anticipation
b. Mosaicism
c. Uniparental disomy
d. Genomic imprinting
e. Mitochondrial inheritance

## Question 27

Apart from macroscopic changes seen in patients with Alzheimer's disease, there have been numerous histopathological changes as well. These include the following, with the exception of
a. Neuronal loss
b. Reactive astrocytosis
c. Neurofibrillary tangles located intracellularly
d. Neuritic plaques located extracellularly
e. Lewy plaques

## Question 28

Which of the following statements regarding Pick's disease is incorrect?
a. Selective asymmetrical atrophy of the anterior temporal lobes and the temporal lobes has been noted.
b. Sulcal widening has been noted.
c. Ventricular enlargement has been noted.
d. In Pick's disease, Pick's bodies, neuronal loss and reactive astrocytosis are noted.
e. The changes usually affect the cerebral cortex, the basal ganglia, the locus coeruleus and the substantia nigra.

## Question 29

A 60-year-old male has disclosed to the community psychiatric nurse following up with him that he is not keen to continue his selective serotonin reuptake inhibitor (SSRI) medications due to its effects on the sexual side of his relationship. Which one of the following medications, when added onto the existing regiment, might help the patient?
a. Bupropion
b. Venlafaxine
c. Imipramine
d. Lithium
e. Risperidone

**Question 30**

The main purpose of twin studies is to identify the relative contributions of genetic and environmental factors to the aetiology of a particular disorder. Which one of the following is not an underlying assumption?

a. Monozygotic twins are considered to be genetically identical as they have developed from the same fertilized ovum.

b. Both monozygotic and dizygotic twins are assumed to share the same environmental risk factors for the disorder to the same degree.

c. The null hypothesis assumes that the risk of the disorder is the same for monozygotic and dizygotic twins.

d. The null hypothesis assumes that the risk of the disorder is the same in twins and singletons.

e. The null hypothesis states that the risk of the disorder is increased when there is an interaction of the environmental risk factors with the underlying genetic risk factors.

**Question 31**

Based on the results of previous studies, it has been estimated that roughly what percentage of people who have committed suicide saw their GP in the week before ending their life?

a. 10%

b. 20%

c. 30%

d. 40%

e. 50%

**Question 32**

As compared to Parkinson's disease, higher densities of Lewy bodies have been found in the following regions, with the exception of

a. Cingulate gyrus

b. Parahippocampal gyrus

c. Temporal cortex

d. Basal ganglia

e. Parietal cortex

**Question 33**

Which of the following is not one of the usual difficulties associated with adoption studies when applied to psychiatric disorders?

a. Few cases would fulfil the criteria for adoption studies.

b. Adoption studies usually take a long time to carry out.

c. Information about the biological father may not necessary be available.

d. Adoption might cause indeterminate psychological sequelae for the adoptees.

e. The process of adoption can be randomized.

## Question 34
The mean age of onset of obsessive-compulsive disorder has been estimated to be around
a. 15 years old
b. 20 years old
c. 25 years old
d. 30 years old
e. More than 30 years old

## Question 35
Which of the following statements about the epidemiology of OCD is incorrect?
a. Females are more affected than males with a gender ratio of 1.5:1.
b. For men: checking rituals and ruminations are more common.
c. For women: obsessional doubts are more common.
d. It has been estimated that around 50% of the OCD patients are unmarried.
e. There has been an association between OCD disorder and the following diseases: pediatric autoimmune neuropsychiatric disorders associated with streptococcal infections (PANDAS), post-encephalitis.

## Question 36
A foundation year trainee has read some books on hypnotherapy and intends to refer a person with anxiety disorder to a hypnotherapist. Which of the following is correct?
a. Hypnosis is recommended by the NICE guidelines for treatment of anxiety disorders or PTSD.
b. Hypnosis is found to be superior to relaxation exercise.
c. Suggestion with hypnosis is found to be superior to suggestion without hypnosis.
d. Sudden removal of symptoms by suggestion under hypnosis can lead to rebound depression and anxiety.
e. Evidence has shown that hypnosis can aid recall in psychotherapy which leads to a better outcome.

## Question 37
Which of the following statements about Creutzfeldt–Jakob disease (CJD) is incorrect?
a. CJD is a disease that is transmitted via infection with a prion.
b. In addition to brain changes, there is associated degeneration in the spinal cord long descending tracts.
c. It usually has a relatively short incubation period.
d. Infection may be transmitted from surgical specimens, post-mortem preparation and also the human pituitary glands.
e. Recently, a new variant of CJD has been reported.

## Question 38

A 35-year-old man presented with dyscalculia, left-right disorientation and digital agnosia. Which area of his brain is affected?

a. Frontal lobe
b. Cerebellum
c. Parietal lobe
d. Temporal lobe
e. Occipital lobe

## Question 39

A 49-year-old woman presents with persistent, severe, distressing pain. Her doctors cannot find any physical disorder despite undergoing multiple tests. What is the lifetime prevalence rate of this disorder?

a. 7%
b. 12%
c. 16%
d. 17%
e. 20%

## Question 40

Which of the following mutations would not result in any alteration in the amino acid residue encoded?

a. Silent mutation
b. Missense mutation
c. Nonsense mutation
d. Transitional mutation
e. Frameshift mutation

## Question 41

Which of the following is false?

a. The DRD3 Ser9Gly polymorphism has been significantly correlated with the development of tardive dyskinesia.
b. The HLA gene has been implicated in the development of agranulocytosis in people taking clozapine.
c. The serotonin transporter-linked polymorphic region has been associated with clinical response to tricyclic antidepressants and SSRIs.
d. The serotonin transporter gene is implicated in the response to methylphenidate among young people with attention deficit hyperactivity disorder.
e. The $5HT_{2A}$ gene has been implicated in the response to electroconvulsive therapy.

## Question 42

Which of the following is false?

a. Phenytoin, valproate and clomipramine are 90%–95% protein bound.
b. Amitriptyline, imipramine, chlorpromazine and diazepam are 95%–99% protein bound.
c. If a drug is highly protein bound, the volume of distribution is reduced and close to the plasma volume.

d. Ionized drugs cross the blood–brain barrier rapidly.
e. The therapeutic window is the range of plasma concentrations which yields therapeutic success.

## Question 43
Which of the following statements about loss of function mutations is incorrect?
a. Loss-of-function mutations result in reduced activity or quantity of the gene product.
b. The mode of inheritance is usually autosomal.
c. The mode of inheritance could also be X-linked.
d. Loss-of-function mutations may not have harmful effects in the heterozygotes state, as 50% of the normal enzyme activity is usually sufficient for normal function.
e. Huntington's disease is a result of a loss-of-function mutation.

## Question 44
Which of the following statements regarding the pharmacokinetics of psychotropic drugs is false?
a. Psychotropic drugs are absorbed from the gastrointestinal tract as they are lipophilic.
b. Psychotropic drugs must reach the central nervous system in adequate amounts to produce therapeutic effects.
c. Psychotropic drugs are mainly metabolized by the liver.
d. Psychotropic drugs are mainly excreted by the liver.
e. Psychotropic drugs are not highly ionized at physiological pH levels.

## Question 45
The pharmacodynamic action of agomelatine involves
a. Alpha agonist
b. Cholinergic agonist
c. Histaminergic agonist
d. Melatonergic antagonist
e. 5-HT$_{2C}$ antagonist

## Question 46
The following neuroanatomical areas demonstrate significant changes before and after antipsychotic treatment in the first episode of schizophrenia, except
a. Amygdala
b. Cerebellum
c. Frontal eye fields
d. Postcentral gyrus
e. Prefrontal cortex

## Question 47
Which of the following is not a feature seen in punch-drunk syndrome, or what is commonly also known as post-traumatic dementia?
a. Cerebral atrophy
b. Ventricular shrinkage

c. Perforation of the cavum septum pellucidum
d. Thinning of the corpus callosum
e. Neuronal loss and neurofibrillary tangles

## Question 48
An 18-year-old woman suffers from borderline personality disorder. She complains of frequent mood swings and poor impulse control. She finds antidepressant treatment is not helpful and is keen to try a mood stabilizer. Her current BMI is 30 kg/m². Which of the following drugs cause weight loss?
  a. Carbamazepine
  b. Gabapentin
  c. Lamotrigine
  d. Topiramate
  e. Valproate

## Question 49
Which of the following statements about the epidemiology of dementia is incorrect?
  a. The prevalence of Alzheimer's disease is 50%, vascular dementia is 20% and Lewy body dementia is 15%.
  b. There is an equal male-to-female ratio.
  c. Risk generally increases with age, with 2% at the age of 65–70 and 20% at the age of 80 and above.
  d. Risk factors include smoking, sedentary lifestyle, high-fat/salt diet and head injury.
  e. Level of education attainment does not play a role in dementia.

## Question 50
Which of the following is considered to be a neuropeptide transmitter?
  a. Noradrenaline
  b. Serotonin
  c. Dopamine
  d. Glutamate
  e. Somatostatin

## Question 51
Antidepressants and antipsychotics might cause dizziness in a minority of patients. This might be attributed to the blockage of which of the following receptors?
  a. Serotonin
  b. Dopamine
  c. Alpha-1 adrenergic
  d. Alpha-2 adrenergic
  e. Beta adrenergic

## Question 52
Down's syndrome is a result of a mutation on which of the following?
  a. DISC-1 and DISC-2 on chromosome 1
  b. 7q gene on chromosome 7

c. APOE gene on chromosome 19

d. Amyloid precursor protein on Chromosome 21

e. COMT gene on chromosome 22

## Question 53

Vasoactive intestinal peptide would help to stimulate the release of adrenocorticotropic hormone, growth hormone and prolactin. It is found in all of the following structures, with the exception of which of the following?

a. Cerebral cortex

b. Hypothalamus

c. Amygdala

d. Hippocampus

e. Cerebellum

## Question 54

It has been estimated that roughly what percentage of patients with late paraphrenia have symptoms resembling paranoid schizophrenia?

a. 20%

b. 40%

c. 60%

d. 80%

e. 90%

## Question 55

Which of the following statements about Huntington's disease is incorrect?

a. This is a condition that results from a mutation of a protein called huntingtin.

b. It is a condition that is characterized by a selective loss of discrete neuronal populations in the brain, along with progressive degeneration of the neurons of the neo-striatum and eventual atrophy.

c. There is noted to be marked atrophy of the corpus stratum.

d. There is noted to be marked atrophy of the cerebral cortex.

e. There is a reduction in size of the lateral and the third ventricles.

## Question 56

Mutation in the following genes would result in schizophrenia, with the exception of

a. DISC-1

b. DISC-2

c. 6p

d. 11p

e. COMT gene

## Question 57

Usage of SSRIs such as fluoxetine on a long-term basis has been known to cause some sexual dysfunction. This is mainly due to the action on which one of the following receptors?

a. Serotonin 5HT1 receptor

b. Serotonin 5HT2 receptors

c. Serotonin 5HT3 receptors
d. Adrenaline receptors
e. Histamine receptors

## Question 58
Which of the following antipsychotics medication has been linked to relatively high incidences of significant agranulocytosis?
a. Haloperidol
b. Risperidone
c. Olanzapine
d. Quetiapine
e. Clozapine

## Question 59
Which of the following is the most common type of cerebral tumours?
a. Gliomas
b. Metastasis
c. Meningeal tumours
d. Pituitary adenoma
e. Neurilemmomas

## Question 60
The older generation of antipsychotics medication might have a high tendency of causing extra-pyramidal side effects. One of these side effects might include tardive dyskinesia. Which of the following statements best explains this side effect?
a. It is due largely to high 5HT2 receptor occupancy.
b. It is due largely to 5HT2 receptor sensitivity.
c. It is due to high D-2 receptor occupancy.
d. It is due to D-2 receptor sensitivity.
e. None of the above.

## Question 61
The gene that is responsible for the development of dementia in patients with Down's syndrome is
a. Amyloid precursor protein gene
b. APOE gene
c. COMT gene
d. DISC-1
e. DISC-2

## Question 62
Which of the following changes is implicated in the neuropathology of obsessive-compulsive disorder?
a. Mesolimbic activation
b. Mesolimbic deactivation
c. Orbitofrontal activation
d. Orbitofrontal deactivation
e. Prefrontal activation

## Question 63
Based on the current understanding about cell division, during which phase of mitosis does the cell replicate its genetic materials prior to undergoing further division?
a. Interphase
b. Prophase
c. Metaphase
d. Anaphase
e. Telophase

## Question 64
In idiopathic Parkinson's disease, Lewy bodies are present in all of the following structures, with the exception of
a. Substantia nigra
b. Hypothalamus
c. Cerebral cortex
d. Olfactory bulb
e. Hippocampus

## Question 65
What is the estimated prevalence of dementia amongst those who are at the age of 80?
a. 5%
b. 10%
c. 15%
d. 20%
e. 25%

## Question 66
A 20-year-old male suffered a head injury following a pub brawl around 2 years ago. Since then, he has had several episodes of epileptic seizures. The neurologist has recommended for him to be started on an anti-epileptic medication. Which one of the following medications would have less of an effect on his cognitive capabilities?
a. Sodium valproate
b. Carbamazepine
c. Phenytoin
d. Lamotrigine
e. Topiramate

## Question 67
Which of the following with regards to switching of antidepressants is incorrect?
a. When switching antidepressants, it would be wise to consider a different SSRI or one of the better-tolerated new-generation antidepressants.
b. Switch over a duration of 2 weeks for drugs with a short half-life.
c. A 2-week wash-out period would be essential when switching from fluoxetine to other antidepressants, or from paroxetine to tricyclic antidepressants.

d. A 2-week wash-out period would also be required if the switch is from other antidepressants to new serotonergic antidepressants or monoamine oxidase inhibitor (MAOI) and from a nonreversible MAOI to other antidepressants.

e. Drugs with shorter half-life usually require a shorter period of switch-over time.

## Question 68

Which of the following statements regarding the neurochemical changes involved in Alzheimer's disease is incorrect?

a. There is a reduction in the amount of acetylcholinesterase.

b. There is a reduction in the amount of choline acetyltransferase.

c. There is an increase in the amount of gamma-aminobutyric acid (GABA).

d. There is a decrease in the amount of GABA.

e. There is a decrease in the amount of noradrenaline.

## Question 69

Which of the following terminology refers to the number of deaths under 1 year old as compared to the number of live births over the course of 1 year?

a. Child mortality rate

b. Infant mortality rate

c. Postnatal mortality rate

d. Neonatal mortality rate

e. Perinatal mortality rate

## Question 70

Which of the following statements about the brain changes in patients with schizophrenia is incorrect?

a. There is a significant reduction in brain mass in schizophrenia as compared to controls.

b. There is a significant reduction in the volumes of the cerebral hemispheres, cerebral cortex and the central grey matter.

c. The volume of the white matter is reduced in patients with schizophrenia.

d. Ventricular enlargement particularly affects the temporal horn.

e. Ventricular enlargement in the temporal lobe is indicative of a temporal lobe neuropathology.

## Question 71

Neuropathological and structural neuroimaging studies have shown hypoplasia of which of the following in individuals with autism?

a. Hippocampus

b. Septal nuclei

c. Cerebellar

d. Mammillary body

e. Amygdala

## Question 72
This refers to the number of deaths in the first 28 days divided by the total number of live births, considered over a total duration of 1 year. Which of the following is true?
a. Child mortality rate
b. Infant mortality rate
c. Postnatal mortality rate
d. Neonatal mortality rate
e. Perinatal mortality rate

## Question 73
A 25-year-old male has a phobia of being judged when he is in crowded place. His psychotherapist has recommended that he be repeatedly exposed to crowds. The psychotherapist is making this recommendation on what basis?
a. Classical conditioning
b. Counter conditioning
c. Extinction
d. Habit reversal
e. Habituation

## Question 74
Which of the following statements about meiosis is incorrect?
a. It usually involves two stages of cell division.
b. Chromosomal division takes place once during meiosis and the resultant gametes are haploid.
c. Recombination takes place during prophase I.
d. There is an interphase in the second stage of cellular division.
e. The following stages are present in both meiosis I and meiosis II: prophase, metaphase, anaphase and telophase.

## Question 75
Which of the following is not a cognitive error usually targeted during cognitive behavioural therapy?
a. Overgeneralization
b. Minimization
c. Magnification
d. Selective abstraction
e. Trial interpretation

## Question 76
A medical student is conducting a research study looking at the number of stillbirths as well as deaths over a 1-year period. Which of the following is the correct mortality index he should be reporting in his research paper?
a. Child mortality rate
b. Infant mortality rate

c. Postnatal mortality rate
d. Neonatal mortality rate
e. Perinatal mortality rate

## Question 77

Which of the following statements about the clinical application of cognitive behavioural therapy (CBT) is incorrect?
  a. CBT is helpful for those with even mild depression.
  b. CBT is of use for those with addiction issues, such as alcohol.
  c. Homework tasks are usually assigned in between the sessions.
  d. CBT focuses on both the cognitive and behavioural aspects.
  e. CBT focuses on changing maladaptive procedural sequences.

## Question 78

This particular statistic helps to express the benefits of an active treatment over a placebo. Which of the following is the correct answer?
  a. Relative risk
  b. Attributable risk
  c. Absolute risk reduction
  d. Relative risk reduction
  e. Number needed to treat

## Question 79

The terminology 'morbid risk', also known as lifetime incidence, is used to express the rates of illness in relatives. Which is the morbid risk of schizophrenia amongst first-degree relatives?
  a. 1.5%
  b. 2.5%
  c. 3.5%
  d. 4.5%
  e. 5.5%

## Question 80

A psychiatry core trainee is being supervised by his psychotherapist for cognitive behaviour therapy for a patient with moderate degree of OCD. Which of the following would be the first recommended step advised by his supervisor?
  a. Taking a detailed history of the current symptoms
  b. Focusing on cognitive distortions
  c. Focusing on basic behavioural techniques such as relaxation
  d. Commencing on exposure and response prevention
  e. Commencing on flooding

## Question 81

A 23-year-old male has been diagnosed with first-episode psychosis. He has been started on medications and the community psychiatric nurse is following up with him. He has been concordant with his medications, but during the home

visit, the nurse noted high levels of expressed emotions. Both he and family are recommended for strategic family therapy. Which of the following is a technique that is commonly used in this particular type of therapy?
a. Classical conditioning
b. Operant conditioning
c. Behavioural experiments
d. Paradoxical interventions
e. Communication skills retraining

## Question 82
What is the estimated morbid risk of depressive disorder amongst first-degree relatives?
a. 3%
b. 6%
c. 9%
d. 12%
e. 15%

## Question 83
Which of the following antipsychotic usually has the lowest risk of inducing sedation?
a. Clozapine
b. Risperidone
c. Olanzapine
d. Aripiprazole
e. Haloperidol

## Question 84
Which of the following psychiatric disorders is contraindicated for brief dynamic psychotherapy?
a. Depressive disorder
b. Anxiety disorders
c. Childhood abuse and trauma
d. Personality disorder
e. Substance abuse disorder

## Question 85
What is the average age of onset of bipolar disorder amongst first-degree relatives based on epidemiological studies?
a. 15
b. 18
c. 19
d. 20
e. 21

### Question 86
Kolberg has previously described the stages of moral development. Which of the following is true with regards to what is described as the conventional stage of morality?
a. It is based entirely on rewards.
b. It is based on classical conditioning.
c. It is based on operant conditioning.
d. It involves obeying what the authority deems to be appropriate.
e. It involves consideration of the individual and weighing the benefits against the risk.

### Question 87
There are several theories of personality being proposed for personality research. Which of the following is not part of the 'Big Five' theory?
a. Openness to experience
b. Neuroticism
c. Extraversion
d. Cautiousness
e. Conscientiousness

### Question 88
What is the estimated morbid risk of a first-degree relative acquiring Alzheimer's disease as compared to the general population?
a. 5%–9%
b. 10%–14%
c. 15%–19%
d. 20%–24%
e. 25%–30%

### Question 89
All of the following are terms that refer to techniques used in psychodynamic psychotherapy, with the exception of which of the following?
a. Establishing a therapeutic alliance
b. Free association by client
c. Interpretation of transference
d. Working through
e. Homework assignment

### Question 90
Client's factors that would render them unsuitable for brief dynamic psychotherapy would include
a. Strong motivation to understand about the influence of the past on current issues
b. Adequate ego strength
c. Ability to tolerate frustration
d. Psychological mindedness
e. Capacity to form but not to sustain relationship

## Question 91
What is the estimated twin (MZ) concordance for schizophrenia?
a. 7%
b. 13%
c. 26%
d. 46%
e. 50%

## Question 92
A 25-year-old male has been started on a new SSRI antidepressant for his depression. He has been complaining that he has been having much difficulty with sleep. Stimulation of which SSRI receptors might cause the sleep disturbances?
a. Serotonin 5-HT1A
b. Serotonin 5-HT2A
c. Serotonin 5-HT3
d. Noradrenaline receptors
e. Histamine receptors

## Question 93
A soccer player missed the most important goal in the season's final and caused his team to lose the championship entirely. He feels that he is definitely not going to score any further goals in the near future and that he has also failed as a husband and a father. Which is the most likely cognitive distortion?
a. Selective abstraction
b. Overgeneralization
c. Minimization
d. Magnification
e. Arbitrary inference

## Question 94
What is the estimated mono-zygotic (MZ) concordance for bipolar disorder?
a. 10%
b. 20%
c. 30%
d. 40%
e. 50%

## Question 95
Which of the following is not a type of adoption study?
a. Adoptee studies
b. Adoptee family studies
c. Cross-fostering studies
d. Adoption studies involving monozygotic twins
e. Adoption studies involving dizygotic twins

**Question 96**

In cognitive analytic therapy, which of the following would the therapist focus upon?

a. Interpersonal role deficits
b. Interpersonal difficulties
c. Cognitive schemas
d. Reciprocal role procedures
e. Automatic cognitive schemas

**Question 97**

A therapist is seeing a patient who has depressive disorder and is using cognitive behaviour therapy to help him with his disorder. Which of the following is not a technique commonly used in cognitive behaviour therapy?

a. Socratic questioning
b. Psycho-education
c. Identification of cognitive errors
d. Identification of rational alternatives
e. Identification of dilemma and snags

**Question 98**

What has been the estimated twin (MZ) concordance for alcohol dependence?

a. 20%
b. 40%
c. 60%
d. 80%
e. 90%

**Question 99**

A 32-year-old male lost his job 5 months ago and has been low in his mood. He has recently increased his usage of alcohol to cope with his problems. He has been admitted to the inpatient unit following an attempt of para-suicide. Which of the following medications would be most helpful for detoxification?

a. Oxazepam
b. Alprazolam
c. Diazepam
d. Lithium
e. Haloperidol

**Question 100**

Which of the following adoption studies compares the adopted children of affected and unaffected biological parents?

a. Adoptee studies
b. Adoptee family studies
c. Cross-fostering studies
d. Adoption studies involving monozygotic twins
e. Adoption studies involving dizygotic twins

## Question 101
Individuals with narcissist personality disorder tend to make use of which one of the following defence mechanisms?
a. Sublimation
b. Humour
c. Regression
d. Projective identification
e. Displacement

## Question 102
There are various aetiological causes for learning disabilities. Which of the following infections acquired intrauterine might not result in learning difficulties?
a. CMV infection
b. Rubella infection
c. Toxoplasma infection
d. Syphilis infection
e. Influenza type B

## Question 103
The five core factors of personality traits proposed by the Big Five theory of personality include all of the following, with the exception of
a. Extraversion
b. Agreeableness
c. Neuroticism
d. Openness to experience
e. Intelligence

## Question 104
Which of the following personality disorders has been known to lead to the most impairment in terms of occupational functioning?
a. Schizoid personality disorder
b. Schizotypal personality disorder
c. Borderline personality disorder
d. Paranoid personality disorder
e. Obsessive-compulsive personality disorder

## Question 105
Which of the following statements with regards to the epidemiology of schizophrenia is incorrect?
a. The point prevalence of the disorder is 1% per year.
b. The lifetime risk of the disorder is 1%.
c. The age of onset is between 25 and 45 years.
d. The age of onset is earlier in men as compared to women.
e. It is most common in social classes IV and V.

**Question 106**
Based on the definition of mortality indexes, which of the following indexes represent the number of deaths in the first 28 days as compared to the total number of live births?
a. Postnatal mortality rate
b. Neonatal morality rate
c. Stillbirth
d. Perinatal mortality rate
e. Child mortality rate

**Question 107**
The average 1-year incidence rate for social phobia in the general population has been estimated to be
a. 2%
b. 4%
c. 6%
d. 8%
e. 10%

**Question 108**
Based on the definition of mortality indexes, which of the following indexes represent the number of stillbirths and deaths which are less than 7 days old, as compared to the total number of live births and stillbirths?
a. Postnatal mortality rate
b. Neonatal mortality rate
c. Stillbirth
d. Perinatal mortality rate
e. Child mortality rate

**Question 109**
The average 1-year incidence rate for panic disorder in the general population has been estimated to be
a. 2%
b. 4%
c. 5%
d. 8%
e. 10%

**Question 110**
Patients who have been commenced on MAOIs for treatment are counselled to watch their dietary intake. In the event that a patient who is on a MAOI happens to consume cheese, a hypertensive reaction might occur. In the emergency services, which of the following medications would be indicated for the treatment of the hypertensive crisis that has resulted?
a. Enalapril
b. Captopril

c. Thiazide diuretics
d. Urgent haemodialysis
e. Phentolamine

# Extended Matching Items (EMIs)

## Theme: Neuropathology
**Options:**
a. Temporal horn ventricular enlargement
b. Hypoplasia of cerebellar vermis
c. Loss of dopaminergic neurons in substantia nigra
d. Selective loss of discrete neuronal population
e. Progressive atrophy of the neostriatum

**Lead in:** Select the most appropriate answer for each of the following. Each option may be used once, more than once or not at all.

**Question 111**
Huntington's disease

**Question 112**
Parkinson disease

**Question 113**
Autism

**Question 114**
Schizophrenia

## Theme: Neurophysiology – action potential
**Options:**
a. Absolute refractory period
b. Relative refractory period
c. Conduction in unmyelinated fibres
d. Conduction in myelinated fibres
e. Excitatory postsynaptic potentials
f. Inhibitory postsynaptic potentials
g. Summation

**Lead in:** Select the most appropriate answer for each of the following. Each option may be used once, more than once or not at all.

**Question 115**
This occurs in the postsynaptic membrane due to the release of an excitatory neurotransmitter.

**Question 116**
This occurs in the postsynaptic membrane due to the release of an inhibitory neurotransmitter.

**Question 117**
It is noted that one excitatory postsynaptic potential might not be enough to give rise to an action potential.

**Question 118**
This refers to the periods in which the initiation of conduction of another action potential is not possible.

**Question 119**
This refers to the period in which the initiation of conduction of another action potential is more difficult.

## Theme: Mood disorder and suicide
**Options:**
  a. Double depression
  b. Depressive stupor
  c. Recurrent brief depression
  d. Masked depression
  e. Seasonal affective disorder
  f. Endogenous depression

**Lead in:** Select the most appropriate answer for each of the following. Each option may be used once, more than once or not at all.

**Question 120**
This form of depression has the following clinical features: motor retardation or agitation, anorexia, excessive guilt, diurnal variation in mood and absence of reactivity of mood, with terminal insomnia.

**Question 121**
This commonly refers to the presence of an additional mood component on top of a background of chronically low mood.

**Question 122**
In this form of depression, after recovery, the patient could then recall the events which have taken place when they are unwell. They are commonly unresponsive when unwell.

**Question 123**
The presence of one or two episodes of mood symptoms per month is characteristic of this condition.

**Question 124**
In this form of depression, depressed mood is not always complained of, rather than other somatic symptoms.

## Theme: Neurology and hormones

**Options:**
  a. ACTH
  b. Follicle-stimulating hormone
  c. Luteinizing hormone
  d. Melanocytes-stimulating hormone
  e. Prolactin
  f. Growth hormone
  g. Thyroid-stimulating hormone

**Lead in:** Select the most appropriate answer for each of the following. Each option may be used once, more than once or not at all.

**Question 125**
The main function of this appears to be with regards to pigmentation.

**Question 126**
This is a single-chain peptide hormone that acts on the mammary glands.

**Question 127**
This is a peptide hormone that stimulates the hepatic secretion of insulin-like growth factor-1.

**Question 128**
The action of this hormone is different for males than for females.

**Question 129**
This stimulates the production of steroid hormones.

## Theme: Arousal and sleep

**Options:**
  a. Stage 0
  b. Stage 1
  c. Stage 2
  d. Stage 3
  e. Stage 4
  f. Stage 5

**Lead in:** Select the most appropriate answer for each of the following. Each option may be used once, more than once or not at all.

**Question 130**
This stage of sleep has increased delta activity (approximately 20%–50%).

**Question 131**
This stage of sleep has increased delta activity (approximately more than 50%).

**Question 132**
These two stages of sleep are commonly referred to as slow-wake sleep.

**Question 133**
In this stage, there is marked alpha activity.

**Question 134**
This stage of sleep is characterized by low-voltage theta activity.

**Question 135**
This stage of sleep is characterized by occasional sleep spindles and K complexes.

## Theme: General principles of psychopharmacology – classification

**Options:**
  a. Moclobemide
  b. Venlafaxine
  c. Reboxetine
  d. Paroxetine
  e. Citalopram
  f. Mirtazapine
  g. Zolpidem
  h. Zopiclone
  i. Diazepam
  j. Temazepam

**Lead in:** Select the most appropriate answer for each of the following. Each option may be used once, more than once or not at all.

**Question 136**
Please select the serotonin–norepinephrine reuptake inhibitor from the aforementioned options.

**Question 137**
Please select the selective nor-adrenaline reuptake inhibitors (NARI) from the aforementioned options.

**Question 138**
Please select the noradrenergic and specific serotonergic antidepressants (NASSA) from the aforementioned options.

**Question 139**
Please select the nonbenzodiazepine hypnotics from the aforementioned options.

**Question 140**
Please select the short-acting benzodiazepine from the aforementioned options.

**Question 141**
Please select the long-acting benzodiazepines from the aforementioned options.

## Theme: General principles of psychopharmacology – concepts

**Options:**
- a. Volume of distribution
- b. Lipid solubility
- c. Phase I metabolism
- d. Phase II metabolism
- e. First-pass effect
- f. Elimination

**Lead in:** Select the most appropriate answer for each of the following. Each option may be used once, more than once or not at all.

**Question 142**
Increased volume of distribution is dependent and associated with this factor. Which factor is this?

**Question 143**
This refers to the theoretical concept that relates the mass of a drug in the body to the blood or plasma concentration.

**Question 144**
This refers to a synthetic reaction that involves the conjugation between a parent drug and a polar endogenous group.

**Question 145**
This refers to a change in the drug molecular structure by non-synthetic reactions.

**Question 146**
This effect varies between individuals and may be reduced by hepatic disease or drugs that increase hepatic blood flow.

## Theme: Other concepts of inheritance

**Options:**
- a. Anticipation
- b. Mosaicism
- c. Uniparental disomy
- d. Genomic imprinting
- e. Mitochondrial inheritance

**Lead in:** Select the most appropriate answer for each of the following. Each option may be used once, more than once or not at all.

**Question 147**
At times, abnormalities in mitosis could give rise to an abnormal cell line. Which concept of inheritance is this?

**Question 148**
This refers to the occurrence of an autonomic dominant disorder at earlier ages of onset or with greater severity in the succeeding generations.

**Question 149**
This refers to the phenomenon in which an individual acquires the same chromosome pair from the same parent.

**Question 150**
This form of inheritance is usually maternally inherited.

**Question 151**
This refers to the phenomenon in which an allele is differentially expressed depending on which parent it is acquired from.

## Theme: Advanced psychology – interviewing techniques

**Options:**
  a. Open-ended questions
  b. Observation
  c. Expression of interests
  d. Set goals
  e. Therapeutic alliance
  f. Affirmation
  g. Praise
  h. Reflective listening
  i. Reassurance and encouragement
  j. Rationalization and reframing

**Lead in:** Select the most appropriate answer for each of the following. Each option may be used once, more than once or not at all.

**Question 152**
This form of questioning confirms the validity of a prior judgement or behaviour.

**Question 153**
This refers to statement of appreciation rendered during the therapy session.

**Question 154**
This refers to repeating patient's own account by paraphrasing or using words that add meaning to what the patient has said.

**Question 155**
This involves providing a logical explanation for an event, situation or outcome.

**Question 156**
This includes both offering acknowledging statements as well as validating feelings.

## Theme: Advanced psychology

**Options:**
- a. Brief psychodynamic psychotherapy
- b. Cognitive behavioural therapy
- c. Dialectical behavioural therapy
- d. Mentalization-based therapy
- e. Cognitive analytic therapy
- f. Interpersonal therapy
- g. Family therapy

**Lead in:** Select the most appropriate answer for each of the following. Each option may be used once, more than once or not at all.

**Question 157**
This form of psychotherapy works on the premise that symptoms of individual family members are a manifestation of the way that the family system is functioning.

**Question 158**
This particular form of psychotherapy has its basis on the attachment theory.

**Question 159**
This particular form of therapy is helpful for borderline personality disorder patients.

**Question 160**
This form of therapy focuses less on transference interpretation, but aim at changing specific patterns of thinking.

**Question 161**
The contraindications for this form of therapy include severe dementia, profound learning disability and delirium and if there is the absence of cognitive errors.

## Theme: Neuroanatomy

**Options:**
- a. Pallium
- b. Corpus striatum
- c. Medullary centre
- d. Thalamus
- e. Subthalamus
- f. Hypothalamus
- g. Habenular gland
- h. Pineal gland
- i. Superior colliculi
- j. Inferior colliculi
- k. Pons

**Lead in:** Please select the most appropriate option for the following questions with regards to the development and organization of the brain.

**Question 162**
The prosencephalon gives rise to the cerebral hemisphere and which THREE of the aforementioned options?

**Question 163**
The epithalamus contains which TWO of the aforementioned structures?

**Question 164**
The mesencephalon gives rise to which TWO of the aforementioned structures?

**Question 165**
The rhombencephalon consists of which ONE of the aforementioned structures?

## Theme: Cranial nerves
**Options:**
   a. Optic nerve
   b. Oculomotor nerve
   c. Trochlear nerve
   d. Trigeminal nerve
   e. Abducens nerve
   f. Facial nerve
   g. Vestibulocochlear nerve
   h. Vagus nerve

**Lead in:** Please select the most appropriate options from the aforementioned options for each of the following questions.

**Question 166**
Inputs from the hypothalamus and even the gastrointestinal tract are received by this nerve. It also supplies the lower respiratory tract and the gastrointestinal tract, to as far as the transverse colon.

**Question 167**
This nerve helps to regulate the actions of the lacrimal gland as well as the salivary glands.

**Question 168**
This is the largest of all the cranial nerves.

## Theme: Neuropathology
**Options:**
   a. Alzheimer's disease
   b. Pick's disease
   c. Lewy body dementia
   d. CJD

e. Punch-drunk syndrome
f. Multi-infarct dementia

**Lead in:** Please select the most appropriate options from the aforementioned options for each of the following questions.

**Question 169**
Macroscopic changes, which include cerebral atrophy, ventricular enlargement, perforation of the cavum septum pellucidum and thinning of the corpus callosum, are observed mainly in this condition.

**Question 170**
In this condition, there is noted to be minimal atrophy of the cerebral cortex for rapidly developing cases.

**Question 171**
Some of the typical macroscopic changes include the presence of multiple cerebral infarcts, local or general brain atrophy and ventricular enlargement.

## Theme: Advanced psychological process and treatment – Yalom's therapeutic factors

**Options:**
  a. Democratization
  b. Instillation of hope
  c. Universality
  d. Permissiveness
  e. Information giving
  f. Reality confrontation
  g. Communalism
  h. Altruism
  i. Corrective recapitulation
  j. Social learning
  k. Interpersonal learning
  l. Catharsis
  m. Existential factors

**Lead in:** Based on your understanding about group therapy and Yalom's therapeutic factors, please select the factors that are in play during each of the stages of group therapy.

**Question 172**
Please select THREE factors that are in play in the early stages of group therapy.

**Question 173**
Please select FOUR factors that are in play in the middle stages of group therapy.

**Question 174**
Please select TWO factors that are in play in the end stage of group therapy.

## GET THROUGH MRCPSYCH PAPER A2: MOCK EXAMINATION

**Question 1 Answer: b, Left-sided lesions are associated with more impaired verbal fluency.**
*Explanation*: It is important to differentiate between left-sided lesions involving the dorsolateral prefrontal cortex and a right-sided lesion. Left-sided lesions are associated with more impaired verbal fluency, whereas right-sided lesions are associated with more impaired nonverbal fluency.

*Reference*: Puri BK, Hall A, Ho R (2014). *Revision Notes in Psychiatry*. London: CRC Press, p. 178.

**Question 2 Answer: e, Hypothalamus**
*Explanation*: All of the aforementioned are structures that are part of the mesial temporal region, with the exception of (e). It is important to note that left-sided lesions can lead to anterograde amnesia affecting verbal information, whereas right-sided lesions can lead to anterograde amnesia affecting nonverbal information. Bilateral lesions would lead to both verbal and non-verbal anterograde amnesia.

*Reference*: Puri BK, Hall A, Ho R (2014). *Revision Notes in Psychiatry*. London: CRC Press, p. 179.

**Question 3 Answer: e, Aripiprazole**
*Explanation*: Based on the existing literature, this is one of the medications that carries the lowest risk of QTc prolongation, lowest risk of sexual dysfunction, EPSE, dyslipidaemia, weight gain and glucose intolerance. It also carries a low risk of hyperprolactinaemia, postural hypotension and sedation.

*Reference*: Puri BK, Hall A, Ho R (2014). *Revision Notes in Psychiatry*. London: CRC Press, p. 367.

**Question 4 Answer: d, Furosemide**
*Explanation*: Furosemide would be indicated in this case. Hypertension should not be treated with diuretics, since thiazide and loop diuretics could reduce lithium excretion and can therefore cause lithium intoxication.

*Reference*: Puri BK, Hall A, Ho R (2014). *Revision Notes in Psychiatry*. London: CRC Press, p. 254.

**Question 5 Answer: b, Lesions on the right side lead to conduction aphasia.**
*Explanation*: It has been shown that lesions on the left side would lead to conduction aphasia, and not lesions on the right side.

*Reference*: Puri BK, Hall A, Ho R (2014). *Revision Notes in Psychiatry*. London: CRC Press, p. 180.

**Question 6 Answer: a, Olanzapine**
*Explanation*: The key findings of the CATIE study done in 2006, which involved more than 1500 patients with schizophrenia, are as follows: (1) the efficacy of first-generation antipsychotics was similar to that of the second-generation antipsychotics; (b2) olanzapine was the most effective in terms of the rates of discontinuation; (3) it is associated with greater weight gain and increases in measures of glucose and lipid metabolism.

*Reference*: Puri BK, Hall A, Ho R (2014). *Revision Notes in Psychiatry*. London: CRC Press, p. 251.

**Question 7 Answer: c, Only males are affected.**
*Explanation*: Both males and females are affected. The phenotype traits are present in all individuals who have the dominant allele in their genes. The phenotypic trait does not skip a generation, and hence vertical transmission could take place. It is of importance to note that both males and females are affected. Male-to-male transmission could potentially take place.

*Reference*: Puri BK, Hall A, Ho R (2014). *Revision Notes in Psychiatry*. London: CRC Press, p. 268.

**Question 8 Answer: d, Hurler's syndrome**
*Explanation*: All of the aforementioned could be inherited in an autosomal dominant manner, with the exception of Hurler's syndrome. Early-onset Alzheimer's disease is considered to be usually inherited in an autosomal dominant manner. The mutations concerned are usually found on either chromosome 14 or chromosome 21.

*Reference*: Puri BK, Hall A, Ho R (2014). *Revision Notes in Psychiatry*. London: CRC Press, p. 269.

**Question 9 Answer: e, Nystagmus**
*Explanation*: Balint's syndrome occurs due to a bilateral lesion involving the occipital lobe. In this condition, the core clinical signs and symptoms would include simultanagnosia, ocular apraxia, psychic gaze paralysis and optic ataxia.

*Reference*: Puri BK, Hall A, Ho R (2014). *Revision Notes in Psychiatry*. London: CRC Press, p. 180.

**Question 10 Answer: b, The more uncommon the disorder, the more unlikely it is that the parents are consanguineous.**
*Explanation*: It is more likely that the parents are related, instead of being unrelated. It is important to note that autosomal recessive disorders usually result from the presence of two abnormal recessive alleles, thus causing the individual to manifest the abnormal phenotypic trait.

*Reference*: Puri BK, Hall A, Ho R (2014). *Revision Notes in Psychiatry*. London: CRC Press, p. 269.

**Question 11 Answer: c, Approximately one third of British women commit suicide by hanging.**
*Explanation*: Based on the findings of epidemiological studies, all of the aforementioned are known to be true, with the exception of (c). It has been found that approximately two thirds of the British men and one third of the British women would commit suicide by hanging or via vehicle exhaust fumes.

*Reference*: Puri BK, Hall A, Ho R (2014). *Revision Notes in Psychiatry*. London: CRC Press, p. 287.

**Question 12 Answer: b, The Goth subculture in the UK is not strongly associated with self-harm.**
*Explanation*: The Goth subculture in the UK has been shown to be strongly associated with self-harm, based on epidemiological findings. All of the other options are true with regards to the epidemiology of deliberate self-harm in the United Kingdom.

*Reference*: Puri BK, Hall A, Ho R (2014). *Revision Notes in Psychiatry*. London: CRC Press, p. 287.

**Question 13 Answer: d, It is made up of four different layers.**
*Explanation*: Based on histology, the hippocampus is made up of three different layers. This would include the molecular layer (outer aspect), the pyramidal layer and the polymorphic layer (inner aspect).

*Reference*: Puri BK, Hall A, Ho R (2014). *Revision Notes in Psychiatry*. London: CRC Press, p. 182.

**Question 14 Answer: e, Females are equally likely to be affected with the X-linked recessive disorders.**
*Explanation*: All of the aforementioned are true with the exception of (e). Hence, the incidence of the disorder is actually very much higher in males as compared to females. Females are more likely to be carriers of the disorder instead.

*Reference*: Puri BK, Hall A, Ho R (2014). *Revision Notes in Psychiatry*. London: CRC Press, p. 269.

**Question 15 Answer: d, 30**
*Explanation*: The age of onset is indeed earlier than that in unipolar depression. The mean age of onset has been estimated to be around 30 years, with a range of 15 to 50 years.

*Reference*: Puri BK, Hall A, Ho R (2014). *Revision Notes in Psychiatry*. London: CRC Press, p. 284.

**Question 16 Answer: d, Fragile X syndrome**
*Explanation*: Fragile X syndrome is an X-linked dominant disorder with low penetrance. The fragile site is located at band q27.3 on the X chromosome. The trinucleotide repeats CGG are found on the long arm of the X chromosome.

*Further reading*: Puri BK, Treasaden I (eds) (2010). *Psychiatry: An Evidence-Based Text*. pp. 1082, 1088, 1091.

**Question 17 Answer: e, Fragile X syndrome**
*Explanation*: All of the aforementioned are considered and classified as autosomal recessive disorders, with the exception of fragile X syndrome. It is important to note that many of the disorders of protein metabolism could be inherited in an autosomal recessive manner.

*Reference*: Puri BK, Hall A, Ho R (2014). *Revision Notes in Psychiatry*. London: CRC Press, p. 269.

**Question 18 Answer: c, The first onset is usually that of a manic episode.**
*Explanation*: It has been noted that the first onset is usually that of a depressive episode. In accordance to the ICD-10 diagnostic criteria, there are repeated episodes of mood disturbances, sometimes elevated and sometimes depressed.

*Reference*: Puri BK, Hall A, Ho R (2014). *Revision Notes in Psychiatry*. London: CRC Press, p. 284.

**Question 19 Answer: b, Delayed sleep phase syndrome**
*Explanation*: The prevalence of delayed sleep phase syndrome is 3 in 2000 with no clear aetiology. Both sleep architecture and total time of sleep are normal. Patients usually feel sleepy in the morning. Depression is a common comorbidity.

Treatment strategies involve adaptation to late-night sleep, regular sleep schedule, good sleep hygiene, light therapy and melatonin.

*Reference*: Puri BK, Hall A, Ho R (2014). *Revision Notes in Psychiatry*. London: CRC Press, p. 613.

### Question 20 Answer: d, Posterior nucleus of the thalamus
*Explanation*: This circuit is responsible for the neuronal mechanism of emotions. The circuit consists of the hippocampus, the hypothalamus, the anterior nucleus of the thalamus and the cingulate gyrus.

*Reference*: Puri BK, Hall A, Ho R (2014). *Revision Notes in Psychiatry*. London: CRC Press, p. 183.

### Question 21 Answer: d, Trigeminal nerve
*Explanation*: The trigeminal nerve has been considered to be the largest of all the cranial nerves. It has four different nuclei, which include the main sensory nucleus, the spinal nucleus, the mesencephalic nucleus and the motor nucleus.

*Reference*: Puri BK, Hall A, Ho R (2014). *Revision Notes in Psychiatry*. London: CRC Press, p. 185.

### Question 22 Answer: e, Myoclonus
*Explanation*: Neuroleptic malignant syndrome is characterized by hyperthermia, fluctuating level of consciousness, muscular rigidity, autonomic dysfunction, tachycardia, labile blood pressure, pallor, sweating and urinary incontinence. In addition, there is elevated creatinine phosphokinase and increased white blood count, and abnormal liver function test. Option (e) is not one of the clinical signs and symptoms commonly observed in neuroleptic malignant syndrome.

*Reference*: Puri BK, Hall A, Ho R (2014). *Revision Notes in Psychiatry*. London: CRC Press, p. 253.

### Question 23 Answer: a, Anticipation
*Explanation*: Anticipation is the correct answer. It refers to the occurrence of an autonomic dominant disorder at earlier ages of onset or with greater severity in the succeeding generations. An example would be Huntington's disease, which has been shown to be caused by expansions of unstable triplet repeat sequences.

*Reference*: Puri BK, Hall A, Ho R (2014). *Revision Notes in Psychiatry*. London: CRC Press, p. 269.

### Question 24 Answer: b, The number of deaths of a specific age divided by the mid-year population of a specific age in 1 year
*Explanation*: The aforementioned is the correct definition for age-specific mortality rate.

*Reference*: Puri BK, Hall A, Ho R (2014). *Revision Notes in Psychiatry*. London: CRC Press, p. 278.

### Question 25 Answer: a, Left frontal cortex

*Explanation*: Depressive disorders are probably the most common psychiatric disorder associated with cerebrovascular disease. Approximately 15%–25% of community-based samples of patients with acute stroke and 30%–40% of patients hospitalized with acute stroke have a clinically diagnosable major or minor depressive disorder. Several studies find that poststroke depression is more likely to be associated with lesions in the left dorsolateral prefrontal cortex and left caudate nucleus.

*Reference*: Sadock BJ, Sadock VA (eds) (2009). *Kaplan and Sadock's Comprehensive Textbook of Psychiatry* (9th edition). Philadelphia, PA: Lippincott, Williams & Wilkins.

### Question 26 Answer: c, Uniparental disomy

*Explanation*: This is the correct explanation for uniparental disomy.

*Reference*: Puri BK, Hall A, Ho R (2014). *Revision Notes in Psychiatry*. London: CRC Press, p. 271.

### Question 27 Answer: e, Lewy plaques

*Explanation*: All of the aforementioned are histopathological changes, with the exception of (e). Other changes would include shrinkage of the dendritic branching as well. There has been a positive correlation between the number of neurofibrillary tangles and plaques and the degree of cognitive impairment.

*Reference*: Puri BK, Hall A, Ho R (2014). *Revision Notes in Psychiatry*. London: CRC Press, p. 195.

### Question 28 Answer: b, There has been noted to be sulcal widening.

*Explanation*: Sulcal widening has been noted for Alzheimer's dementia, and not Pick's disease.

*Reference*: Puri BK, Hall A, Ho R (2014). *Revision Notes in Psychiatry*. London: CRC Press, p. 195.

### Question 29 Answer: a, Bupropion

*Explanation*: Bupropion would be suitable. It is an antidepressant with noradrenergic activity. The main side effects include headache (30%), insomnia, and rash (0.1%). As compared to other antidepressants in the option, it has the least potential to affect sexual functions.

*Reference*: Puri BK, Hall A, Ho R (2014). *Revision Notes in Psychiatry*. London: CRC Press, p. 549.

**Question 30 Answer: e, The null hypothesis states that the risk of the disorder is increased when there is an interaction of the environmental risk factors with the underlying genetic risk factors.**

*Explanation*: All of the aforementioned are the assumptions that twin studies are based on, with the exception of (e). The null hypothesis for twin studies states two major assumptions: (1) the risk of the disorder is the same in twins and singletons; (2) the risk of the disorder is the same for monozygotic and dizygotic twins.

*Reference*: Puri BK, Hall A, Ho R (2014). *Revision Notes in Psychiatry*. London: CRC Press, p. 273.

**Question 31 Answer: d, 40%**

*Explanation*: It has been estimated that around two in five people who committed suicide saw their GP in the week preceding their death, according to a study done by Power in 1997.

*Reference*: Puri BK, Hall A, Ho R (2014). *Revision Notes in Psychiatry*. London: CRC Press, p. 288.

**Question 32 Answer: d, Basal ganglia**

*Explanation*: Lewy bodies are also found in Parkinson's disease. The density of Lewy bodies is much higher in all of the aforementioned regions, with the exception of the basal ganglia.

*Reference*: Puri BK, Hall A, Ho R (2014). *Revision Notes in Psychiatry*. London: CRC Press, p. 196.

**Question 33 Answer: e, The process of adoption can be randomized.**

*Explanation*: All of the aforementioned are problems associated with the use of adoption studies, with the exception of (e). Option (e) is incorrect as the process of adoption cannot be randomized. The fact that randomized is not possible makes it one of the core difficulties when adoption studies are conducted.

*Reference*: Puri BK, Hall A, Ho R (2014). *Revision Notes in Psychiatry*. London: CRC Press, p. 273.

**Question 34 Answer: b, 20 years old**

*Explanation*: The mean age of onset of the disorder is around 20 years, with at least 70% of the patients having it before the age of 25 years. Approximately 70% have their first episode before the age of 25 years and the remaining 15% would have their onset after the age of 35 years.

*Reference*: Puri BK, Hall A, Ho R (2014). *Revision Notes in Psychiatry*. London: CRC Press, p. 291.

**Question 35 Answer: c, For women, obsessional doubts are more common.**
*Explanation*: It has been noted that for women, compulsive washing and avoidance are more common. However, it should be noted that, for males, it is the checking rituals and the ruminations that are more common.

*Reference*: Puri BK, Hall A, Ho R (2014). *Revision Notes in Psychiatry*. London: CRC Press, p. 291.

**Question 36 Answer: d, Sudden removal of symptoms by suggestion under hypnosis can lead to rebound depression and anxiety.**
*Explanation*: Hypnosis is not commonly used in psychiatry and not recommended by the NICE guidelines to treat psychiatric disorders. Hypnosis is not found to be superior to other psychological treatments.

*Further Reading*: Puri BK, Treasaden I (eds) (2010). *Psychiatry: An Evidence-Based Text*. p. 141.

**Question 37 Answer: c, It usually has a relatively short incubation period.**
*Explanation*: The incubation period of CJD is usually for many years. CJD is transmitted by infection with a prion. In addition to the brain changes, it is known to be associated with degeneration in the spinal cord long descending tracts. Infection may be transmitted from surgical specimens, postmortem preparations (such as corneal grafts) and human pituitary gland; the latter have been used to produce the human somatotropin for clinical use. In 1995, a new variant of CJD has been reported.

*Reference*: Puri BK, Hall A, Ho R (2014). *Revision Notes in Psychiatry*. London: CRC Press, p. 196.

**Question 38 Answer: c, Parietal lobe**
*Explanation*: The man suffered from Gerstmann's syndrome, which affects the dominant parietal lobe. Individuals present with the following:

- Dyscalculia
- Finger agnosia
- Left-right disorientation
- Agraphia

*Reference*: Sadock BJ, Sadock VA (eds) (2009). *Kaplan and Sadock's Comprehensive Textbook of Psychiatry* (9th edition). Philadelphia, PA: Lippincott, Williams & Wilkins.

**Question 39 Answer: b, 12%**
*Explanation*: This woman has somatoform pain disorder. The lifetime prevalence rate is 12.3%, and the 6-month prevalence rate is 5.4%. The disorder is common in general medical practice. It is diagnosed almost twice as frequently in females as in males. Onset can occur at any age but is most frequent in the thirties and forties.

*References*: Grabe HJ, Meyer C, Hapke U et al. (2003). Somatoform pain disorder in the general population. *Psychother Psychosom*, 72: 88–94; Puri BK, Treasaden I, eds. (2010). *Psychiatry: An Evidence-Based Text*. London: Hodder Arnold, pp. 675–677, 840.

**Question 40 Answer: a, Silent mutation**
*Explanation*: Silent mutation would not result in any alteration in the amino acid encoded. Silent mutation is also classified as part of a substitution mutation.

*Reference*: Puri BK, Hall A, Ho R (2014). *Revision Notes in Psychiatry*. London: CRC Press, p. 261.

**Question 41 Answer: d, The serotonin transporter gene is implicated in the response to methylphenidate among young people with ADHD.**
*Explanation*: Option (d) is false as the dopamine transporter gene is implicated. The genes related to the dopaminergic function are implicated such as the dopamine receptor D4 gene, the dopamine transporter (DAT1) gene, the alpha 2A gene, norepinephrine transporter gene and the COMT gene.

*Reference*: Puri BK, Hall A, Ho R (2014). *Revision Notes in Psychiatry*. London: CRC Press, p. 631.

**Question 42 Answer: d, Ionized drugs cross the blood–brain barrier rapidly.**
*Explanation*: Ionised drugs (highly basic or acidic) cross the blood–brain barrier slowly. For option (e), therapeutic window refers to 'toxic dose' divided by 'therapeutic dose'.

*Reference*: Basant K. Puri, Annie Hall & Roger Ho (2014). *Revision Notes in Psychiatry*. London: CRC Press, p. 243.

**Question 43 Answer: e, Huntington's disease is a result of a loss-of-function mutation.**
*Explanation*: All of the aforementioned statements about loss-of-function mutations are true, with the exception of the disease example (Huntington's disease). Usually inborn errors of metabolism are a result of a loss-of-function mutation. Huntington's disease is an example of a gain-of-function mutation.

*Reference*: Puri BK, Hall A, Ho R (2014). *Revision Notes in Psychiatry*. London: CRC Press, p. 261.

**Question 44 Answer: d, Psychotropic drugs are mainly excreted by the liver**
*Explanation*: Psychotropic drugs are mainly excreted by the kidneys.

*Reference*: Puri BK, Hall A, Ho R (2014). *Revision Notes in Psychiatry*. London: CRC Press, pp. 243–244.

**Question 45 Answer: e, 5-HT$_{2C}$ antagonist**
*Explanation*: Agomelatine is an antidepressant which resynchronizes the circadian rhythm. It is a melatonergic agonist at MT$_1$ and MT$_2$ receptors and a 5-HT$_{2C}$ antagonist. It has no affinity for alpha-, beta-, adrenergic, histaminergic, cholinergic, dopaminergic and benzodiazepine receptors.

*Reference*: Puri BK, Hall A, Ho R (2014). *Revision Notes in Psychiatry*. London: CRC Press, p. 614.

**Question 46 Answer: d, Postcentral gyrus**
*Explanation*: The postcentral gyrus is the somatosensory cortex and shows the least change in activity after antipsychotic treatment. Changes in prefrontal and amygdala activity during olanzapine treatment have been reported in people with schizophrenia and these areas are involved in emotional processing. Increased activation in both frontal eye fields and the cerebellum can signify improvement in attentional and sensorimotor systems after antipsychotic treatment.

*References*: Blasi G, Popolizio T, Taurisano P (2009). Changes in prefrontal and amygdala activity during olanzapine treatment in schizophrenia. *Psychiatry Res*, 173: 31–38; Keedy SK, Rosen C, Khine T (2009). An fMRI study of visual attention and sensorimotor function before and after antipsychotic treatment in first-episode schizophrenia. *Psychiatry Res*, 172: 16–23.

**Question 47 Answer: b, Ventricular shrinkage**
*Explanation*: This is a common form of dementia usually affecting boxers, and also those who have been involved in repeated head injury. Macroscopic changes usually show the presence of ventricular enlargement.

*Reference*: Puri BK, Hall A, Ho R (2014). *Revision Notes in Psychiatry*. London: CRC Press, p. 197.

**Question 48 Answer: d, Topiramate**
*Explanation*: Amongst all the aforementioned mood stabilizers, topiramate is the one that would induce weight loss.

*Further Reading*: Puri BK, Treasaden I (eds) (2010). *Psychiatry: An Evidence-Based Text*. pp. 538, 699, 905, 910.

**Question 49 Answer: e, Level of educational attainment does not play a role in dementia.**
*Explanation*: All of the aforementioned with regards to the epidemiology of dementia are correct, with the exception of (e). Other risk factors include smoking, sedentary lifestyle, taking in a high-fat/salt diet and prior head injury. Those with a family history of Down's syndrome and Parkinson's disease also have an increased risk of acquiring dementia.

*Reference*: Puri BK, Hall A, Ho R (2014). *Revision Notes in Psychiatry*. London: CRC Press, p. 300.

### Question 50 Answer: e, Somatostatin
*Explanation*: Somatostatin is considered to be a neuropeptide transmitter that has largely inhibitory effects on the growth hormone secretion. With regards to its clinical relevance, a decrease in the CSF concentration has been noted in both unipolar and bipolar depression. It is also noted to be decreased in conditions such as Alzheimer's dementia.

*Reference*: Puri BK, Hall A, Ho R (2014). *Revision Notes in Psychiatry*. London: CRC Press, p. 234.

### Question 51 Answer: c, Alpha-1 adrenergic
*Explanation*: It has been shown that some TCAs and also antipsychotics would cause sedation and postural hypotension as a result of blockage of the alpha-1 receptors.

*Reference*: Puri BK, Hall A, Ho R (2014). *Revision Notes in Psychiatry*. London: CRC Press, p. 226.

### Question 52 Answer: d, Amyloid precursor protein on chromosome 21
*Explanation*: A mutation involving the amyloid precursor protein on chromosome 21 results in Down's syndrome. Approximately 94% of the cases are caused by meiotic nondisjunction or trisomy 21 (thus resulting in 47 chromosomes). Five per cent of the cases are caused by translocation that results in a fusion between chromosomes 21 and 14 (thus resulting in a net total of 46 chromosomes).

*Reference*: Puri BK, Hall A, Ho R (2014). *Revision Notes in Psychiatry*. London: CRC Press, p. 258.

### Question 53 Answer: e, Cerebellum
*Explanation*: Option (e) is incorrect. It is also found in the autonomic ganglia, and intestinal and respiratory tracts.

*Reference*: Puri BK, Hall A, Ho R (2014). *Revision Notes in Psychiatry*. London: CRC Press, p. 234.

### Question 54 Answer: c, 60%
*Explanation*: Around 60% of patients with late paraphrenia have symptoms that resemble paranoid schizophrenia. It is of importance to note that first onset of schizophrenia after the age of 60 is actually very rare. Only 1.5% of all individuals with schizophrenia have an onset after the age of 60.

*Reference*: Puri BK, Hall A, Ho R (2014). *Revision Notes in Psychiatry*. London: CRC Press, p. 300.

**Question 55 Answer: e, There is a reduction in size of the lateral and the third ventricles.**
*Explanation*: In this condition, the lateral and the third ventricles are increased in size. Macroscopic changes also include smaller brain with a reduction in mass.

*Reference*: Puri BK, Hall A, Ho R (2014). *Revision Notes in Psychiatry*. London: CRC Press, p. 201.

**Question 56 Answer: d, 11p**
*Explanation*: Mutations of all of the aforementioned genes would result in schizophrenia, with the exception of 11p. The gene 11p has been associated with brain-derived neurotrophic factor gene and bipolar affective disorder.

*Reference*: Puri BK, Hall A, Ho R (2014). *Revision Notes in Psychiatry*. London: CRC Press, p. 258.

**Question 57 Answer: b, Serotonin 5HT2 receptors**
*Explanation*: It has been shown that 5HT2A receptor agonism has been associated with circadian rhythm disturbances as well as sexual disturbances.

*Reference*: Puri BK, Hall A, Ho R (2014). *Revision Notes in Psychiatry*. London: CRC Press, p. 230.

**Question 58 Answer: e, Clozapine**
*Explanation*: Clozapine has the highest tendency to induce agranulocytosis and it is more common amongst Jews.

*Reference*: Puri BK, Hall A, Ho R (2014). *Revision Notes in Psychiatry*. London: CRC Press, p. 367.

**Question 59 Answer: a, Gliomas**
*Explanation*: Gliomas are usually tumours derived from the glial cells and their precursors and might include astrocytomas, oligodendrocytomas, and ependymomas. The relative frequencies of cerebral tumours are in the following order: gliomas, metastases, meningeal tumour, pituitary adenomas, neurilemmomas, haemangioblastomas and medulloblastomas.

*Reference*: Puri BK, Hall A, Ho R (2014). *Revision Notes in Psychiatry*. London: CRC Press, p. 197.

**Question 60 Answer: d, It is due to D-2 receptor sensitivity.**
*Explanation*: The major categories of adverse drug reactions caused by antipsychotics are due to antagonist action on the following receptors: dopamine, acetylcholine–muscarinic receptors, adrenaline and noradrenaline and the histamine receptors.

*Reference*: Puri BK, Hall A, Ho R (2014). *Revision Notes in Psychiatry*. London: CRC Press, p. 252.

**Question 61 Answer: a, Amyloid precursor protein gene**
*Explanation*: Individuals with Down syndrome tend to develop early-onset Alzheimer's disorder. This is due to the presence of an extra copy of the amyloid precursor protein gene on chromosome 21. People with Down syndrome are thus at a higher risk to develop Alzheimer's disease. Over the age of 40, there is a high incidence of neurofibrillary tangles and plaques with an increase in the P300 latency.

*Reference*: Puri BK, Hall A, Ho R (2014). *Revision Notes in Psychiatry*. London: CRC Press, p. 258.

**Question 62 Answer: c, Orbitofrontal activation**

*Reference*: Drummond LM, Finberg NA (2007). Phobias and obsessive-compulsive disorder, in Stein G, Wilkinson G (eds) *Seminars in General Adult Psychiatry*. London: Gaskell.

**Question 63 Answer: a, Interphase**
*Explanation*: It is during interphase that the cell replicates its genetic material prior to undergoing cellular division.

*Reference*: Puri BK, Hall A, Ho R (2014). *Revision Notes in Psychiatry*. London: CRC Press, p. 259.

**Question 64 Answer: e, Hippocampus**
*Explanation*: Lewy bodies are present in all of the aforementioned, with the exception of the hippocampus. They are also found in other areas such as the dorsal motor nucleus of the vagus nerve, the hypothalamus, the nucleus basalis of Meynert and the raphe nuclei.

*Reference*: Puri BK, Hall A, Ho R (2014). *Revision Notes in Psychiatry*. London: CRC Press, p. 200.

**Question 65 Answer: d, 20%**
*Explanation*: The risk has been estimated to double every 5 years. It has been estimated that around 20% of elderly at the age of 80 would have dementia.

*Reference*: Puri BK, Hall A, Ho R (2014). *Revision Notes in Psychiatry*. London: CRC Press, p. 300.

**Question 66 Answer: d, Lamotrigine**
*Explanation*: Lamotrigine might have a reduced effect on cognitive capabilities. The medication works via the inhibition of glutamate release.

*Reference*: Puri BK, Hall A, Ho R (2014). *Revision Notes in Psychiatry*. London: CRC Press, p. 247.

**Question 67 Answer: b, Switch over a duration of 2 weeks for drugs with a short half-life.**
*Explanation*: For drugs with a short half-life, it would only be necessary to switch over a period of 1 week. It is essential to be cognizant that a 2-week wash-out period is essential when switching from paroxetine to TCA and from an SSRI to a MAOI antidepressant.

*Reference*: Puri BK, Hall A, Ho R (2014). *Revision Notes in Psychiatry*. London: CRC Press, p. 391.

**Question 68 Answer: c, There is an increase in the amount of GABA.**
*Explanation*: There is an overall reduction in the amount of GABA based on neurochemical studies.

*Reference*: Puri BK, Hall A, Ho R (2014). *Revision Notes in Psychiatry*. London: CRC Press, p. 195.

**Question 69 Answer: b, Infant mortality rate**
*Explanation*: Infant mortality rate has been estimated to be around 4.9/1000 in the United Kingdom. It refers to the number of deaths under 1 year old divided by the number of live births, considered over the duration of 1 year.

*Reference*: Puri BK, Hall A, Ho R (2014). *Revision Notes in Psychiatry*. London: CRC Press, p. 278.

**Question 70 Answer: c, The volume of the white matter is reduced in patients with schizophrenia.**
*Explanation*: The volume of white matter did not differ significantly between normal control and those with schizophrenia.

*Reference*: Puri BK, Hall A, Ho R (2014). *Revision Notes in Psychiatry*. London: CRC Press, p. 198.

**Question 71 Answer: c, Cerebellar**
*Explanation*: Studies have shown that there is hypoplasia of the cerebellar vermis in people with autism. In addition, around 30% of individuals have nonspecific EEG abnormalities. MRI is not routinely done, but ventricular enlargement is found in 20%–25% of people with autism.

*Reference*: Puri BK, Hall A, Ho R (2014). *Revision Notes in Psychiatry*. London: CRC Press, p. 200.

**Question 72 Answer: d, Neonatal mortality rate**
*Explanation*: This is the definition of neonatal mortality rate.

*Reference*: Puri BK, Hall A, Ho R (2014). *Revision Notes in Psychiatry*. London: CRC Press, p. 278.

**Question 73 Answer: c, Extinction**
*Explanation*: By being repeatedly exposed to the crowds, extinction would take place. Extinction refers to the gradual disappearance of the conditioned response (fear in this case).

*Reference*: Puri BK, Hall A, Ho R (2014). *Revision Notes in Psychiatry*. London: CRC Press, p. 25.

**Question 74 Answer: d, There is an interphase stage in the second stage of cellular division.**
*Explanation*: There is no interphase stage in the second stage of cellular division.

*Reference*: Puri BK, Hall A, Ho R (2014). *Revision Notes in Psychiatry*. London: CRC Press, p. 259.

**Question 75 Answer: e, Trial interpretation**
*Explanation*: All of the aforementioned are commonly targeted cognitive errors, with the exception of (e). Other errors might include personalization, arbitrary inference, dichotomous thinking, catastrophic thinking and labelling.

*Reference*: Puri BK, Hall A, Ho R (2014). *Revision Notes in Psychiatry*. London: CRC Press, p. 388.

**Question 76 Answer: e, Perinatal mortality rate**
*Explanation*: Perinatal mortality rate takes into consideration the number of stillbirths and deaths divided by the number of live births and stillbirths over a 1-year period.

*Reference*: Puri BK, Hall A, Ho R (2014). *Revision Notes in Psychiatry*. London: CRC Press, p. 278.

**Question 77 Answer: e, CBT focuses on changing maladaptive procedural sequences.**
*Explanation*: The key objective of CBT is to help alleviate symptoms such as anxiety and depression by helping the client to identify and challenge negative cognitions. CBT is suitable for clients with depressive disorder as well as substance abuse. Homework tasks are usually assigned in between the sessions. Both cognitive and behavioural techniques are being used. Answer (e) is what cognitive analytical therapy would focus upon.

*Reference*: Puri BK, Hall A, Ho R (2014). *Revision Notes in Psychiatry*. London: CRC Press, p. 337.

### Question 78 Answer: e, Number needed to treat

*Explanation*: The number needed to treat expresses the benefits of an active treatment as compared to a placebo. It can be used to summarize the results of a trial and also in medical decision-making.

*Reference*: Puri BK, Hall A, Ho R (2014). *Revision Notes in Psychiatry*. London: CRC Press, p. 279.

### Question 79 Answer: c, 3.5%

*Explanation*: The morbid risk, also known as lifetime incidence, is computed from the number of affected relatives divided by the total number of relatives. The incidence of morbid risk for schizophrenia amongst first-degree relatives has been estimated to be 3.5%.

*Reference*: Puri BK, Hall A, Ho R (2014). *Revision Notes in Psychiatry*. London: CRC Press, p. 272.

### Question 80 Answer: a, Taking a detailed history of the current symptoms

*Explanation*: Taking a detailed history of the current symptoms would be essential. It has been proposed that in the early phase (sessions 1–4), there is a need to educate the client about the model of CBT and set goals for psychotherapy. This needs to be done prior to the identification of negative automatic thoughts and further assessment by questioning.

*Reference*: Puri BK, Hall A, Ho R (2014). *Revision Notes in Psychiatry*. London: CRC Press, p. 337.

### Question 81 Answer: d, Paradoxical interventions

*Explanation*: This methodology is being used at times when direct methods fail or when there is strong resistance in some family members. The therapist will reverse the vector and adopt a bottom-up approach from children to parents. It is noted that change and improvement usually take place as family members cannot tolerate the paradoxical pattern. Family therapy is usually indicated when there are changes in the family, for example a family member being recently diagnosed with an illness that could be terminal or causes a significant change in role (for example cancer in one parent).

*Reference*: Puri BK, Hall A, Ho R (2014). *Revision Notes in Psychiatry*. London: CRC Press, p. 344.

### Question 82 Answer: c, 9%

*Explanation*: The estimated morbid risk of depressive disorder is around 9%.

*Reference*: Puri BK, Hall A, Ho R (2014). *Revision Notes in Psychiatry*. London: CRC Press, p. 272.

**Question 83 Answer: d, Aripiprazole**
*Explanation*: As compared to the rest of the antipsychotics, aripiprazole has the lowest risk of sedation. In addition, it also carries the lowest risk of QTc prolongation, low risk of sexual dysfunction, low risk for EPSE and low risk of postural hypotension.

*Reference*: Puri BK, Hall A, Ho R (2014). *Revision Notes in Psychiatry*. London: CRC Press, p. 367.

**Question 84 Answer: e, Substance abuse disorder**
*Explanation*: Depressive disorder, anxiety disorder, childhood abuse and trauma, relationship problem and personality disorder are indications for brief dynamic psychotherapy. Disorders that are contraindicated include schizophrenia, delusional disorder, high tendency for serious self-harm and very poor insight.

*Reference*: Puri BK, Hall A, Ho R (2014). *Revision Notes in Psychiatry*. London: CRC Press, p. 333.

**Question 85 Answer: e, 21**
*Explanation*: The average age of onset of bipolar disorder amongst first-degree relatives has been estimated to be 21 years.

*Reference*: Puri BK, Hall A, Ho R (2014). *Revision Notes in Psychiatry*. London: CRC Press, p. 272.

**Question 86 Answer: d, It involves obeying what the authority deems to be appropriate.**
*Explanation*: In the conventional stage of morality, children tend to adopt the good girl/good boy orientation, in which rules are conformed in order to avoid the disapproval of others. In addition, they also adopt what is known as authority orientation, whereby laws and social rules are upheld in order to avoid the censure of authorities and because of the guilt about not doing one's duty.

*Reference*: Puri BK, Hall A, Ho R (2014). *Revision Notes in Psychiatry*. London: CRC Press, p. 69.

**Question 87 Answer: d, Cautiousness**
*Explanation*: Based on Eysenck's theory, the following are part of what he has proposed: neuroticism/stability, extroversion/introversion, psychoticism/stability and intelligence.

*Reference*: Puri BK, Hall A, Ho R (2014). *Revision Notes in Psychiatry*. London: CRC Press, p. 437.

**Question 88 Answer: c, 15%–19%**
*Explanation*: The morbid risk associated with a first-degree individual acquiring Alzheimer's disease has been estimated to be 15%–19%. This is around three times the risk for the general population.

*Reference*: Puri BK, Hall A, Ho R (2014). *Revision Notes in Psychiatry*. London: CRC Press, p. 272.

**Question 89 Answer: e, Homework assignment**
*Explanation*: All of the aforementioned are commonly used techniques in psychodynamic psychotherapy, with the exception of (e). Other techniques include focusing on internal conflicts since childhood, enactment, modifying and avoiding maladaptive defences.

*Reference*: Puri BK, Hall A, Ho R (2014). *Revision Notes in Psychiatry*. London: CRC Press, p. 333.

**Question 90 Answer: e, Capacity to form but not to sustain relationship**
*Explanation*: Client's factors that need to be considered prior to engaging them in brief dynamic psychotherapy include all of the following: strong motivation to understand about the influence of the past, adequate ego strength, tolerance to frustration, capacity to form and sustain relationship, psychological mindedness and good response to trial interpretation.

*Reference*: Puri BK, Hall A, Ho R (2014). *Revision Notes in Psychiatry*. London: CRC Press, p. 333.

**Question 91 Answer: d, 46%**
*Explanation*: The estimated twin (MZ) concordance for schizophrenia has been estimated to be around 46%.

*Reference*: Puri BK, Hall A, Ho R (2014). *Revision Notes in Psychiatry*. London: CRC Press, p. 358.

**Question 92 Answer: b, Serotonin 5-HT2A**
*Explanation*: Serotonin 5-HT2A would inhibit DA release upon binding to 5-HT. 5-HT2A receptor antagonism leads to anxiolytic effects. 5-HT2A receptor agonism is associated with circadian rhythm disturbances and sexual dysfunction.

*Reference*: Puri BK, Hall A, Ho R (2014). *Revision Notes in Psychiatry*. London: CRC Press, p. 230.

**Question 93 Answer: b, Overgeneralization**
*Explanation*: This is an example of over-generalization, a cognitive distortion.

*Reference*: Puri BK, Hall A, Ho R (2014). *Revision Notes in Psychiatry*. London: CRC Press, p. 387.

**Question 94 Answer: d, 40%**
*Explanation*: The estimated concordance rate is around 40%.

*Reference*: Puri BK, Hall A, Ho R (2014). *Revision Notes in Psychiatry*. London: CRC Press, p. 273.

**Question 95 Answer: e, Adoption studies involving dizygotic twins**
*Explanation*: All of the aforementioned are common methodologies of adoption studies, with the exception of adoption studies involving dizygotic twins. Adoptee studies compare the adopted children of affected and unaffected biological parents. Adoptee family studies compare the MR in the biological and adoptive families of affected adoptees. In cross-fostering studies, the risk of the disorder is compared in adoptees who have affected biological parents.

*Reference*: Puri BK, Hall A, Ho R (2014). *Revision Notes in Psychiatry*. London: CRC Press, p. 274.

**Question 96 Answer: d, Reciprocal role procedures**
*Explanation*: The main objective of this model is to aim at changing maladaptive procedural sequences. It also focuses on specific patterns of thinking and less on interpersonal behaviour. It focuses less on transference interpretation. In addition, in cognitive analytic therapy, there is a need to formulate a procedural sequence model. The model tries to understand the aim-directed action (such as formulating an aim, evaluating environmental plans, planning actions and evaluating results of actions). There is also a need to identify faulty procedures. These faulty procedures include traps, dilemma and snag.

*Reference*: Puri BK, Hall A, Ho R (2014). *Revision Notes in Psychiatry*. London: CRC Press, p. 339.

**Question 97 Answer: e, Identification of dilemma and snags**
*Explanation*: All of the aforementioned are true, with the exception of (e). Cognitive techniques include cognitive restructuring, which will help the client to identify negative thoughts, dysfunctional assumptions and maladaptive core beliefs related to their underlying problems. Behavioural techniques are also used in the therapy.

*Reference*: Puri BK, Hall A, Ho R (2014). *Revision Notes in Psychiatry*. London: CRC Press, p. 337.

**Question 98 Answer: c, 60%**
*Explanation*: The estimated twin concordance rate is around 60%.

*Reference*: Puri BK, Hall A, Ho R (2014). *Revision Notes in Psychiatry*. London: CRC Press, p. 273.

**Question 99 Answer: a, Oxazepam**
*Explanation*: For those with suspected liver damage, it would be wiser to consider using short-acting benzodiazepines such as oxazepam.

*Reference*: Puri BK, Hall A, Ho R (2014). *Revision Notes in Psychiatry*. London: CRC Press, p. 513.

### Question 100 Answer: a, Adoptee studies
*Explanation*: Adoptee studies compare the adopted children of affected and unaffected biological parents. An improved version of this design also incorporates the affection status of the adoptive parents.

*Reference*: Puri BK, Hall A, Ho R (2014). *Revision Notes in Psychiatry*. London: CRC Press, p. 274.

### Question 101 Answer: d, Projective identification
*Explanation*: In projective identification, the subject not only sees the other as possessing aspects of the self that have been repressed but constraints the other to take on those aspects. It is considered a primitive form of projection. Most theories state that people with this personality disorder develop narcissism in response usually to their inherent low self-esteem. They tend to have thus inflated self-esteem and would seek information that confirms their illusory bias.

*Reference*: Puri BK, Hall A, Ho R (2014). *Revision Notes in Psychiatry*. London: CRC Press, pp. 136, 450.

### Question 102 Answer: e, Influenza type B
*Explanation*: Congenital infections have been associated with the development of learning disabilities. Rubella, measles, influenza type B, Japanese encephalitis, cytomegalovirus, syphilis, HIV and toxoplasmosis have been implicated in the causation of learning disabilities.

*Reference*: Puri BK, Hall A, Ho R (2014). *Revision Notes in Psychiatry*. London: CRC Press, p. 664.

### Question 103 Answer: e, Intelligence
*Explanation*: (e) is incorrect. This is based on Eysneck's theory. Based on the theory and factor analysis of the rating scale data, it yields the dimensions including neuroticism/stability, extroversion/introversion, psychoticism/stability and intelligence.

*Reference*: Puri BK, Hall A, Ho R (2014). *Revision Notes in Psychiatry*. London: CRC Press, p. 437.

### Question 104 Answer: c, Borderline personality disorder
*Explanation*: A 15-year follow-up of 100 patients with borderline personality disorder showed that 75% are no longer diagnosed as borderline. However, there is a high risk of suicide, with 8.5% committing suicide in the 15-year follow-up. Poor prognosis is usually associated with early childhood sexual abuse, early first psychiatric contract, chronic symptoms and high affective instability. The impulsivity symptoms tend to improve significantly over time. However, the affective symptoms have the least amount of improvement.

*Reference*: Puri BK, Hall A, Ho R (2014). *Revision Notes in Psychiatry*. London: CRC Press, p. 447.

**Question 105 Answer: c, The age of onset is between 25 and 45 years.**
*Explanation*: The age of onset is usually between 15 and 45 years, and it is equally common in both males and females. Schizophrenia usually occurs much earlier in males as compared to females. There is a much higher incidence amongst those who are not married. It is also essential to take note that the prevalence of the disorder varies in accordance to the geographical location.

*Reference*: Puri BK, Hall A, Ho R (2014). *Revision Notes in Psychiatry*. London: CRC Press, p. 281.

**Question 106 Answer: b, Neonatal mortality rate**
*Explanation*: Neonatal mortality rate refers to the number of deaths in the first 28 days divided by the total number of life births over a period of 1 year.

*Reference*: Puri BK, Hall A, Ho R (2014). *Revision Notes in Psychiatry*. London: CRC Press, p. 280.

**Question 107 Answer: c, 6%**
*Explanation*: The average 1-year prevalence rate for social phobia in the general population has been estimated to be around 6%. The lifetime prevalence has been estimated to be 6%. For children and adolescents, the prevalence of social phobia is 1%. The prevalence of simple phobia and specific phobia is 2%–9% and 3%, respectively.

*Reference*: Puri BK, Hall A, Ho R (2014). *Revision Notes in Psychiatry*. London: CRC Press, p. 291.

**Question 108 Answer: d, Perinatal mortality rate**
*Explanation*: This is commonly referred to as the perinatal mortality rate. It takes into account the number of stillbirths and deaths that are less than 7 days old over the total number of live births as well as stillbirths.

*Reference*: Puri BK, Hall A, Ho R (2014). *Revision Notes in Psychiatry*. London: CRC Press, p. 280.

**Question 109 Answer: e, 10%**
*Explanation*: The estimated 1-year prevalence rate of panic disorders in the general population has been estimated to be around 10%. Based on Ham et al. (2005) research, it has been noted that approximately 25% of those who present to the emergency department with chest pain do fulfil the criteria for pain disorder. Panic disorder typically affects more females than males, and there is noted to be a bimodal peak in occurrence, with a peak at 15–24 years and another at 45–54 years. Medical conditions such as COPD, hypertension as well as irritable bowel syndrome have been found to be associated with panic disorder.

*Reference*: Puri BK, Hall A, Ho R (2014). *Revision Notes in Psychiatry*. London: CRC Press, p. 291.

### Question 110 Answer: e, Phentolamine

*Explanation*: Phentolamine is considered to be an alpha-adrenergic antagonist that can help to immediately lower the elevated blood pressure. The inhibition of peripheral pressor amines, particularly dietary tyramine, by MAOIs can lead to a hypertensive crisis when foods rich in tyramine are eaten.

*Reference*: Puri BK, Hall A, Ho R (2014). *Revision Notes in Psychiatry*. London: CRC Press, p. 255.

# Extended Matching Items (EMIs)

## Theme: Neuropathology

### Question 111 Answer: d, Selective loss of discrete neuronal population and (e) progressive atrophy of the neostriatum

*Explanation*: Huntington's disease results from a mutation of the protein huntingtin and is characterized by a selective loss of discrete neuronal populations in the brain with progressive degeneration of efferent neurons of the neostriatum and sparing of the dopaminergic afferents, resulting in progressive atrophy of the neostriatum.

### Question 112 Answer: c, Loss of dopaminergic neurons in substantia nigra

*Explanation*: Idiopathic Parkinson's disease is characterized by a loss of dopaminergic neurons in the substantia nigra.

### Question 113 Answer: b, Hypoplasia of cerebellar vermis

*Explanation*: Both neuropathological and structural neuroimaging studies have indicated that hypoplasia of the cerebellar vermis as well as hypoplasia of the cerebellar hemispheres occurs in some subjects with autism.

### Question 114 Answer: a, Temporal horn ventricular enlargement

*Explanation*: In schizophrenia, the ventricular enlargement particularly affects the temporal horn, indicating temporal lobe neuropathology.

*Reference*: Puri BK, Hall A, Ho R (2014). *Revision Notes in Psychiatry*. London: CRC Press, pp. 198–199.

## Theme: Neurophysiology – action potential

### Question 115 Answer: e, Excitatory postsynaptic potentials

*Explanation*: Excitatory postsynaptic potentials occur in the postsynaptic membrane following the release of an excitatory neurotransmitter from the presynaptic neuron at central excitatory synapses.

**Question 116 Answer: f, Inhibitory postsynaptic potentials**
*Explanation*: These occur in the postsynaptic membrane following the release of an inhibitory neurotransmitter from the presynaptic neurons at central inhibitory synapses.

**Question 117 Answer: g, Summation**
*Explanation*: One EPSP on its own is not usually sufficient to initiate an action potential. However, temporal and/or spatial summation may allow the degree of depolarization to reach the critical threshold, as shown in Figure 16.2. IPSPs, on summating with EPSPs, however, counter the effect of the latter.

**Question 118 Answer: a, Absolute refractory period**
*Explanation*: This is the period during which the active part of the neuronal membrane has a reversed polarity so that conduction or initiation of another action potential is not possible in it.

**Question 119 Answer: b, Relative refractory period**
*Explanation*: This is the period of repolarization after an action potential, during which hyperpolarization occurs, making it more difficult for stimulation to allow the membrane potential to reach the critical threshold.

*Reference*: Puri BK, Hall A, Ho R (2014). *Revision Notes in Psychiatry*. London: CRC Press, pp. 209–210.

## Theme: Mood disorder and suicide

**Question 120 Answer: f, Endogenous depression**
*Explanation*: The endogenous form of depression is commonly thought to be of biological origin, with the symptoms of motor retardation or agitation, agitation and weight loss, diurnal variation, excessive guilt, absence of reactivity of mood, anhedonia and terminal insomnia. In comparison, the reactive form is thought to be of psychological origin and the mood still remains reactive with predominance of initial insomnia.

**Question 121 Answer: a, Double depression**
*Explanation*: This is a major depression superimposed upon dysthymia.

**Question 122 Answer: b, Depressive stupor**
*Explanation*: The person is unresponsive, akinetic, mute and fully conscious. Following an episode, the patient can recall the events that took place at that time. Episode of excitement can occur between the episodes of stupor.

**Question 123 Answer: c, Recurrent brief depression**
*Explanation*: The diagnostic criterion for this condition is the presence of dysphoric mood or loss of interest for a duration of less than 2 weeks, with at least four of the following: poor appetite, sleep problems, agitation, loss of interest, fatigue, feeling of worthlessness, difficulty concentrating and suicidal ideations. One or two episodes per month for at least 1 year are characteristic of this condition.

**Question 124 Answer: d, Masked depression**
*Explanation*: In masked depression, depressed mood is not always complained of, rather somatic or other complaints. It is more common in the underdeveloped world and in those who are unable to articulate their emotions. The presence of biological symptoms is helpful in making the diagnosis. Diurnal variation in abnormal behaviour may mirror diurnal variation in mood.

*Reference*: Puri BK, Hall A, Ho R (2014). *Revision Notes in Psychiatry*. London: CRC Press, p. 380.

## Theme: Neurology and hormones

**Question 125 Answer: d, Melanocytes-stimulating hormone**
*Explanation*: MSH does not appear to be found in the anterior pituitary. Its function in relation to pigmentation appears to have been taken over by ACTH and also beta-lipotropin.

**Question 126 Answer: e, Prolactin**
*Explanation*: This is a single-chain peptide hormone that acts on the mammary glands to stimulate the secretion of milk. It also inhibits the activity of the testes and ovaries.

**Question 127 Answer: f, Growth hormone**
*Explanation*: GH is a peptide hormone that stimulates the hepatic secretion of IGF-1. In turn, binding of IGF-1 to widespread IGF-binding proteins leads to the stimulation of anabolism and widespread biosynthesis of proteins and collagen. Another important action of IGF-1 is in terms of opposing the action of insulin.

**Question 128 Answer: c, Luteinizing hormone**
*Explanation*: LH consists of two peptide chains. In males, LH stimulates the testicular Leydig cells to produce testosterone. In females, it stimulates the ovaries to produce androgens.

**Question 129 Answer: a, ACTH**
*Explanation*: This is a single-chain peptide that stimulates the production of the steroid hormone cortisol by the adrenal glands.

*Reference*: Puri BK, Hall A, Ho R (2014). *Revision Notes in Psychiatry*. London: CRC Press, pp. 211–212.

## Theme: Arousal and sleep

**Question 130 Answer: d, Stage 3**
*Explanation*: This is a stage of sleep that occurs during the normal NREM sleep (in which there is reduced neuronal activity). Stage 3 sleep is characterized by deep sleep, with increased delta activity of 20–50%.

**Question 131 Answer: e, Stage 4**
*Explanation*: This is also a stage of sleep that occurs during the normal NREM sleep. Stage 4 sleep is characterized by deep sleep, with increased delta activity of more than 50%.

**Question 132 Answer: d, Stage 3 and Stage 4**
*Explanation*: Stage 3 and Stage 4 sleep are classified as slow-wave sleep.

**Question 133 Answer: a, Stage 0**
*Explanation*: Stage 0 sleep is characterized by quiet wakefulness and shut eyes, and the EEG would show alpha activity.

**Question 134 Answer: b, Stage 1**
*Explanation*: The EEG for stage 1 sleep would show reduction in alpha activity and low-voltage theta activity.

**Question 135 Answer: c, Stage 2**
*Explanation*: Stage 2 is considered to be light sleep and the EEG would be around 2–7 Hz, with occasional sleep spindles and K complexes.

*Reference*: Puri BK, Hall A, Ho R (2014). *Revision Notes in Psychiatry*. London: CRC Press, p. 216.

## Theme: General principles of psychopharmacology – classification

**Question 136 Answer: b, Venlafaxine**
*Explanation*: Venlafaxine belongs to the class of SNRI antidepressants.

**Question 137 Answer: c, Reboxetine**
*Explanation*: Reboxetine belongs to the class of the NARI antidepressants.

**Question 138 Answer: f, Mirtazapine**
*Explanation*: Mirtazapine belongs to the class of NASSA antidepressants.

**Question 139 Answer: g, Zolpidem, and h, Zopiclone**
*Explanation*: These short-acting hypnotics are less likely to cause dependency than benzodiazepines and may be used for the short-term relief of insomnia.

**Question 140 Answer: j, Temazepam**
*Explanation*: Temazepam and lorazepam are considered to be short-acting benzodiazepines.

**Question 141 Answer: i, Diazepam**
*Explanation*: The long-acting benzodiazepines include diazepam, chlordiazepoxide and nitrazepam.

*Reference*: Puri BK, Hall A, Ho R (2014). *Revision Notes in Psychiatry*. London: CRC Press, p. 239.

**Question 142 Answer: b, Lipid solubility**
*Explanation*: Increased lipid solubility is associated with an increased volume of distribution. This is the common case for most psychotropic drugs at physiological pH.

**Question 143 Answer: a, Volume of distribution**
*Explanation*: Volume of distribution refers to the mass of a drug in the body at a given time over the concentration of the drug at that time in the blood or the plasma.

**Question 144 Answer: d, Phase II metabolism**
*Explanation*: This is the synthetic reaction that involves the conjugation between a parent drug/drug metabolite/endogenous substance and a polar endogenous molecule or group. Examples of the latter would include sulphate and glycine.

**Question 145 Answer: c, Phase 1 metabolism**
*Explanation*: Phase I metabolism refers to the change in the drug molecular structure by the following nonsynthetic reactions: oxidation, hydrolysis and reduction.

**Question 146 Answer: e, First-pass effect**
*Explanation*: The first-pass effect is the metabolism undergone by an orally absorbed drug during its passage from the hepatic portal system through the liver before reaching the systematic circulation. It varies between individuals and may be reduced by hepatic disease, food or drugs that increase hepatic blood flow.

*Reference*: Puri BK, Hall A, Ho R (2014). *Revision Notes in Psychiatry*. London: CRC Press, p. 244.

## Theme: Other concepts of inheritance

**Question 147 Answer: b, Mosaicism**
*Explanation*: Abnormalities in mitosis can give rise to an abnormal cell line. Such mosaicism may affect somatic cells or germ cells.

**Question 148 Answer: a, Anticipation**
*Explanation*: Anticipation refers to the occurrence of an autonomic dominant disorder at earlier ages of onset or with greater severity in the succeeding generations. In Huntington's disease, it has been shown to be caused by expansions of unstable triplet repeat sequences.

**Question 149 Answer: c, Uniparental disomy**
*Explanation*: This refers to the phenomenon in which an individual inherits both homologues of a chromosome pair from the same parent.

**Question 150 Answer: e, Mitochondrial inheritance**
*Explanation*: Since mitochondrial DNA is essential maternally inherited, mitochondrial inheritance may explain some of the disorders that affect both males and females but that are transmitted through females only and not through males.

**Question 151 Answer: d, Genomic imprinting**
*Explanation*: Genomic imprinting refers to the phenomenon in which an allele is differentially expressed depending on whether it is maternally or paternally derived.

*Reference*: Puri BK, Hall A, Ho R (2014). *Revision Notes in Psychiatry*. London: CRC Press, p. 271.

## Theme: Advanced psychology – interviewing techniques

### Question 152 Answer: f, Affirmation
*Explanation*: Affirmation confirms the validity of a prior judgement or behaviour, for example the therapist might say this: 'I must say, if I were in your position, I might have a hard time dealing with those difficult people in your company'.

### Question 153 Answer: g, Praise
*Explanation*: Praise refers to compliments, statements of appreciation and understanding. Praise could help to reinforce positive behaviours and seek feedback from the client to ensure acceptance of praise.

### Question 154 Answer: h, Reflective listening
*Explanation*: Reflective listening refers to repeating patient's own account by paraphrasing or using words that add meaning to what the client has said. For example, the client complains that she does not like the way that her partner comments on how she handles her children. The therapist could say, 'It seems that you are a bit annoyed by your partner's comments'.

### Question 155 Answer: j, Rationalization and reframing
*Explanation*: Rationalization and reframing involve providing a logical *Explanation* for an event, situation or outcome. Reframing involves providing an alternative way to look at a situation.

### Question 156 Answer: c, Expression of interests
*Explanation*: Expression of interests refers to offering acknowledging statements and validating feelings.

*Reference*: Puri BK, Hall A, Ho R (2014). *Revision Notes in Psychiatry*. London: CRC Press, pp. 329–330.

## Theme: Advanced psychology

### Question 157 Answer: g, Family therapy
*Explanation*: Milan developed the family therapy that emphasizes that the family system is more than the sum of its components and the system as a whole is the focus of therapy. Symptoms of individual family members are a manifestation of the way that the family system is functioning.

**Question 158 Answer: f, Interpersonal therapy**
*Explanation*: Interpersonal therapy is based on the attachment theory. The objective is to create a therapeutic environment with meaningful therapeutic relationship and recognize the client's underlying attachment needs. It also helps to develop an understanding of the client's communication difficulties and attachment style both inside and outside of therapy.

**Question 159 Answer: c, Dialectical behavioural therapy, d, Mentalization-based therapy**
*Explanation*: For DBT, it helps the client to build a life that is worth living. It helps to reduce self-harm and/or suicidal behaviour and helps to reduce or stop therapy-interfering behaviour. It reduces or stops the serious quality of life-interfering behaviour. For metallization-based therapy, it helps the client with BPD to develop the capacity to realize that a person has an agentive mind and to recognize the importance of mental state in other people.

**Question 160 Answer: e, Cognitive analytical therapy**
*Explanation*: Cognitive analytical therapy aims at changing maladaptive procedural sequences and focuses on specific patterns of thinking and less on interpersonal behaviour. CAT focuses less on transference interpretation.

**Question 161 Answer: b, Cognitive behavioural therapy**
*Explanation*: The objective of cognitive behavioural therapy is to alleviate symptoms such as anxiety and depression by helping the client to identify and challenging the negative cognitions. It helps to develop alternative and flexible schemas. It helps to rehearse new cognitive and behavioural responses in a difficult situation.

*Reference*: Puri BK, Hall A, Ho R (2014). *Revision Notes in Psychiatry*. London: CRC Press, pp. 330–341.

## Theme: Neuroanatomy
**Question 162 Answer: a, Pallium, b, Corpus striatum, c, Medullary centre**
*Explanation*: Apart from the aforementioned three structures, it also gives rise to the rhinencephalon.

**Question 163 Answer: g, Habenular gland, h Pineal gland**
*Explanation*: The epithalamus is derived from the diencephalon. It contains both (g) and (h). Other derivatives include the thalamus, subthalamus and hypothalamus.

**Question 164 Answer: i, Superior colliculi, j, Inferior colliculi**
*Explanation*: It consists of the tectum, and the tectum consists of the corpora quadrigemina, which includes both (i) and (j). The red nucleus is also part of the structure.

**Question 165 Answer: k, Pons**
*Explanation*: It consists of the pons, the oral part of the medulla oblongata as well as the cerebellum.

*Reference*: Puri BK, Hall A, Ho R (2014). *Revision Notes in Psychiatry*. London: CRC Press, p. 176.

## Theme: Cranial nerves

**Question 166 Answer: h, Vagus nerve**
*Explanation*: The vagus nerve has three nuclei: the main motor nucleus, the parasympathetic nuclei and the sensory nucleus. It does receive input from the hypothalamus, the heart, the lower respiratory tract as well as the gastrointestinal tract to as far as that of the transverse colon. In addition, it also supplies the involuntary muscle of the heart, the lower respiratory tract and the gastrointestinal tract as far as the distal one-third of the transverse colon.

**Question 167 Answer: f, Facial nerve**
*Explanation*: The facial nerve has three nuclei: the main motor nucleus, the parasympathetic nuclei as well as the sensory nucleus. The parasympathetic nuclei are responsible for supplying the neuronal inputs to the lacrimal gland as well as the salivary glands.

**Question 168 Answer: d, Trigeminal nerve**
*Explanation*: This is considered to be the largest cranial nerve. It has four nuclei: the main sensory nucleus, the spinal nucleus, the mesencephalic nucleus as well as the motor nucleus.

*Reference*: Puri BK, Hall A, Ho R (2014). *Revision Notes in Psychiatry*. London: CRC Press, p. 184.

## Theme: Neuropathology

**Question 169 Answer: e, Punch-drunk syndrome**
*Explanation*: These are characteristic macroscopic changes for patients with punch-drunk syndrome. In addition to this syndrome occurring in boxers, it also affects individuals who are involved in contact sports, who might have sustained repeated head injuries.

**Question 170 Answer: d, CJD**
*Explanation*: There is no noted atrophy of the cerebral cortex for rapidly developing cases. Those who survive longer might have selective cerebellar atrophy, generalized cerebral atrophy and ventricular enlargement.

**Question 171 Answer: f, Multi-infarct dementia**
*Explanation*: This is also known as vascular dementia. In this condition, there are arteriosclerotic changes in major arteries, in addition to the presence of the aforementioned.

*Reference*: Puri BK, Hall A, Ho R (2014). *Revision Notes in Psychiatry*. London: CRC Press, p. 196.

## Theme: Advanced psychological process and treatment – Yalom's therapeutic factors

**Question 172 Answer: b, Instillation of hope, c, Universality, e, Information giving**
*Explanation*: Instillation of hope refers to the sense of optimism about the progress and improvement. Universality refers to how one member's problems also occur in other members. Hence, the member is not alone. In information giving, it refers to how members would receive information on their illness and associated problems.

**Question 173 Answer: h, Altruism, i, Corrective recapitulation, j, Social learning, k, Interpersonal learning**
*Explanation*: Altruism refers to how one member feels better by helping other members and sharing their solutions. Corrective recapitulation refers to how the group mirrors one's own family and provides a chance for self-exploration of past family conflicts. Social learning refers to how social skills could be improved by means of social learning. Interpersonal learning is established by corrective experience in social microcosm.

**Question Answer: l, Catharsis, m, Existential factors**
*Explanation*: Catharsis refers to how group members feel encouraged and supported by expressing emotionally laden materials. With regards to existential factors, after group therapy, group members have more self-understanding and insight into responsibility and capriciousness of existence.

*Reference*: Puri BK, Hall A, Ho R (2014). *Revision Notes in Psychiatry*. London: CRC Press, p. 345.

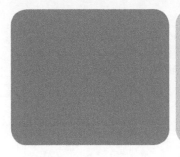
## GET THROUGH MRCPSYCH PAPER A2: MOCK EXAMINATION

Total number of questions: 167 (125 MCQs, 42 EMIs)
Total time provided: 180 minutes

**Question 1**
Cytoarchitectural abnormalities have been reported in the entorhinal cortex in schizophrenia. The changes that are suggestive of disturbed development include all of the following, with the exception of
  a. Aberrant invaginations of the surface
  b. Disruption of the cortical layers
  c. Heterotopic displacement of neurons
  d. Paucity of neurons in superficial layers
  e. Increased density of neurons in the deeper layer

**Question 2**
A neurologist has been called to the emergency service to assess a 70-year-old man. It was noted that the man was unable to speak and comprehend speech. Which terminology best describes this?
  a. Alexia
  b. Agraphia
  c. Apraxia
  d. Aphasia
  e. Amusia

**Question 3**
A 22-year-old male has been started on a new medication known as quetiapine to help him with his symptoms. He has been measuring his blood pressure daily and he has noted that his blood pressure is now lower when he takes the medication. This is due to the effect of
  a. Blockage of the serotonin receptors
  b. Blockage of the alpha-1 adrenergic receptors
  c. Blockage of the alpha-2 adrenergic receptors
  d. Blockage of the dopamine-1 receptors
  e. Blockage of the dopamine-2 receptors

### Question 4
A couple is considering adopting a child after multiple failures with artificial fertilization. They found a 2-year-old boy whom they were keen to adopt. However, they realized that the child's biological parents were alcoholic. What is the risk ratio of the child having similar alcohol dependence?
a. At least two times more
b. At least three times more
c. At least four times more
d. At least five times more
e. At least six times more

### Question 5
Based on epidemiological studies, roughly what percentage of patients with late paraphrenia would resemble that with paranoid schizophrenia?
a. 10%
b. 20%
c. 40%
d. 60%
e. 80%

### Question 6
The ICD-10 and the DSM-5 both have a specific constellation of symptoms for the diagnosis of borderline personality disorder. Which of the following clinical signs and symptoms would improve over time?
a. Irritability
b. Impulsiveness
c. Affective instability
d. Self-harm
e. Unstable relationships

### Question 7
A 6-year-old child was lost whilst he was out shopping with his mother. Initially, he showed marked signs of distress when he realized that he was lost, but when his mother returned, he began to ignore her. Based on Ainsworth's theory, what particular type of attachment would this be?
a. Secure attachment
b. Anxious ambivalent
c. Avoidant
d. Disorganized
e. Atypical

### Question 8
Based on epidemiological studies, roughly what percentage of people with schizophrenia would have an onset older than 60 years?
a. 0.5%
b. 1.0%
c. 1.5%

d. 2.0%

e. 3.0%

## Question 9

Antidepressants that act on which one of the following receptors might cause weight gain?

a. Histamine

b. Serotonin 5HT-1

c. Serotonin 5HT-3

d. Dopamine D1

e. Dopamine D2

## Question 10

Which of the following statements about serotonin is incorrect?

a. Serotonin is synthesized from dietary amino acid L-tryptophan.

b. Depletion of serotonin could be achieved by inhibiting tryptophan hydroxylase, removing L-tryptophan from the diet or adding natural amino acids such as alanine to compete for the transport process with L-tryptophan.

c. The release of 5-HT is dependent on calcium ions.

d. When depressed patients take SSRI, it would not lead to a reduction in 5-HT levels in the platelets.

e. Serotonin is taken back into the neurons and degraded by monoamine oxidase (MAO)-A.

## Question 11

The consultant psychiatrist has decided to start one of his patients on a MAO-I antidepressant in order to help him with his mood symptoms. He cautions the patient to be wary of his dietary intake. Which of the following should the patient avoid?

a. Food with artificial colourings

b. Cheese

c. Crackers

d. Nuts

e. Dried fruits

## Question 12

All of the following disorders are caused by trisomy, with the exception of

a. Edward's syndrome

b. Patau's syndrome

c. Down's syndrome

d. Cri-du-chat syndrome

e. Warkany syndrome 2

## Question 13

Epidemiological studies have shown which of the following findings to be incorrect for bipolar disorder?

a. Bipolar disorder is equally common in both males and females.

b. Rapid cycling disorder is more common in males.

c. The age of onset of bipolar disorder is much earlier as compared to unipolar depression.

d. There is a significant comorbidity with substance misuse and this has been estimated to be as high as 50%.

e. On average, around 25%–50% of bipolar patients commit suicide.

## Question 14

Which of the following theories explains how a child learns about what is considered to be gender appropriate for his or her anatomical sex?

a. Klein's theory

b. Kolberg's theory

c. Freud's theory

d. Social learning theory

e. Attachment theory

## Question 15

Long-acting benzodiazepines would include all of the following, with the exception of

a. Diazepam

b. Chlordiazepoxide

c. Nitrazepam

d. Temazepam

e. Clonazepam

## Question 16

A consultant psychiatrist decides to start a patient on a combination of clozapine and carbamazepine. The pharmacist reviewed the prescription and decides to call upon the consultant as she is worried about the patient developing which one of the following?

a. Neuroleptic malignant syndrome

b. Serotonin syndrome

c. Extrapyramidal side effects

d. Reduced total white blood cell count

e. Hypokalaemia

## Question 17

Which of the following is a known mechanism of placebo effect?

a. Homeostatic mechanism

b. Classical conditioning

c. Operant conditioning

d. Cognitive affective behavioural self-control

e. All of the aforementioned

### Question 18
Children with autism are believed to have impaired developments of their theory of mind. At roughly what age would children develop a theory of the mind?
a. 1 year old
b. 2 years old
c. 3 years old
d. 4 years old
e. 5 years old

### Question 19
In borderline personality disorder, it is known that impulsivity improves significantly over time. Poorer prognosis has been associated with all of the following, with the exception of?
a. Early childhood abuse
b. Early first psychiatric contact
c. Chronicity of symptoms
d. High affective instability
e. Chronic depression

### Question 20
Which of the following statements about the biosynthesis and metabolism of GABA is incorrect?
a. GABA is derived from glutamic acid via the action of glutamic acid decarboxylase.
b. It would require pyridoxal phosphate that is a vitamin B6 co-factor.
c. In schizophrenia, there is an increased expression of the messenger RNA for the enzyme in the prefrontal cortex.
d. The metabolic breakdown of GABA to glutamic acid involves the action of GABA transaminase.
e. GABA transaminase is often the target for anticonvulsants and inhibitor of this enzyme would lead to an increase in the GABA levels and prevent convulsions.

### Question 21
Clomipramine, imipramine and trimipramine belong to which specific class of tricyclic antidepressant?
a. Dibenzocycloheptanes
b. Iminodibenzyls
c. Diiminodibenzyls
d. Triiminodibenzyls
e. Phenothiazines

**Question 22**

Fragile X syndrome is due to

a. Failure of FMR1 gene transcription due to hypermethylation
b. Splicing errors
c. Failure of t-RNA to bind to the correct amino acids
d. Loss-of-function mutations
e. Gain-of-function mutations

**Question 23**

What is the estimated increase in risk of a child developing alcoholism if his father is dependent on alcohol?

a. 10%
b. 20%
c. 40%
d. 60%
e. 80%

**Question 24**

In this form of therapy, the therapy focuses on four core areas, including role transitions, interpersonal difficulties, interpersonal deficits and grief. Which one of the following best describes the therapy?

a. Interpersonal therapy
b. Cognitive behavioural therapy
c. Cognitive analytical therapy
d. Psychodynamic therapy
e. Strategic family therapy

**Question 25**

Which of the following is a rate-limiting enzyme in the synthesis of dopamine?

a. COMT
b. Dopamine (DOPA) decarboxylase
c. MAO
d. Phenylalamine hydroxylase
e. Tyrosine hydroxylase

**Question 26**

Which of the following statements about the rate of absorption is incorrect?

a. The rate of absorption is dependent on the particular form of the drug.
b. The rate of absorption is dependent on the $pK_a$ of the drug.
c. The rate of absorption is dependent on the particle size of the drug.
d. The rate of absorption is independent of the ambient pH.
e. The rate of absorption is dependent on the rate of blood flow through the tissue.

## Question 27

It has been shown that mania in patients with human immunodeficiency virus (HIV) indicates poor prognosis and would affect the adherence to anti-retroviral drugs. Which one of the following statements about the application of mood stabilizers in HIV-infected patients is incorrect?

a. Lithium is usually well tolerated.
b. When lithium is used, it is necessary to monitor closely for neurotoxicity and gastrointestinal side effects.
c. Sodium valproate is effective in treating mania in patients infected with HIV.
d. The usage of carbamazepine would result in an elevated risk of pancytopenia in HIV-infected patients.
e. It is important to note that carbamazepine would induce its own metabolism and this would decrease not only its own levels, but that of other drugs as well.

## Question 28

The cognitive component of cognitive behavioural therapy usually involves all of the following, with the exception of

a. Identification of negative automatic cognitions
b. Finding evidence for the cognitions identified
c. Identification of common cognitive errors
d. Restructuring underlying cognitive assumptions
e. Social skills training

## Question 29

Which of the following personality disorders is known to be the most common amongst inpatients?

a. Paranoid personality disorder
b. Borderline personality disorder
c. Histrionic personality disorder
d. Narcissistic personality disorder
e. Avoidant personality disorder

## Question 30

A patient presents to the emergency services with the following symptoms: unilateral pupil that is moderately dilated, with poor reaction to light and slow reaction to accommodation. Which of the following is the correct clinical diagnosis?

a. Holmes–Adie pupil
b. Hutchison's pupil
c. Argyll Robertson pupil
d. Horner's syndrome
e. Papilloedema

### Question 31

A core trainee has been asked to assess a patient who was opioid dependent in the emergency department. He is unsure what drugs are commonly used for the treatment of opioid dependence. Based on your understanding, which of the following is incorrect due to its potential side effects?

a. Methadone
b. Lofexidine
c. Naltrexone
d. Buprenorphine
e. Levo-alpha-acetylmethadol (LAAM)

### Question 32

Which of the following statements about Huntington's disease is incorrect?

a. It is an autosomal recessive disease
b. It is a progressive, inherited neurodegenerative disease
c. The clinical features include abnormal involuntary movements and cognitive deterioration.
d. There might be further progression to death and dementia over a course of 10–20 years.
e. The gene responsible is located on the short arm of chromosome 4.

### Question 33

Which of the following personality disorders is considered to be relatively uncommon in outpatients?

a. Paranoid personality disorder
b. Schizoid personality disorder
c. Antisocial personality disorder
d. Borderline personality disorder
e. Obsessive-compulsive personality disorder

### Question 34

A psychotherapist mentions to his client, 'If I were in your position, I might have a hard time dealing with those difficult people in your company'. Which particular type of interviewing technique is he using?

a. Affirmation
b. Praise
c. Reassurance
d. Encouragement
e. Rationalization

### Question 35

Which of the following statements is correct?

a. Adenine always pairs with guanine.
b. Introns are not expressed in the final protein product.
c. Telomeres play a key role in chromosome assortment during cell division.

d. The lagging strand is formed continuously, moving in the 5′ to 3′ direction during DNA replication.
e. The leading strand is formed in blocks during DNA replication.

## Question 36
A core trainee wants to consider referring one of the patients he has seen and diagnosed with depressive disorder for brief psychodynamic psychotherapy. He wonders which one of the following psychiatric conditions would not benefit from brief dynamic psychotherapy intervention?
a. Anxiety disorder
b. Childhood abuse and trauma
c. Relationship problems
d. Personality problems
e. Severe dependence on substances

## Question 37
Adoption studies for depressive disorder have shown that there is an increase in the rate for affective disorder among the relatives of index adoptees by roughly what percentage?
a. 2%
b. 4%
c. 6%
d. 8%
e. 10%

## Question 38
There is an association between schizophrenia and the following genes, with the exception of which one of the following?
a. Dopamine D3 receptor gene
b. Dopamine D2 receptor gene
c. 5-HT2A receptor gene
d. COMT gene
e. Dysbindin and neuregulin

## Question 39
This is a clinical condition involving a pupil due to rapidly increasing unilateral intracranial pressures. Which of the following is the correct clinical diagnosis?
a. Holmes–Adie pupil
b. Hutchison's pupil
c. Argyll Robertson pupil
d. Horner's syndrome
e. Papilloedema

## Question 40

A drug addict was involved in a gang fight and sustained an open laceration of his elbow. He believes that one of the drugs which he has been abusing might help to relieve his pain. Which one of the following drugs does have pain-relieving properties?

a. Alcohol
b. Amphetamine
c. Lysergic acid diethylamide (LSD)
d. Cocaine
e. Heroin

## Question 41

The female-to-male ratio for post traumatic stress disorder (PTSD) has been estimated to be

a. 5:1
b. 1:5
c. 2:1
d. 1:2
e. 1:1

## Question 42

Body dysmorphic disorder tends to affect females more than males. The comorbid psychiatric disorder includes all of the following, with the exception of

a. Depression
b. Trichotillomania
c. Social phobia
d. OCD
e. Eating disorders

## Question 43

Which of the following is not one of the factors that would render a client suitable for brief dynamic psychotherapy?

a. Client has strong motivation to understand more about the influence of the past on the presence.
b. Client has sufficient ego strength to deal with the topics that are discussed.
c. Client has the ability to tolerate frustration.
d. Client does not have the capacity to sustain previous relationships.
e. Client is psychologically minded.

## Question 44

A 55-year-old black African man suffers from hypertension and bipolar disorder. His GP wants to consult you about the safest diuretic to prescribe, as he takes lithium. Your recommendation is

a. Amiloride
b. Bendroflumethiazide
c. Chlorthalidone

d. Furosemide
e. Indapamide

## Question 45
A 35-year-old woman with agoraphobia is gradually exposed to crowded areas while relaxed. The periods of exposure gradually become longer and longer until she can confidently go to the market without an anxious response. This phenomenon is known as
a. Desensitization
b. Extinction
c. Flooding
d. Habituation
e. Sensitization

## Question 46
The big five factors of personality do not include which of the following?
a. Agreeableness
b. Carelessness
c. Conscientiousness
d. Extraversion
e. Neuroticism

## Question 47
Which of the following is not a relative contraindication for brief dynamic psychotherapy?
a. Schizophrenia
b. Delusional disorder
c. High tendency of serious self-harm
d. Partial insight
e. Severe dependence on substance

## Question 48
It has been shown that inheritance plays a significant role in the transmission of bipolar disorder. What is the estimated heritability of bipolar disorder?
a. 10%
b. 20%
c. 40%
d. 60%
e. 80%

## Question 49
For patients who have been diagnosed with normal-pressure hydrocephalus, which of their symptoms would improve after shunting?
a. Visual impairments
b. Cognitive impairments

c. Gait disturbances
d. Urinary disturbances
e. Judgments

## Question 50
Which of the following is not one of the factors that could help to optimize a patient's compliance?
a. Educating the patient about his or her medications
b. Reducing the number of tablets to be taken
c. Reducing the dosage frequency
d. Considering using parental or depot administration
e. Allowing the patient and not the family members to take ownership

## Question 51
The clinical features of fragile X syndrome are due to the failure of FMR1 gene transcription due to hypermethylation, thus resulting in the absence of the FMR1 gene protein. In addition, associated changes have been found such as the presence of a sequence of repeats. Which of the following sequence is being repeated?
a. ACG
b. GCG
c. CGG
d. CAG
e. AAG

## Question 52
Which of the following is not one of the risk factors for depression that has been proposed previously by Brown and Harris in their study?
a. Having three or more children under the age of 11 years old
b. Unemployment
c. Recent separation
d. Lack of a confiding relationship
e. Bereavement

## Question 53
During a session of brief dynamic psychotherapy, the client is silent when asked to speak about his previous experiences. Which one of the following negative reactions is this considered to be?
a. Resistance
b. Acting out
c. Acting in
d. Negative therapeutic reaction
e. Positive therapeutic reaction

## Question 54
Based on the experiments conducted by H. Wimmer and J. Perner, the theory of mind develops after the age of
a. 6 months
b. 1 year
c. 2 years
d. 4 years
e. 6 years

## Question 55
Which of the following statements about the Hayling and Brixton Test is false?
a. People with frontal lobe impairment perform poorly on the Hayling and Brixton Test.
b. The Hayling and Brixton Test was developed by Paul Burgess and Tim Shallice.
c. The Brixton Test is a spatial awareness Test.
d. The Brixton Test is a response initiation and response suppression test.
e. The Hayling Test is a sentence completion test.

## Question 56
A 14-year-old female adolescent develops non-epileptic fits when she is stressed. Her response was initially reinforced by attention from her teachers and peers. The non-epileptic fit is subsequently ignored until the non-epileptic fits no longer occur. This phenomenon is known as
a. Desensitization
b. Extinction
c. Flooding
d. Habituation
e. Sensitization

## Question 57
During a session of brief dynamic psychotherapy, the client decided to explore more about the therapist's personal and private information. Which of the following negative reactions is this considered to be?
a. Resistance
b. Acting in
c. Acting out
d. Negative therapeutic reaction
e. None of the aforementioned

## Question 58
The neuroanatomical area involved in face recognition is
a. Angular gyrus
b. Fusiform gyrus
c. Heschl gyrus

d. Postcentral gyrus
e. Precentral gyrus

## Question 59
Which of the following statements regarding the Camberwell Family Interview is false?
a. Both verbal responses and nonverbal cues are used to assess expressed emotion.
b. It has five components: critical comments, hostility, emotional overinvolvement, warmth and positive comments.
c. It is used to assess expressed emotion.
d. The interview is audio taped.
e. The Camberwell Family Interview does not measure the perception of the patient.

## Question 60
Which of the following is not part of Beck's cognitive model of depression?
a. Core beliefs
b. Cognitive distortions
c. Effect of early experiences
d. Attachment issues
e. Automatic thoughts

## Question 61
Specific reading disorder has been defined as a child having a score on reading or comprehension that is at least two standard deviations below that expected for the child's chronological age and intelligence. What is the estimated prevalence of this condition amongst the 9–1-year-olds in the United Kingdom?
a. 1%
b. 2%
c. 3%
d. 4%
e. 5%

## Question 62
A core trainee was asked to review an intravenous drug abuser. He noted that the patient seemed to have marked impairments in his memory, especially with regards to word finding difficulties. Which one of the following might be the most likely diagnosis?
a. HIV dementia
b. Mild cognitive impairment
c. Mixed dementia
d. Opioid intoxication
e. Opioid withdrawal

## Question 63
A 15-year-old boy was brought into the emergency department presenting with raised blood pressure, palpitations, and enlarged pupils. He was agitated and

shouting that he saw spirits chasing after him. His friend who accompanied him mentioned that he had been ingesting 'bath salts' in the pub. Which of the following mechanisms does 'bath salts' act upon that could have accounted for the boy's presentation?

a. Blocks N-methyl-D-aspartate (NMDA) receptors
b. Empties presynaptic serotonin stores
c. Enhances dopamine and serotonin reuptake
d. Inhibits dopamine and norepinephrine reuptake
e. Provokes release of dopamine in the mesolimbic system

## Question 64
Which of the following statements about meiosis is incorrect?

a. It usually involves two stages of cell divisions.
b. Chromosomal division takes place once during meiosis, and the resultant gametes are haploid.
c. Recombination takes place during prophase I.
d. There is an interphase stage in the second stage of cellular division.
e. The following stages are present in both meiosis I and meiosis II: prophase, metaphase, anaphase and telophase.

## Question 65
What has been believed to be the estimated prevalence of personality disorder in the general practice setting?

a. 10%
b. 20%
c. 30%
d. 40%
e. 50%

## Question 66
Which of the following statements about the objectives of cognitive behavioural therapy is incorrect?

a. It helps to alleviate symptoms such as anxiety and depression by helping clients to identify negative cognitions.
b. It helps to enable clients to challenge negative cognitions.
c. It helps them to develop alternative and flexible schema.
d. It helps them to rehearse new cognitive and behavioural responses to difficult situations.
e. It helps individuals to identify faculty procedures.

## Question 67
Tardive dyskinesia is associated with supersensitivity of which of the following receptors?

a. $D_1$
b. $D_2$
c. $D_3$

d. $D_4$

e. $D_5$

## Question 68

A 30-year-old man with a dual diagnosis of schizophrenia and alcohol dependence is admitted to hospital. He presents with tender hepatomegaly and jaundice. The level of aspartate transaminase (AST) is 250 IU/L (normal value: 3–35 IU/L), and the level of alanine transaminase (ALT) is 150 IU/L (normal value: 3–35 IU/L). He is disturbed by third-person auditory hallucinations and a delusion of persecution. The medical consultant would like to consult you about which antipsychotic to prescribe. Your recommendation is

a. Amisulpride

b. Chlorpromazine

c. Haloperidol

d. Risperidone

e. Quetiapine

## Question 69

A core trainee is asked to list down what he thinks are the typical characteristics of cognitive behavioural therapy (CBT). Which one of the following statements is incorrect as it is not one of the core characteristics of CBT?

a. This is a therapy that focuses on specific issues.

b. Homework is usually assigned.

c. It is a time-limited therapy.

d. It focuses entirely on the here and now.

e. Outcomes can be measured only by physiological measures, standardized instruments and self-report measures.

## Question 70

A 22-year-old nurse suffers from depression and she needs to work night shifts. She does not like to take medications on a daily basis. Which of the following antidepressants is the most suitable for her?

a. Amitriptyline

b. Citalopram

c. Fluoxetine

d. Mirtazapine

e. Paroxetine

## Question 71

Which of the following statements regarding duloxetine is true?

a. Duloxetine induces cytochrome P450 enzymes.

b. Duloxetine is safe to be co-administered with a monoamine oxidase inhibitor (MAOI).

c. Duloxetine is beneficial to people with urinary stress incontinence.

d. Its half-life is 4 hours.

e. There is clear evidence that duloxetine offers efficacy benefits over tricyclic antidepressants in the treatment of depression.

## Question 72

What is believed to be the estimated prevalence of personality disorder amongst the psychiatric inpatients?

a. 10%
b. 20%
c. 30%
d. 40%
e. 50%

## Question 73

Based on genetic studies, which of the following genes have been associated with Alzheimer's disease, with the exception of?

a. Presenilin 2 on chromosome 1
b. Presenilin 1 on chromosome 14
c. Apolipoprotein E (APOE) gene on chromosome 19
d. Amyloid precursor protein on chromosome 21
e. Disrupted in schizophrenia (DISC) gene on chromosome 4

## Question 74

Which of the following statements about cognitive impairment and dementia is incorrect?

a. Early cognitive impairments occur in around 10% of patients infected with HIV.
b. Cognitive symptoms include poor memory, concentration impairment, and mental slowing.
c. Behavioural symptoms include apathy, reduced spontaneity, and social withdrawal.
d. Motor symptoms include loss of balance, poor coordination, clumsiness, and leg weakness.
e. The onset of AIDS-associated dementia is usually insidious and occurs later in the course of the illness when there is significant immunosuppression.

## Question 75

Which of the following statements about factors affecting the absorption of drugs from the gastrointestinal tract is incorrect?

a. Absorption is dependent on then gastric pH.
b. Absorption is dependent on the intestinal motility.
c. The presence of food enhances absorption.
d. Absorption rate is dependent on the area of absorption.
e. Absorption rate is dependent on the blood flow.

## Question 76

With regards to the genetics of Down's syndrome, approximately what percentage are a result of translocation involving chromosomes?

a. 1%
b. 2%
c. 3%

d. 4%

e. 5%

## Question 77

Kleptomania is an impulse control disorder that is characterized by repeated failure to resist the impulse to steal, in which the tension is relieved by stealing. What is the gender ratio for kleptomania (females:males)

a. 1:1

b. 1:2

c. 2:1

d. 1:4

e. 4:1

## Question 78

A 30-year-old American woman suffering from depression asks to take reboxetine as her British friend has recommended this medication. Which of the following statements regarding reboxetine is true?

a. Based on previous study findings, there is clear evidence that reboxetine offers efficacy benefits over other antidepressants in the treatment of depression.

b. Reboxetine does not have anticholinergic effects.

c. Reboxetine exerts more influence on serotonin reuptake than on noradrenaline reuptake.

d. Reboxetine is metabolized by cytochrome P450 3A4.

e. Reboxetine is available in the United States.

## Question 79

The heritability of bipolar disorder is

a. 55%

b. 65%

c. 75%

d. 85%

e. 95%

## Question 80

All of the following are contraindications for cognitive behavioural therapy, with the exception of

a. Severe dementia

b. Learning disability

c. Delirium

d. Impulse control disorders

e. No evidence for cognitive errors

## Question 81

What is the estimated prevalence of learning disability (which is defined as having an IQ of less than 70) in the general population in the United Kingdom?

a. 1%

b. 2%

c. 3%

d. 4%

e. 5%

## Question 82

Translocation involving certain chromosomes might lead to the development of Down's syndrome. Exchange of chromosomal substance occurs between chromosome 21 and all of the following chromosomes, with the exception of

a. Chromosome 13

b. Chromosome 14

c. Chromosome 15

d. Chromosome 21

e. Chromosome 19

## Question 83

Huntington's disease is a result of which one of the following proteins?

a. Huntingtin

b. Hirano

c. Pick's

d. Lewy

e. Neuritic

## Question 84

A 22-year-old male has just taken some cannabis that his friend recommended him to try. For how long would the cannabis that he has taken be present and detectable in the blood after just a single dose?

a. 5 hours

b. 10 hours

c. 15 hours

d. 20 hours

e. 25 hours

## Question 85

With regards to DNA replication, which one of the following statements is incorrect?

a. Replication usually occurs from the 5′ to the 3′ direction.

b. New nucleotides are added to the 3′ end.

c. One strand is formed continuously and is known as the leading strand.

d. The other strand is known as the lagging strand and is composed of 100–1000 nucleotides.

e. The process is continuous as both the DNA strands are synthesized.

## Question 86

In order to fulfil the diagnosis of learning disability, the age of onset must be before the age of

a. 5

b. 8

c. 12
d. 16
e. 18

## Question 87

Based on the Isle of Wight study, what has been estimated to be the overall prevalence of child psychiatric disorder in middle childhood?
a. 2%
b. 4%
c. 6%
d. 8%
e. 10%

## Question 88

Which of the following disorders, based on the Isle of Wight study, is known to be the most common amongst middle childhood children?
a. Emotional disorder
b. Depressive disorder
c. Anxiety disorder
d. Conduct disorder
e. Hyperkinetic disorder

## Question 89

A 32-year-old woman suffering from depression is currently 35 weeks pregnant and she needs to take antidepressant treatment. Which of the following antidepressants is the most likely to cause withdrawal in the neonate after birth?
a. Duloxetine
b. Mirtazapine
c. Paroxetine
d. Sertraline
e. Trazodone

## Question 90

A medical student is interested in mirtazapine and she wants to find out more about its pharmacodynamics. Which of the following is the mechanism of action of mirtazapine?
a. $\alpha_2$ receptor antagonism
b. $5HT_{1A}$ receptor antagonism
c. $5HT_{2A}$ receptor agonism
d. $5HT_{2C}$ receptor agonism
e. $5HT_3$ receptor agonism

## Question 91

Which of the following statements regarding the epidemiology of delusional disorder is incorrect?
a. The estimated lifetime risk is between 0.05% and 1.0%.
b. The mean age of onset is 35 years for males and 45 years for females.

c. Onset tends to be gradual.
d. Remission rate is 60%.
e. There is equal sex ratio of sufferers.

## Question 92
With regards to DNA transcription, which of the following statements is false?
  a. Transcription is the process in which information from the DNA molecule is transcribed onto a primary RNA transcript.
  b. Transcription starts in the upstream locus control region.
  c. Reverse transcription would commence in the downstream locus control region.
  d. Transcription factors are essential as they have specific structural domains such as zinc fingers that could bind to the locus control region.
  e. Concealed strands of DNA would be unfolded and then prepared for transcription.

## Question 93
Research studies (such as that by Weinberger et al.) have looked into the regional cerebral blood flow at rest and during specific neuropsychological testing of schizophrenic patients. Impaired performance on specific task is due to the reduced blood flow to which area of the brain?
  a. Prefrontal cortex
  b. Parietal cortex
  c. Occipital cortex
  d. Hippocampus
  e. Temporal cortex

## Question 94
It has been estimated that the risk of dementia is increased amongst first-degree relatives by approximately what incidence?
  a. 1%
  b. 3%
  c. 6%
  d. 10%
  e. 15%

## Question 95
Which of the following neuroanatomical areas is associated with OCD?
  a. Dorsolateral prefrontal cortex
  b. Inferior frontal gyrus
  c. Orbitofrontal cortex
  d. Prefrontal cortex
  e. Primary motor cortex

## Question 96

A 20-year-old woman is admitted to the ward and she suffers from borderline personality disorder. Her parents want to know which of the following symptoms is the easiest to treat with medication or psychotherapy. Your answer is

a. Demandingness and manipulativeness
b. Impulsive acts and self-mutilation
c. Identity disturbance and hostility
d. Irritability and moodiness
e. Mercuriality and substance misuse

## Question 97

Newly synthesized polypeptide chains could be further modified. All of the following are common posttranslational modification processes, with the exception of

a. Formation of disulfide bonds
b. Cleavage of certain transport polypeptides
c. Hydroxylation
d. Phosphorylation
e. Hydrolysis

## Question 98

Which one of the following statements about the neurochemistry of panic disorder is incorrect?

a. There has been shown to be hypersensitivity of the presynaptic alpha-2 receptors and a resultant increase in the adrenergic activity.
b. There is increased sensitivity of the serotonin receptors and exaggerated postsynaptic receptor response.
c. There is a reduction in the GABA receptor sensitivity.
d. Cholecystokinin would cause panic attack.
e. Sodium lactate has been implicated in the induction of panic attack.

## Question 99

What is the estimated prevalence of depressive symptoms amongst the elderly population in the UK?

a. 1%
b. 2%
c. 5%
d. 10%
e. 15%

## Question 100

A 20-year-old male was involved in a fight in the pub and suffered head injuries. He was taken to the hospital and was treated. He was noted to have disinhibited and antisocial behaviour after the incident. He is likely to have had suffered a head injury involving which part of his cerebral cortex?

a. Left frontal lobe
b. Right frontal lobe

c. Left temporal lobe
d. Right parietal lobe
e. Left parietal lobe

## Question 101

Which of the following statements regarding the MacArthur Competence Assessment (MacCAT-CA) is false?

a. The assessment begins with a vignette of a hypothetical offence.
b. The MacCAT-CA comprises 30 items that are organized into five sections.
c. The MacCAT-CA differs notably from earlier competence assessment instruments (e.g. Competence to Stand Trial Assessment Instrument, Interdisciplinary Fitness Interview [IFI] and Fitness Interview Test [FIT]).
d. The MacCAT-CA is used to assess a defendant's competence to stand trial.
e. The respondents are asked to make judgements about their own cases and explain their reasoning.

## Question 102

A 26-year-old man was involved in a fight in the pub and has suffered head injuries. He was taken to the hospital and has been treated. Thereafter, his mother noted that he had non-fluent speech and seemed to be more depressed. He is likely to have suffered a head injury involving which part of the cortex?

a. Left frontal lobe
b. Right frontal lobe
c. Left temporal lobe
d. Right temporal lobe
e. Bilateral parietal cortex

## Question 103

Which one of the following neurochemicals would be capable of affecting one's food intake?

a. Cholecystokinin
b. Serotonin
c. Dopamine
d. Vasopressin
e. Prolactin

## Question 104

Based on existing epidemiological studies, what has been estimated to be the prevalence of deliberate self-harm among young people in the United Kingdom?

a. 2%
b. 3%
c. 6%
d. 10%
e. 20%

**Question 105**

Translation is the process in genetic expression whereby mRNA would serve as a template allowing the genetic code to be deciphered, and in turn allowing for the formation of a peptide chain. At which location does this take place?
a. Nucleus
b. Smooth endoplasmic reticulum
c. Rough endoplasmic reticulum
d. Liposome
e. Endosome

**Question 106**

Neuroimaging studies involving structural MRI have shown which of the following structural changes in patients with panic disorder?
a. Increase in frontal lobe volume
b. Reduction in frontal lobe volume
c. Increase in medial temporal lobe volume
d. Reduction in medial temporal lobe volume
e. Increase in ventricular sizes

**Question 107**

This is a concept that refers to the occurrence of an autonomic dominant disorder at earlier ages of onset or with greater severity in the succeeding generations. Which concept is this?
a. Anticipation
b. Mosaicism
c. Uniparental disomy
d. Genomic imprinting
e. Mitochondrial inheritance

**Question 108**

Previous epidemiological studies have identified that there is a high prevalence of self-harm among the Goth subculture in the United Kingdom. What is the estimated incidence of lifetime self-harm in that particular subculture?
a. 10%
b. 20%
c. 30%
d. 40%
e. 50%

**Question 109**

Which of the following cell types is responsible for the secretion of prolactin?
a. Somatotrope
b. Mammotrope
c. Gonadotrope

d. Corticotrope

e. Thyrotrope

## Question 110

Rapid cycling bipolar disorder tends to affect roughly what percentage of patients?

a. 5%

b. 10%

c. 20%

d. 40%

e. 50%

## Question 111

This is a concept that refers to the phenomenon in which an individual inherits both homologues of a chromosome pair from the same parent. Which concept is this?

a. Anticipation

b. Mosaicism

c. Uniparental disomy

d. Genomic imprinting

e. Mitochondrial inheritance

## Question 112

The old age psychiatrist has diagnosed Mr Smith with mild cognitive impairment. Mrs Smith, the caregiver, wants to know how this is different from dementia. Which one of the following statements is representative of the most important difference?

a. Patients with mild cognitive impairment tend to have a higher MMSE score as compared to those with dementia.

b. Patients with dementia tend to complain of more subjective memory loss.

c. Patients with dementia tend to have more objective evidence of cognitive impairment.

d. Patients with mild cognitive impairment tend to have preserved basic ADL and are able to still live independently.

e. Patients with dementia would have more significant decline from previously normal level of functioning.

## Question 113

It has been known that vascular dementia accounts for what proportion of all the dementia in the United Kingdom?

a. 10%

b. 15%

c. 20%

d. 30%

e. 50%

## Question 114

What has been estimated to be the life-time risk for adults in the general population of acquiring bipolar disorder?

a. 0.5%

b. 1.5%

c. 2.0%
d. 3.0%
e. 3.5%

## Question 115
One of the following cell types has been described as the macrophages of the central nervous system. Which one of the following is the correct option?
a. Microglia
b. Astrocytes
c. Oligodendrocytes
d. Ependymal cells
e. Satellite cells

## Question 116
Which of the following is the function of the ribosome?
a. It helps to provide cellular energy.
b. It is the main site of DNA storage.
c. It helps in the post-translational modification process of the proteins.
d. It helps with the synthesis of new proteins.
e. It helps with the transcription process of DNA to mRNA.

## Question 117
Creutzfeldt–Jakob disease (CJD) has been known to be a very rare cause of a rapidly progressive dementia. Which one of the following causes the characteristic spongiform appearance that could be detected in this condition?
a. Vacuolar changes in the grey matter, especially in the cerebral and cerebellar cortex
b. The loss of nerve cells
c. Reactive astrocytosis
d. The presence of prion proteins
e. Mutations of the prion proteins

## Question 118
When people with Down's syndrome reach the age of 40 years, they have a high risk of developing Alzheimer's disease. The gene that accounts for this association is
a. Amyloid precursor protein
b. Apolipoprotein E
c. Neuregulin
d. Presenilin1
e. Presenilin 2

## Question 119
Functions of astrocytes include the following, except
a. Forming the myelin sheath
b. Maintaining the blood–brain barrier

c. Providing metabolic support to the brain
d. Providing structural support to the brain
e. Phagocytosis of injured nerve cells

## Question 120
The ventral tegmental area is located in the
a. Locus coeruleus
b. Medulla
c. Midbrain
d. Pons
e. Reticular formation

## Question 121
Which of the following enzymes are involved in the metabolism of serotonin?
a. COMT and tyrosine hydroxylase
b. Dopa decarboxylase and sulfotransferase
c. GABA transaminase and glutamic acid decarboxylase
d. MAO-A and aldehyde dehydrogenase
e. Phenylalanine hydroxylase and tyrosine hydroxylase

## Question 122
Which of the following is a type of glutamate receptor?
a. Amino-3-hydroxy-5- methylisoxazole propionic acid (AMPA) receptor
b. Cannabinoid (CB) receptor
c. γ-Aminobutyric acid (GABA) receptor
d. 3,4-Methylenedioxymethamphetamine (MDMA) receptor
e. Sigma-1 ($\sigma_1$) receptor

## Question 123
A 24-year-old man with schizophrenia complains of third-person auditory hallucinations. Which of the following gyri is involved?
a. Angular gyrus
b. Heschl gyrus
c. Inferior frontal gyrus
d. Postcentral gyrus
e. Supramarginal gyrus

## Question 124
A 30-year-old woman with borderline personality disorder wants to find out more about dialectical behaviour therapy (DBT). Which of the following statements regarding DBT is true?
a. DBT uses thinking and techniques drawn from Shinto philosophy emphasizing harmony with the environment.
b. DBT does not promote the use of metaphor as DBT is strongly influenced by cognitive behaviour therapy.

c. DBT does not promote the judicious use of humour or irreverence to reinforce the boundary between the therapist and the patient.
d. Dialectical thinking refers to the way of thinking that emphasizes the limitations of linear ideas about causation.
e. Out-of-therapy telephone contact by a case manager is usually available on a 24-hour basis to prevent self-harm.

### Question 125
The following symptoms found in patients with bulimia nervosa are the focus of interpersonal therapy (IPT) except:
a. Binge eating, guilt and self-induced vomiting
b. Conflict avoidance and difficulty with role expectations
c. Confusion regarding the needs for closeness and distance
d. Difficulty in managing negative emotions
e. Social anxiety, sensitivity to conflict and rejection

# Extended Matching Items (EMIs)

## Theme: Drugs and effects on EEG
**Options:**
a. Antidepressants
b. Antipsychotics
c. Anxiolytics
d. Lithium

**Lead in:** Select the most appropriate answer for each of the following. Each option may be used once, more than once or not at all.

### Question 126
Which of the aforementioned medications would cause increased delta activity?

### Question 127
Which of the aforementioned medications would cause a decreased alpha activity, but an increased beta activity?

### Question 128
This particular class of medication would cause an increase in the low-frequency delta activity.

### Question 129
This particular class of medication would lead to only small EEG changes that are likely to be missed on recordings.

## Theme: Neurochemistry – serotonin and psychiatric disorders
**Options:**
a. Anxiety disorder
b. OCD

c. Depressive disorder
d. Manic disorder
e. Schizophrenia
f. Alzheimer's disorder
g. Cloninger's type 1 alcoholism
h. Cloninger's type 2 alcoholism

**Lead in:** Select the most appropriate answer for each of the following. Each option may be used once, more than once or not at all.

**Question 130**
It is noted that 5-HT transmission from the caudal raphe nuclei and rostral raphe nuclei is increased in patients with this condition.

**Question 131**
It is noted that in this condition, when there is an excess of 5-HT, there will be a reduction in the availability of DA. This might give rise to some of the symptoms such as reduced interest and withdrawal. Which condition is this?

**Question 132**
It is noted that in this condition, the 5HT transmission from the rostral raphe nuclei to the temporal lobe is reduced.

**Question 133**
Presynaptic 5HT dysfunction is considered to be a state marked in this condition.

## Theme: Neurochemistry – neuropeptides
**Options:**
a. Corticotrophin-releasing factor
b. Somatostatin
c. Thyrotropin-releasing factor
d. Cholecystokinin
e. Vasoactive intestinal peptide

**Lead in:** Select the most appropriate answer for each of the following. Each option may be used once, more than once or not at all.

**Question 134**
This neuropeptide has an inhibitory effect on the growth hormone release.

**Question 135**
This is considered to be the smallest brain peptide, but it has the ability to reverse sedation caused by drugs.

**Question 136**
This neuropeptide is involved in appetite and feeding, as well as emotional behaviour.

**Question 137**
This neuropeptide could be found in multiple locations, which include the cerebral cortex, hypothalamus, amygdala, hippocampus, autonomic ganglia and intestinal and respiratory tracts.

**Question 138**
Injections of this neuropeptide might lead to depressive symptoms such as reduced appetite and sex drive.

## Theme: Psychotropic drugs and adverse drug reactions
**Options:**
  a. Causal relationship
  b. Intolerance
  c. Idiosyncratic reactions
  d. Allergic reactions
  e. Pharmacokinetic interactions
  f. Pharmacodynamic interactions

**Lead in:** Select the most appropriate answer for each of the following. Each option may be used once, more than once or not at all.

**Question 139**
These adverse drug reactions are consistent with the known pharmacological actions of the drug.

**Question 140**
These adverse drug reactions are not characteristic and predictable.

**Question 141**
These adverse drug reactions involve the body's immune system.

**Question 142**
Enzyme inhibition and enzyme induction are part of this process.

## Theme: Genetics – gene and psychiatric disorder
**Options:**
  a. Chromosome 1
  b. Chromosome 2
  c. Chromosome 4
  d. Chromosome 8
  e. Chromosome 13
  f. Chromosome 14
  g. Chromosome 17
  h. Chromosome 18

**Lead in:** Select the most appropriate answer for each of the following. Each option may be used once, more than once or not at all.

**Question 143**
This chromosome is involved in Edward's syndrome.

**Question 144**
This chromosome is involved in Alzheimer's disease.

**Question 145**
This chromosome is involved in Patau's syndrome and Wilson's disease.

**Question 146**
Neuregulin is encoded on this chromosome.

**Question 147**
This chromosome is involved in autism.

## Theme: Advanced psychology – dynamic therapies
**Options:**
a. Brief focal psychotherapy
b. Time-limited psychotherapy
c. Short-term dynamic psychotherapy

**Lead in:** Select the most appropriate answer for each of the following. Each option may be used once, more than once or not at all.

**Question 148**
The focus of this form of dynamic therapy is to clarify the nature of the defences and its relationship to anxiety and impulses.

**Question 149**
The focus of this form of therapy is on the triangular conflict.

**Question 150**
The focus of this form of dynamic therapy is to focus on the present.

## Theme: Genetics
**Options:**
a. Deletion
b. Insertion
c. Frame shift
d. Missense mutation
e. Nonsense mutation
f. Regulatory (transcription) mutations
g. RNA processing mutation
h. Silent mutation
i. Substitution
j. Transition
k. Transversion

**Lead in:** Select the aforementioned mutations to match the following descriptions.

## Question 151
This mutation involves a change to a single nucleotide. (Choose one option.)

## Question 152
Substitution of a purine for a purine. (Choose one option.)

## Question 153
Owing to the degeneracy of the genetic code, this mutation does not alter the amino acid being encoded. (Choose one option.)

## Question 154
This mutation results in the substitution of one amino acid for another. (Choose one option.)

## Question 155
This mutation creates a new stop codon (UAA, UPG or UGA) and results in premature termination of translation. (Choose one option.)

## Question 156
The mutation usually results in a shortened (truncated) protein product. (Choose one option.)

## Theme: Genetics
**Options:**
   a. Adoption studies
   b. Association studies
   c. Family studies
   d. Segregation analysis
   e. Twin studies

**Lead in:** Select the aforementioned options to the match the following descriptions. Each option may be used only once.

## Question 157
The morbid risk of the illness is determined within families, and rates of occurrence in the different degrees of relatives are compared with those in the general population. (Choose one option.)

## Question 158
It compares the concordance rates of diagnosis in twins, both monozygotic and dizygotic, thus allowing researchers the possibility of dissecting the role of genes from that of the environment. (Choose one option.)

## Question 159
Genetic study to delineate inherited and environmental factors. (Choose one option.)

## Question 160

It compares the likelihood for the observed frequency of illness in a pedigree with multiple cases of affective disorder with those that can be predicted by different modes of transmission. (Choose one option.)

## Theme: Genetics

**Options:**
a. Chromosome 1
b. Chromosome 4
c. Chromosome 5
d. Chromosome 6
e. Chromosome 7
f. Chromosome 8
g. Chromosome 9
h. Chromosome 10
i. Chromosome 15
j. Chromosome 17
k. Chromosome 22

**Lead in:** Select the chromosome that is affected in each of the following presentations. Each option might be used once, more than once or not at all.

## Question 161

A 10-year-old girl presents with a small head, happy face, jerk movement and ataxia. She is known to have a history of epilepsy and learning disability. (Choose one option.)

## Question 162

A 14-year-boy is referred to the early psychosis service. He has features of a round face, cleft palate, low-set ears, learning disability and congenital heart disease with frequent infections. (Choose one option.)

## Question 163

A 7-year-old girl is admitted to the paediatric ward for self-injury. She also presents with hyperactivity, severe learning disability, attention-seeking and sleep disturbance. The mother reports that she cried like a cat at birth. (Choose one option.)

## Theme: Basic neurosciences

**Options:**
a. Diffuse slow activity with episodic, bilaterally synchronous and symmetrical bursts of rhythmic waves
b. Unusual appearance of episodic discharges, recurring every 1–3 seconds and variable focal slow waves over the temporal areas
c. Periodic stereotyped repetitive discharges at a rate of 1 per second
d. High-amplitude, repetitive, bilaterally synchronous and symmetrical, polyphasic sharp-wave and slow-wave complexes, occurring every 4–15 seconds

**Lead in:** Match the EEG patterns to the following conditions. Each option might be used once, more than once or not at all.

**Question 164**
Acute encephalitis. (Choose one option.)

**Question 165**
Creutzfeldt–Jakob disease. (Choose one option.)

**Question 166**
Herpes simplex encephalitis. (Choose one option.)

**Question 167**
Subacute Sclerosing panencephalitis. (Choose one option.)

## GET THROUGH MRCPSYCH PAPER A2: MOCK EXAMINATION

**Question 1 Answer: e, Increased density of neurons in the deeper layer**
*Explanation*: Arnold et al. (1991) have proposed that all of the aforementioned are responsible for the disturbed development that has led to the onset of schizophrenia with the exception of option (e). It has also been proposed that schizophrenic post-mortem brains had a smaller neuron size in the hippocampal regions of the subiculum, CAI and layer II of the entorhinal cortex.

*Reference*: Puri BK, Hall A, Ho R (2014). *Revision Notes in Psychiatry*. London: CRC Press, p. 198.

**Question 2 Answer: d, Aphasia**
*Explanation*: Dysphasia, paraphasia or aphasia refers to disturbances in the comprehension and expression of speech as a result of the underlying brain lesions. It is important to know the following speech and language areas: Broca's area is involved in coordinating the organs of speech in order to produce coherent sounds; Wernicke's area is involved in making sense of speech and language.

*Reference*: Puri BK, Hall A, Ho R (2014). *Revision Notes in Psychiatry*. London: CRC Press, p. 105.

**Question 3 Answer: b, Blockage of the alpha-1 adrenergic receptors**
*Explanation*: It has been shown that some TCAs and also antipsychotics would cause sedation and postural hypotension as a result of blockage of the alpha-1 receptors.

*Reference*: Puri BK, Hall A, Ho R (2014). *Revision Notes in Psychiatry*. London: CRC Press, p. 226.

**Question 4 Answer: c, At least four times more**
*Explanation*: Adoption studies have found that there is at least a four times increase in the risk of the children being alcoholic, given that the parents are alcoholic.

*Reference*: Puri BK, Hall A, Ho R (2014). *Revision Notes in Psychiatry*. London: CRC Press, p. 300.

**Question 5 Answer: d, 60%**

*Explanation*: It has been estimated that around 60% of patients with paraphrenia actually resemble those with paranoid schizophrenia.

*Reference*: Puri BK, Hall A, Ho R (2014). *Revision Notes in Psychiatry*. London: CRC Press, p. 302.

**Question 6 Answer: d, Impulsiveness**

*Explanation*: With regards to the course and prognosis of borderline personality disorder, it has been noted that the impulsiveness tends to improve significantly over time. Affective instability usually is associated with the least amount of improvement.

*Reference*: Puri BK, Hall A, Ho R (2014). *Revision Notes in Psychiatry*. London: CRC Press, p. 447.

**Question 7 Answer: c, Avoidant**

*Explanation*: For a child with avoidant attachment, it has been noted that a distance is usually kept from the mother, who sometimes might be entirely ignored. Clinically, avoidant attachment style in children might lead to poor social functioning in later life and might also result in aggressive behaviour.

*Reference*: Puri BK, Hall A, Ho R (2014). *Revision Notes in Psychiatry*. London: CRC Press, p. 64.

**Question 8 Answer: c, 1.5%**

*Explanation*: It has been estimated that roughly 1.5% of all people with schizophrenia have an onset older than 60 years.

*Reference*: Puri BK, Hall A, Ho R (2014). *Revision Notes in Psychiatry*. London: CRC Press, p. 302.

**Question 9 Answer: a, Histamine**

*Explanation*: Blockade of the histamine H1 receptors can lead to both weight gain and drowsiness.

*Reference*: Puri BK, Hall A, Ho R (2014). *Revision Notes in Psychiatry*. London: CRC Press, p. 252.

**Question 10 Answer: d, When depressed patients take SSRI, it would not lead to a reduction of 5-HT in the platelets.**

*Explanation*: It is essential to note that most of the peripheral 5-HTs are stored in the platelets. When depressed patients take SSRI, it would lead to a reduction of 5-HT in the platelets but an increase in the net plasma 5-HT levels.

*Reference*: Puri BK, Hall A, Ho R (2014). *Revision Notes in Psychiatry*. London: CRC Press, p. 228.

**Question 11 Answer: b, Cheese**
*Explanation*: Cheese should be avoided. It has been shown that the inhibition of peripheral pressor amines, particularly dietary tyramine, by MAOIs can lead to a hypertensive crisis when food rich in tyramine are eaten.

*Reference*: Puri BK, Hall A, Ho R (2014). *Revision Notes in Psychiatry*. London: CRC Press, p. 246.

**Question 12 Answer: d, Cri-Du-Chat syndrome**
*Explanation*: Cri-Du-Chat syndrome results from the partial deletion of the short arm of chromosome 5. The main clinical feature is high-pitched cry.

*Reference*: Puri BK, Hall A, Ho R (2014). *Revision Notes in Psychiatry*. London: CRC Press, p. 259.

**Question 13 Answer: b, Rapid cycling disorder is more common in males.**
*Explanation*: This is incorrect. Rapid cycling is usually more prevalent in females.

*Reference*: Puri BK, Hall A, Ho R (2014). *Revision Notes in Psychiatry*. London: CRC Press, p. 286.

**Question 14 Answer: d, Social learning theory**
*Explanation*: Social learning theory refers to learning via observation, imitation and also operant conditioning.

*Reference*: Puri BK, Hall A, Ho R (2014). *Revision Notes in Psychiatry*. London: CRC Press, p. 60.

**Question 15 Answer: d, Temazepam**
*Explanation*: All of the aforementioned are considered to be long-acting benzodiazepines, with the exception of lorazepam and temazepam.

*Reference*: Puri BK, Hall A, Ho R (2014). *Revision Notes in Psychiatry*. London: CRC Press, p. 239.

**Question 16 Answer: d, Reduced total white blood cells counts**
*Explanation*: The combination might lead to a reduction in the total white blood cell count. Agranulocytosis is the most common in Jews.

*Reference*:Puri BK, Hall A, Ho R (2014). *Revision Notes in Psychiatry*. London: CRC Press, p. 367.

**Question 17 Answer: e, All of the aforementioned**
*Explanation*: All of the aforementioned are mechanisms of placebo effect. In addition, it is important to consider also the doctor's attitude, the patient's expectations as well as the transitional object phenomena.

*Reference*: Puri BK, Hall A, Ho R (2014). *Revision Notes in Psychiatry*. London: CRC Press, p. 240.

**Question 18 Answer: d, 4 years old**
*Explanation*: Theory of the mind refers to the capacity to attribute independent mental states to oneself and to others, thereby allowing one to predict and explain actions. It usually develops at the age of 4 years.

*Reference*: Puri BK, Hall A, Ho R (2014). *Revision Notes in Psychiatry*. London: CRC Press, p. 625.

**Question 19 Answer: e, Chronic depression**
*Explanation*: In addition to the aforementioned, other factors would include aggression and also substance use disorder. It has been noted that those patients with chronic depression, good motivation and a stable environment are most responsive to treatment.

*Reference*: Puri BK, Hall A, Ho R (2014). *Revision Notes in Psychiatry*. London: CRC Press, p. 447.

**Question 20 Answer: c, In schizophrenia, there is an increased expression of the messenger RNA for the enzyme in the prefrontal cortex.**
*Explanation*: Based on current research, there is a decreased expression, instead of an increased expression, of the enzymes in the prefrontal cortex. Hence, in schizophrenia, there is a net increment in the GABA activity. For generalized anxiety disorder, there is a reduction in the GABA activity.

*Reference*: Puri BK, Hall A, Ho R (2014). *Revision Notes in Psychiatry*. London: CRC Press, p. 229.

**Question 21 Answer: b, Iminodibenzyls**
*Explanation*: All of the aforementioned tricyclic antidepressants belong to the class of the iminodibenzyls.

*Reference*: Puri BK, Hall A, Ho R (2014). *Revision Notes in Psychiatry*. London: CRC Press, p. 238.

**Question 22 Answer: a, Failure of FMR1 gene transcription due to hypermethylation**
*Explanation*: Fragile X syndrome is due to the failure of FMR1 gene as a result of hypermethylation, thus leading to the absence of the FMR1 gene protein.

*Reference*: Puri BK, Hall A, Ho R (2014). *Revision Notes in Psychiatry*. London: CRC Press, p. 260.

**Question 23 Answer: e, 80%**
*Explanation*: It has been estimated that a child has 80% chance of developing alcohol misuse. Hence, the risk is around four times higher than a child whose father is not dependent on alcohol.

*Reference*: Puri BK, Hall A, Ho R (2014). *Revision Notes in Psychiatry*. London: CRC Press, p. 298.

**Question 24 Answer: a, Interpersonal therapy**
*Explanation*: In interpersonal therapy, the following areas are covered: grief, interpersonal disputes, role transitions and interpersonal role deficits.

*Reference*: Puri BK, Hall A, Ho R (2014). *Revision Notes in Psychiatry*. London: CRC Press, p. 343.

**Question 25 Answer: e, Tyrosine hydroxylase**
*Explanation*: Dopamine synthesis commences with the amino acid phenylalanine being converted by phenylalanine hydroxylase to tyrosine. It then becomes DOPA with the action of tyrosine hydroxylase. DOPA decarboxylase then decarboxylates DOPA to form dopamine. COMT, mostly an extracellular enzyme, and MAO, mostly an intracellular enzyme, metabolize dopamine.

*Reference*: Kaufman DM, Milstein MJ. (2013). *Kaufman's Clinical Neurology for Psychiatrists* (7th edition). Philadelphia, PA: Saunders, p. 501.

**Question 26 Answer: d, The rate of absorption is independent of the ambient pH.**
*Explanation*: (d) is incorrect as the solubility of the drug is influenced by the pH of the surroundings.

*Reference*: Puri BK, Hall A, Ho R (2014). *Revision Notes in Psychiatry*. London: CRC Press, p. 241.

**Question 27 Answer: a, Lithium is usually well tolerated.**
*Explanation*: It is important to note that lithium carbonate is poorly tolerated, especially for those with HIV nephropathy. It is thus very important to monitor closely for neurotoxicity as well as gastrointestinal side effects.

*Reference*: Puri BK, Hall A, Ho R (2014). *Revision Notes in Psychiatry*. London: CRC Press, p. 483.

**Question 28 Answer: e, Social skills training**
*Explanation*: All of the aforementioned options are part of the cognitive component of cognitive behavioural therapy with the exception of (e). In addition, clients are encouraged to formulate alternative positive belief and rate the impact of the maladaptive belief on emotions.

*Reference*: Puri BK, Hall A, Ho R (2014). *Revision Notes in Psychiatry*. London: CRC Press, p. 337.

### Question 29 Answer: b, Borderline personality disorder

*Explanation*: The incidence of borderline personality disorder is 20% and it is the most common personality disorder amongst the inpatients.

*Reference*: Puri BK, Hall A, Ho R (2014). *Revision Notes in Psychiatry*. London: CRC Press, p. 435.

### Question 30 Answer: a, Holmes–Adie pupil

*Explanation*: 80% of the cases are unilateral in onset. The common symptoms of Holmes–Adie pupil are as aforementioned. The pupils appear to be moderately dilated, with poor reaction to light, and slow reaction to accommodation. It is associated with diminished and also absent knee jerk.

*Reference*: Puri BK, Hall A, Ho R (2014). *Revision Notes in Psychiatry*. London: CRC Press, p. 161.

### Question 31 Answer: e, LAAM

*Explanation*: All of the aforementioned are drugs that are commonly used in the treatment of opioid dependence, with the exception of LAAM. LAAM (levo-alpha-acetylmethadol) is a synthetic opioid that can block the effects of heroin for up to 72 hours. The frequency of usage has been estimated to be three times per week due to its long duration of action. However, it should be noted that its use is associated with torsades de pointes.

*Reference*: Puri BK, Hall A, Ho R (2014). *Revision Notes in Psychiatry*. London: CRC Press, p. 531.

### Question 32 Answer: a, It is an autosomal recessive disorder.

*Explanation*: It is classified and genetic studies have found out that it is an autosomal dominant disorder. It is important also to note that the relative age of onset is determined largely by the number of repeat units.

*Reference*: Puri BK, Hall A, Ho R (2014). *Revision Notes in Psychiatry*. London: CRC Press, p. 266.

### Question 33 Answer: b, Schizoid personality disorder

*Explanation*: Schizoid personality disorder is considered to be relatively uncommon amongst outpatients.

*Reference*: Puri BK, Hall A, Ho R (2014). *Revision Notes in Psychiatry*. London: CRC Press, p. 435.

### Question 34 Answer: a, Affirmation

*Explanation*: The particular technique that is in use is affirmation. It helps to confirm the validity of a prior judgement or behaviour.

*Reference*: Puri BK, Hall A, Ho R (2014). *Revision Notes in Psychiatry*. London: CRC Press, p. 330.

**Question 35 Answer: b, Introns are not expressed in the final protein product.**
*Explanation*: Adenine pairs with thymine, while guanine pairs with cytosine. The centromere plays a key role in chromosome assortment during cell division. The leading strand is formed continuously, moving in the 5′ to 3′ direction during DNA replication. The leading strand (Okazaki fragments) is formed in blocks during DNA replication.

*Further Reading*: Puri BK, Treasaden I (eds) (2010). *Psychiatry: An Evidence-Based Text*. London: Hodder Arnold, p. 467.

**Question 36 Answer: e, Severe dependence on substances**
*Explanation*: Brief dynamic psychotherapy is indicated for all of the aforementioned conditions. It helps to improve self-understanding by enabling individuals to develop a capacity for self-reflection. It helps to increase awareness of maladaptive defences and modify such defences. It helps to understand the relationship between the past and the present. The contraindications for this modality of treatment are schizophrenia, delusional disorder, high tendency for serious self-harm, severe dependence on substances and very poor insight.

*Reference*: Puri BK, Hall A, Ho R (2014). *Revision Notes in Psychiatry*. London: CRC Press, p. 331.

**Question 37 Answer: d, 8%**
*Explanation*: An eightfold increment in the rate of affective disorder has been shown among relatives of index adoptees with affective disorder.

*Reference*: Puri BK, Hall A, Ho R (2014). *Revision Notes in Psychiatry*. London: CRC Press, p. 272.

**Question 38 Answer: b, Dopamine D2 receptor gene**
*Explanation*: All of the aforementioned genes have been found to be associated with the development of schizophrenia, with the exception of (b).

*Reference*: Puri BK, Hall A, Ho R (2014). *Revision Notes in Psychiatry*. London: CRC Press, p. 266.

**Question 39 Answer: b, Hutchinson's pupil**
*Explanation*: Due to the rapidly rising unilateral intracranial pressure, most often due to intra-cerebral haemorrhage, the pupils would appear dilated and unreactive on the side of the intracranial mass lesion due to compression of the oculomotor nerve (CNIII) on the ipsilateral side.

*Reference*: Puri BK, Hall A, Ho R (2014). *Revision Notes in Psychiatry*. London: CRC Press, p. 161.

**Question 40 Answer: d, Cocaine**
*Explanation*: Cocaine blocks the dopamine reuptake at the dopamine reuptake site. Hence, the extracellular levels of dopamine are markedly increased. Dopaminergic activity, particularly at the nucleus accumbens, has been found to have a major role in the pleasurable and reinforcing effects of cocaine.

*Reference*: Puri BK, Hall A, Ho R (2014). *Revision Notes in Psychiatry*. London: CRC Press, p. 541.

**Question 41 Answer: c, 2:1**
*Explanation*: The female-to-male ratio for PTSD has been estimated to be around 2:1.

*Reference*: Puri BK, Hall A, Ho R (2014). *Revision Notes in Psychiatry*. London: CRC Press, p. 291.

**Question 42 Answer: e, Eating disorders**
*Explanation*: All of the aforementioned are common comorbid conditions, with the exception of eating disorders. It also includes substance misuse and suicide attempt.

*Reference*: Puri BK, Hall A, Ho R (2014). *Revision Notes in Psychiatry*. London: CRC Press, p. 291.

**Question 43 Answer: d, Client does not have the capacity to sustain previous relationship.**
*Explanation*: All of the aforementioned factors would render a client suitable for therapy, with the exception of (d). Client must have the capacity to form and sustain relationships. Client must also have good response to trial interpretation.

*Reference*: Puri BK, Hall A, Ho R (2014). *Revision Notes in Psychiatry*. London: CRC Press, p. 331.

**Question 44 Answer: a, Amiloride**
*Explanations*: Potassium-sparing diuretics (e.g. amiloride) are recommended, as potassium depletion may induce lithium toxicity. There is an unpredictable rise in the lithium concentration when it is combined with thiazide diuretics (e.g. bendroflumethiazide, chlorthalidone and indapamide). Loop diuretics (e.g. furosemide) are not very useful in treating hypertension and may lead to lithium toxicity.

*Reference*: Taylor D. Paton C, Kapur S (2009). *The Maudsley Prescribing Guidelines* (10th edition). London: Informa Healthcare.

**Question 45 Answer: a, Desensitization**
*Explanation*: In systematic desensitization, the patient is successfully exposed (in reality or in imagination) to stimuli in the hierarchy, beginning with the least anxiety-provoking one, each exposure being paired with relaxation.

*Reference*: Puri BK, Hall A, Ho R (2014). *Revision Notes in Psychiatry*. London: CRC Press, p. 28.

### Question 46 Answer: b, Carelessness
*Explanation*: The factors included are neuroticism/stability, extroversion/introversion, psychoticism/stability and intelligence.

*Further Reading*: Puri BK, Treasaden I (eds) (2010). *Psychiatry: An Evidence-Based Text*. London: Hodder Arnold, pp. 79, 282.

### Question 47 Answer: d, Partial insight
*Explanation*: All of the aforementioned are contraindications for therapy, with the exception of the patient having partial insight. A patient with poor insight is contraindicated for brief dynamic psychotherapy.

*Reference*: Puri BK, Treasaden I (eds) (2010). *Psychiatry: An Evidence-Based Text*. London: Hodder Arnold, pp. 79, 282.

### Question 48 Answer: e, 80%
*Explanation*: The estimated heritability of bipolar disorder has been estimated to be between 79% and 93%.

*Reference*: Puri BK, Hall A, Ho R (2014). *Revision Notes in Psychiatry*. London: CRC Press, p. 284.

### Question 49 Answer: c, Gait disturbances
*Explanation*: The presentation is usually an insidious onset of dementia, with psychomotor retardation, unsteady gait and urinary incontinence. The onset is usually in the 60s or the 70s. Behavioural disturbances, hallucinations and paranoia are typically uncommon. The diagnosis is usually made on the basic of clinical presentation with a CT scan of the brain revealing dilated ventricles (especially for the third ventricle) without cortical atrophy and with normal CSF pressures. The shunt would help with the drainage of the CSF from the ventricles to the heart.

*Reference*: Puri BK, Hall A, Ho R (2014). *Revision Notes in Psychiatry*. London: CRC Press, p. 704.

### Question 50 Answer: e, Allow the patient and not the family members to take ownership.
*Explanation*: It is important to have the family members involved with regards to concordance to medications.

*Reference*: Puri BK, Hall A, Ho R (2014). *Revision Notes in Psychiatry*. London: CRC Press, p. 240.

### Question 51 Answer: c, CGG
*Explanation*: Fragile X is associated with the repetition of CGG sequence.

*Reference*: Puri BK, Hall A, Ho R (2014). *Revision Notes in Psychiatry*. London: CRC Press, p. 260.

### Question 52 Answer: e, Bereavement
*Explanation*: All of the aforementioned are factors that have been proposed by Brown and Harris in their study to account for the onset of depression. Bereavement has not been previously proposed.

*Reference*: Puri BK, Hall A, Ho R (2014). *Revision Notes in Psychiatry*. London: CRC Press, p. 284.

### Question 53 Answer: a, Resistance
*Explanation*: Resistance is with regards to the client being ambivalent about getting help and may oppose attempts from the therapist who offers help. Resistance may manifest in the form of silence, avoidance or even absences. It can also help to reveal much about the significant relationship in the past.

*Reference*: Puri BK, Hall A, Ho R (2014). *Revision Notes in Psychiatry*. London: CRC Press, p. 331.

### Question 54 Answer: d
*Explanation*: Research on children suggests that at the age of 3 years, children do not acknowledge false belief as they have difficulty differentiating belief from the world. Formulating a theory of mind appears not to be inevitable, but relies on cognitive changes that occur at the age of 4. It has been suggested that a failure to acquire a theory of mind is associated with disorders such as autism.

*Further Reading*: Puri BK, Treasaden I (eds) (2010). *Psychiatry: An Evidence-Based Text*. London: Hodder Arnold, pp. 22, 290–291, 974, 1089.

### Question 55 Answer: d
*Explanation*: The Hayling Test is a response initiation and response suppression test. The assessor would read each sentence and the subject has to simply complete the sentence.

*Further Reading*: Puri BK, Treasaden I (eds) (2010). *Psychiatry: An Evidence-Based Text*. London: Hodder Arnold, p. 516.

### Question 56 Answer: b, Extinction
*Explanation*: Extinction also occurs in operant conditioning when positive reinforcement (i.e. attention from others) is removed.

*Further Reading*: Puri BK, Treasaden I (eds) (2010). *Psychiatry: An Evidence-Based Text*. London: Hodder Arnold, pp. 208, 503.

### Question 57 Answer: b, Acting in
*Explanation*: This clearly refers to acting in behaviour. This refers to the exploration of the therapist's personal and private information by the client or even presenting a symbolic gift to the therapist.

*Reference*: Puri BK, Hall A, Ho R (2014). *Revision Notes in Psychiatry*. London: CRC Press, p. 332.

**Question 58 Answer: b, Fusiform gyrus**
*Explanation*: It is also believed that the underactivity of the fusiform gyrus would lead to autistic disorder.

*Further Reading*: Puri BK, Treasaden I (eds) (2010). *Psychiatry: An Evidence-Based Text*. London: Hodder Arnold, pp. 332–335.

**Question 59 Answer: e, The Camberwell Family Interview does not measure the perception of the patient.**
*Explanation*: The Camberwell Family Interview rates the patient's perception of how his family feels about him and the disorder, although the patient is absent when the family is interviewed.

*Reference*: Vaughn C, Leff J (1976). The measurement of expressed emotion in the families of psychiatric patients. *British Journal of Social and Clinical Psychology*, 15: 157–165.

**Question 60 Answer: d, Attachment issues**
*Explanation*: Beck's cognitive triad would include the effect of early experiences, core beliefs, underlying assumptions, cognitive distortions, automatic thoughts and the negative cognitive triad.

*Reference*: Puri BK, Hall A, Ho R (2014). *Revision Notes in Psychiatry*. London: CRC Press, p. 334.

**Question 61 Answer: d, 4%**
*Explanation*: The prevalence has been estimated to be around 4%. Serious reading difficulty refers to a reading impairment that significantly interferers with academic achievements or ADL.

*Reference*: Puri BK, Hall A, Ho R (2014). *Revision Notes in Psychiatry*. London: CRC Press, p. 642.

**Question 62 Answer: a, HIV Dementia**
*Explanation*: Given the profile of the patient, it is highly likely that the patient has underlying HIV-associated dementia. In the later stages of HIV dementia, there is global deterioration of cognitive functions, which is usually manifested as word finding difficulties. Patients might also exhibit psychomotor retardation and even mutism. Speech might be slow and monotonous. Neurological examination might reveal that the patient has difficulties associated with walking as a result of paraparesis.

*Reference*: Puri BK, Hall A, Ho R (2014). *Revision Notes in Psychiatry*. London: CRC Press, p. 483.

**Question 63 Answer: d, Inhibits dopamine and norepinephrine reuptake**
*Explanation*: 'Bath salts' are a group of stimulants that are also called 'Ivory Wave' or 'White Horse'. The active ingredient is methylenedioxypyrovalerone, which inhibits dopamine and norepinephrine reuptake. They therefore can cause cocaine-like effects that include sympathetic overstimulation (hypertension, tachycardia, enlarged pupils, etc.), psychosis (hallucinations, persecutory delusions) and complications such as stroke and myocardial infarction.

*Reference*: Kaufman DM, Milstein MJ. (2013). *Kaufman's Clinical Neurology for Psychiatrists* (7th edition). Philadelphia, PA: Saunders, p. 513.

**Question 64 Answer: d, There is an interphase stage in the second stage of cellular division.**
*Explanation*: There is no interphase stage in the second stage of cellular division.

*Reference*: Puri BK, Hall A, Ho R (2014). *Revision Notes in Psychiatry*. London: CRC Press, p. 259.

**Question 65 Answer: b, 20%**
*Explanation*: The approximate prevalence of personality disorder in the general practice setting has been estimated to be around 20%.

*Reference*: Puri BK, Hall A, Ho R (2014). *Revision Notes in Psychiatry*. London: CRC Press, p. 435.

**Question 66 Answer: e, It helps individuals to identify faulty procedures.**
*Explanation*: All of the aforementioned are the objectives of cognitive behavioural therapy, with the exception of (e). Identification of faulty procedures usually occurs in cognitive analytic therapy.

*Reference*: Puri BK, Hall A, Ho R (2014). *Revision Notes in Psychiatry*. London: CRC Press, p. 334.

**Question 67 Answer: b**
*Explanation*: The prevalence of tardive dyskinesia increases with age and is more common in women. The length of treatment is more strongly related than the absolute dose.

*Further Reading*: Puri BK, Treasaden I (eds) (2010). *Psychiatry: An Evidence-Based Text*. London: Hodder Arnold, pp. 604, 903.

**Question 68 Answer: a, Amisulpride**
*Explanation*: This man suffers from moderate alcohol hepatitis. Amisulpride is predominantly excreted by the kidneys and dosage reduction is not necessary as this man is floridly psychotic.

*Reference and Further Reading*: Taylor D, Paton C, Kapur S (2009). *The Maudsley Prescribing Guidelines* (10th edition). London: Informa Healthcare; Puri BK, Treasaden I (eds) (2010). *Psychiatry: An Evidence-Based Text*. London: Hodder Arnold, p. 425.

**Question 69 Answer: e, Outcomes can be measured only by physiological measures, standardized instruments and self-report measures.**
*Explanation*: Outcomes can also be determined by means of direct observation. It is true that CBT focuses on specific issues and homework is assigned. It is time-limited and it focuses on the here and now.

*Reference*: Puri BK, Hall A, Ho R (2014). *Revision Notes in Psychiatry*. London: CRC Press, p. 336.

**Question 70 Answer: c, Fluoxetine**
*Explanation*: Fluoxetine is less sedative compared with other antidepressants and has a long half-life. Hence, fluoxetine is suitable for this patient as it can be taken every other day.

*Further Reading*: Puri BK, Treasaden I (eds) (2010). *Psychiatry: An Evidence-Based Text*. London: Hodder Arnold, pp. 698, 708, 724, 762.

**Question 71 Answer: c, Duloxetine is beneficial to people with urinary stress incontinence.**
*Explanation*: Duloxetine does not induce cytochrome P450 enzymes. Co-administered with an MAOI may lead to potentially serious drug interactions. Its half-life is 12 hours, and there is no clear evidence that it offers benefits over tricyclic antidepressants in efficacy.

*Further Reading*: Puri BK, Treasaden I (eds) (2010). *Psychiatry: An Evidence-Based Text*. London: Hodder Arnold, p. 907.

**Question 72 Answer: d, 40%**
*Explanation*: The estimated prevalence of personality disorder amongst the psychiatric inpatients has been estimated to be around 40%.

*Reference*: Puri BK, Hall A, Ho R (2014). *Revision Notes in Psychiatry*. London: CRC Press, p. 435

**Question 73 Answer: e, DISC gene on chromosome 4**
*Explanation*: All of the aforementioned have been linked to Alzheimer's disease, with the exception of option (e).

*Reference*: Puri BK, Hall A, Ho R (2014). *Revision Notes in Psychiatry*. London: CRC Press, p. 258.

**Question 74 Answer: a, Early cognitive impairments occur in around 10% of patients infected with HIV.**
*Explanation*: Early cognitive impairment occurs in 20% of patients affected with HIV. It can be classified into cognitive, behavioural and motor symptoms. The overall prevalence of dementia in patients suffering from HIV is around 25%. The onset of AIDS-associated dementia is insidious and occurs later in the course of the illness when there is significant immunosuppression.

*Reference*: Puri BK, Hall A, Ho R (2014). *Revision Notes in Psychiatry*. London: CRC Press, p. 483.

**Question 75 Answer: c, The presence of food enhances absorption. It has been noted that the presence of food would delay gastric emptying.**
*Explanation*: It has been noted that the presence of food delays gastric emptying and hence it would influence the rate of absorption of the drug.

*Reference*: Puri BK, Hall A, Ho R (2014). *Revision Notes in Psychiatry*. London: CRC Press, p. 241.

**Question 76 Answer: d, 4%**
*Explanation*: The most common cause of Down's syndrome is trisomy 21. Approximately 4% has resulted from translocation involving chromosome 21.

*Reference*: Puri BK, Hall A, Ho R (2014). *Revision Notes in Psychiatry*. London: CRC Press, p. 258.

**Question 77 Answer: e, 4:1**
*Explanation*: The gender ratio of kleptomania has been estimated to be around 4:1.

*Reference*: Puri BK, Hall A, Ho R (2014). *Revision Notes in Psychiatry*. London: CRC Press, p. 719.

**Question 78 Answer: d, Reboxetine is metabolized by cytochrome P450 3A4.**
*Explanation*: Reboxetine is an ineffective and potentially harmful antidepressant. It has anticholinergic properties and does not inhibit serotonin reuptake. At the time of writing, reboxetine is not licensed in the United States.

*Reference and Further Reading*: Eyding D, Lelgemann M, Grouven U (2010). Reboxetine for acute treatment of major depression: Systematic review and meta-analysis of published and unpublished placebo and selective serotonin reuptake inhibitor controlled trials. *British Medical Journal*, 341: c4737; Puri BK, Treasaden I (eds) (2010). *Psychiatry: An Evidence-Based Text*. London: Hodder Arnold, pp. 425, 907.

**Question 79 Answer: d, 85%**
*Explanation*: The heritability for bipolar disorder is 85% and that of depression 60%. There are gender differences. Men are at risk of depression if there is a family history of alcoholism and antisocial behaviour. Women are at risk if there is a family history of anxiety disorder.

*Further Reading*: Puri BK, Treasaden I (eds) (2010). *Psychiatry: An Evidence-Based Text*. London: Hodder Arnold, p. 468.

**Question 80 Answer: d, Impulse control disorders**
*Explanation*: Impulse control disorders are indicated for treatment using cognitive behavioural therapy approaches. The other indications include mood disorders, generalized anxiety disorder, phobia, eating disorders, impulse control disorders, schizophrenia, personality disorders, and in patients with chronic pain, chronic fatigue and also with physical illnesses.

*Reference*: Puri BK, Hall A, Ho R (2014). *Revision Notes in Psychiatry*. London: CRC Press, p. 334.

**Question 81 Answer: d, 4%**
*Explanation*: The prevalence of learning disability, which is defined as having an IQ of less than 70, has been estimated to be around 3.7%, and hence option (d) would be the most appropriate answer.

*Reference*: Puri BK, Hall A, Ho R (2014). *Revision Notes in Psychiatry*. London: CRC Press, p. 659.

**Question 82 Answer: e, Chromosome 19**
*Explanation*: Exchange of chromosomal substance between chromosome 21 and chromosome 13, 14, 15, 21 and 22 might result in Down's syndrome.

*Reference*: Puri BK, Hall A, Ho R (2014). *Revision Notes in Psychiatry*. London: CRC Press, p. 258.

**Question 83 Answer: a, Huntingtin**
*Explanation*: Huntington's disease or chorea results usually from a mutation of the protein huntingtin, and is characterized by a selective loss of discrete neuronal populations in the brain with progressive degeneration of efferent neurons of the neostriatum and sparing of the dopaminergic afferents, resulting in the progressive atrophy of the neostriatum.

*Reference*: Puri BK, Hall A, Ho R (2014). *Revision Notes in Psychiatry*. London: CRC Press, p. 201.

**Question 84 Answer: d, 20 hours**
*Explanation*: The active component in cannabis is 9-THC. It is derived from cannabis salve. It is known to be highly lipophilic, and so it can be detected in the blood for at least 20 hours following a single dose.

*Reference*: Puri BK, Hall A, Ho R (2014). *Revision Notes in Psychiatry*. London: CRC Press, p. 534.

**Question 85 Answer: e, The process is continuous as both the 2 DNA strands are synthesized.**
*Explanation*: The process is not continuous. It is described as semi-discontinuous due to the different ways in which the two DNA strands are being synthesized.

*Reference*: Puri BK, Hall A, Ho R (2014). *Revision Notes in Psychiatry*. London: CRC Press, p. 260.

**Question 86 Answer: e, 18**
*Explanation*: The age of onset is usually before the age of 18 in order for the diagnosis to be made.

*Reference*: Puri BK, Hall A, Ho R (2014). *Revision Notes in Psychiatry*. London: CRC Press, p. 659.

**Question 87 Answer: c, 6%**
*Explanation*: The Isle of Wright study has demonstrated that the point prevalence of child psychiatric disorder is estimated to be around 6.8%.

*Reference*: Puri BK, Hall A, Ho R (2014). *Revision Notes in Psychiatry*. London: CRC Press, p. 619.

**Question 88 Answer: d, Conduct disorder**
*Explanation*: Conduct disorder has been estimated to have 4% prevalence.

*Reference*: Puri BK, Hall A, Ho R (2014). *Revision Notes in Psychiatry*. London: CRC Press, p. 619.

**Question 89 Answer: c, Paroxetine**
*Explanation*: Paroxetine has a shorter half-life compared with other antidepressants and is associated with discontinuation syndrome.

*Further Reading*: Puri BK, Treasaden I (eds) (2010). *Psychiatry: An Evidence-Based Text*. London: Hodder Arnold, p. 717.

**Question 90 Answer: a, $\alpha_2$ receptor antagonism**
*Explanation*: The mechanism of action of mirtazapine includes $5HT_{1A}$ agonism, $5HT_{2A}$ antagonism, $5HT_{2C}$ antagonism and $5HT_3$ antagonism.

*Further Reading*: Puri BK, Treasaden I (eds) (2010). *Psychiatry: An Evidence-Based Text*. London: Hodder Arnold, pp. 426, 661, 907, 1110–1111.

### Question 91 Answer: d, Remission rate is 60%

*Explanation*: Based on previous studies done by Munro (1991), the mean age of onset is 35 for males and 45 for females. The onset is gradual and unremitting in 62%. It is incorrect that the remission rate is 60%.

*Reference*: Puri BK, Hall A, Ho R (2014). *Revision Notes in Psychiatry*. London: CRC Press, p. 373.

### Question 92 Answer: c, Reverse transcription would commence in the downstream locus control region.

*Explanation*: All of the aforementioned are true with regards to the processes involved in transcription, with the exception of (c).

*Reference*: Puri BK, Hall A, Ho R (2014). *Revision Notes in Psychiatry*. London: CRC Press, p. 260.

### Question 93 Answer: a, Prefrontal cortex

*Explanation*: Impaired task performance by schizophrenic patients has been linked to a reduction in the blood flow especially to the prefrontal cortex. Cognitive impairment is common in schizophrenic patients, and the cognitive deficits include learning and memory, working memory, executive functioning, attentional deficits and functional deficits.

*Reference*: Puri BK, Hall A, Ho R (2014). *Revision Notes in Psychiatry*. London: CRC Press, p. 361.

### Question 94 Answer: b, 3%

*Explanation*: The risk of dementia is increased amongst first-degree relatives by approximately 3%.

*Reference*: Puri BK, Hall A, Ho R (2014). *Revision Notes in Psychiatry*. London: CRC Press, p. 302.

### Question 95 Answer: c, Orbitofrontal cortex

*Explanation*: Diffuse-tensor imaging shows decreased cortico-striato-thalamo-striato-cortical circuitry. FMRI studies show increased orbitofrontal cortex, anterior cingulate cortex and striatum involvement.

*Further Reading*: Puri BK, Treasaden I (eds) (2010). *Psychiatry: An Evidence-Based Text*. London: Hodder Arnold, pp. 333, 1181.

**Question 96 Answer: b, Impulsive acts and self-mutilation**
*Explanation*: Impulsivity improves significantly over time. Affective symptoms in borderline personality disorder have the least improvement.

*Reference and Further Reading*: Stone MH (2010). Recovery from borderline personality disorder. *American Journal of Psychiatry*, 167: 618–619; Puri BK, Treasaden I (eds) (2010). *Psychiatry: An Evidence-Based Text*. London: Hodder Arnold, pp. 707, 709.

**Question 97 Answer: e, Hydrolysis**
*Explanation*: All of the aforementioned are common posttranslational modifications, with the exception of option (e). In fact, phosphorylation is crucial as it helps in signal transduction.

*Reference*: Puri BK, Hall A, Ho R (2014). *Revision Notes in Psychiatry*. London: CRC Press, p. 261.

**Question 98 Answer: b, There is an increased sensitivity of the serotonin receptors and exaggerated postsynaptic receptor response.**
*Explanation*: Studies have shown there is a sub-sensitivity of the receptors, instead of an increase in the sensitivity of the receptors.

*Reference*: Puri BK, Hall A, Ho R (2014). *Revision Notes in Psychiatry*. London: CRC Press, p. 414.

**Question 99 Answer: e, 15%**
*Explanation*: The prevalence of depressive symptoms has been estimated to be 15%. Elderly women have a higher prevalence.

*Reference*: Puri BK, Hall A, Ho R (2014). *Revision Notes in Psychiatry*. London: CRC Press, p. 302.

**Question 100 Answer: b, Right frontal lobe**
*Explanation*: The left frontal lobe is involved in controlling language-related movement whereas the right frontal love is involved in non-verbal abilities. Damage to the right frontal lobe would lead to disinhibition and also antisocial behaviours.

*Reference*: Puri BK, Hall A, Ho R (2014). *Revision Notes in Psychiatry*. London: CRC Press, p. 110.

**Question 101 Answer: b, The MacCAT-CA comprises 30 items that are organized into five sections.**
*Explanation*: The MacCAT-CA comprises 22 items that are organized into three sections. The first section, Understanding, assesses defendants' ability

to understand general information about the legal system and the process of adjudication. The second section, Reasoning, evaluates defendants' ability to discern the legal relevance of information and their capacity to reason about specific choices that confront defendants during the course of a typical criminal proceeding. The third section, Appreciation, assesses defendants' ability to appreciate the meaning and consequences of their own legal circumstances.

*Reference*: Pinals DA, Tillbrook CE, Mumley DL (2006). Practical application of the MacArthur Competence Assessment Tool–Criminal Adjudication (MacCAT-CA) in a public sector forensic setting. *The Journal of the American Academy of Psychiatry and the Law*, 34(2): 179–188.

### Question 102 Answer: a, Left frontal lobe
*Explanation*: The left frontal lobe is involved in controlling language-related movement. Left frontal lobe damage would lead to non-fluent speech as well as depression.

*Reference*: Puri BK, Hall A, Ho R (2014). *Revision Notes in Psychiatry*. London: CRC Press, p. 110.

### Question 103 Answer: a, Cholecystokinin
*Explanation*: Cholecystokinin regulates the postprandial release of bile locally in the gut and helps to control the appetite in the central nervous system.

*Reference*: Puri BK, Hall A, Ho R (2014). *Revision Notes in Psychiatry*. London: CRC Press, p. 234.

### Question 104 Answer: d, 10%
*Explanation*: The incidence of deliberate self-harm amongst young people in the UK has been estimated to be between 7% and 14% based on previous studies by Hawton and James in 2005.

*Reference*: Puri BK, Hall A, Ho R (2014). *Revision Notes in Psychiatry*. London: CRC Press, p. 286.

### Question 105 Answer: c, Rough endoplasmic reticulum
*Explanation*: This process which involves the presence of t-RNA molecules usually occurs in the rough endoplasmic reticulum.

*Reference*: Puri BK, Hall A, Ho R (2014). *Revision Notes in Psychiatry*. London: CRC Press, p. 261.

### Question 106 Answer: d, Reduction in medial temporal lobe volume
*Explanation*: Studies have shown that there is a net reduction in the medial temporal lobe volume on structural MRI. Functional MRI studies have shown an increased hemodynamic response in the amygdala, hippocampus and also the insula.

*Reference*: Puri BK, Hall A, Ho R (2014). *Revision Notes in Psychiatry*. London: CRC Press, p. 410.

**Question 107 Answer: a, Anticipation**
*Explanation*: This refers to the concept of anticipation. Huntington's disease is a disease that has been shown to be caused by expansions of unstable triplet repeat sequences and to occur at earlier ages and with greater severity in the succeeding generation.

*Reference*: Puri BK, Hall A, Ho R (2014). *Revision Notes in Psychiatry*. London: CRC Press, p. 269.

**Question 108 Answer: e, 50%**
*Explanation*: The estimated prevalence of self-harm amongst the Goth subculture has been estimated to be around 53%.

*Reference*: Puri BK, Hall A, Ho R (2014). *Revision Notes in Psychiatry*. London: CRC Press, p. 286.

**Question 109 Answer: b, Mammotrope**
*Explanation*: Mammotrope is the cell type that is responsible for the secretion of prolactin. They are also one of the most commonly involved cells in pituitary adenomas.

*Reference*: Puri BK, Hall A, Ho R (2014). *Revision Notes in Psychiatry*. London: CRC Press, p. 197.

**Question 110 Answer: c, 20%**
*Explanation*: Rapid cycling bipolar disorder tends to affect 13%–30% of bipolar patients, based on a previous study done by Hajek et al. (2008).

*Reference*: Puri BK, Hall A, Ho R (2014). *Revision Notes in Psychiatry*. London: CRC Press, p. 283.

**Question 111 Answer: c, Uniparental disomy**
*Explanation*: This is the concept of uniparental disomy.

*Reference*: Puri BK, Hall A, Ho R (2014). *Revision Notes in Psychiatry*. London: CRC Press, p. 269.

**Question 112 Answer: d, Patients with mild cognitive impairment tend to have preserved basic ADL and are still able to live independently.**
*Explanation*: There are a number of differences between MCI and dementia, but option (d) would be indicative of the most significance difference. Patients with MCI tend to have MMSE scores of 24–30, both subjective and objective complaints

of memory loss, and a decline too from their previous normal level of functioning. However, they are still able to have intact-level ADLs.

*Reference*: Puri BK, Hall A, Ho R (2014). *Revision Notes in Psychiatry*. London: CRC Press, p. 688.

### Question 113 Answer: c, 20%
*Explanation*: It has been estimated that vascular dementia accounts for around 20% of the dementia in the UK. The most common dementia would be Alzheimer's dementia, followed by vascular dementia and then Lewy body dementia.

*Reference*: Puri BK, Hall A, Ho R (2014). *Revision Notes in Psychiatry*. London: CRC Press, p. 300.

### Question 114 Answer: b, 1.5%
*Explanation*: The life-time risk for adults in the general population acquiring bipolar disorder has been estimated to be 1%–1.5%.

*Reference*: Puri BK, Hall A, Ho R (2014). *Revision Notes in Psychiatry*. London: CRC Press, p. 283.

### Question 115 Answer: a, Microglia
*Explanation*: They have been considered to be the smallest neuroglial cells and are the most abundant in the grey matter. Their key function would include acting as scavenger cells at the main sites of CNS injury.

*Reference*: Puri BK, Hall A, Ho R (2014). *Revision Notes in Psychiatry*. London: CRC Press, p. 177.

### Question 116 Answer: d, It helps with the synthesis of new proteins.
*Explanation*: Ribosomes are the primary sites at which translation occurs, and they are actively involved in the synthesis of proteins.

*Reference*: Puri BK, Hall A, Ho R (2014). *Revision Notes in Psychiatry*. London: CRC Press, p. 269.

### Question 117 Answer: a, Due to vacuolar changes in the grey matter, especially in the cerebral and cerebellar cortex
*Explanation*: The characteristic spongiform appearance is ldue to vacuolar changes in the grey matter, largely in the cerebral and the cerebellar cortex. In CJD there is rapid brain shrinkage and reduction in size due to diffuse and focal atrophy and neuronal loss.

*Reference*: Puri BK, Hall A, Ho R (2014). *Revision Notes in Psychiatry*. London: CRC Press, p. 704.

**Question 118 Answer: a, Amyloid precursor protein**
*Explanation*: The amyloid precursor protein gene is located on chromosome 21.

*Further Reading*: Puri BK, Treasaden I (eds) (2010). *Psychiatry: An Evidence-Based Text*. London: Hodder Arnold, pp. 473, 1104.

**Question 119 Answer: a, Formation of the myelin sheath**
*Explanation*: Oligodendrocytes form the myelin sheath.

*Further Reading*: Puri BK, Treasaden I (eds) (2010). *Psychiatry: An Evidence-Based Text*. London: Hodder Arnold, p. 436.

**Question 120 Answer: c, Midbrain**
*Explanation*: The ventral tegmental area is part of the mesolimbic dopamine pathway.

*Further Reading*: Puri BK, Treasaden I (eds) (2010). *Psychiatry: An Evidence-Based Text*. London: Hodder Arnold, p. 997.

**Question 121 Answer: d, Monoamine oxidase A (MAO-A) and aldehyde dehydrogenase**
*Explanation*: With regards to the degradation of 5-HT, the 5-HT is taken back into the neurons and degraded by MAO-A. SSRI blocks the 5-HT reuptake. This will lead to mood improvement in depressed patients, but nausea and impaired sexual functioning may arise as possible side effects.

*Further Reading*: Puri BK, Treasaden I (eds) (2010). *Psychiatry: An Evidence-Based Text*. London: Hodder Arnold, pp. 413–414.

**Question 122 Answer: a, Amino methylisoxazole propionic acid (AMPA) receptor**
*Explanation*: There are three main types of glutamate receptors: AMPA receptors, kainite receptors and *N*-methyl-D-aspartic acid (NMDA) receptors.

*Further Reading*: Puri BK, Treasaden I (eds) (2010). *Psychiatry: An Evidence-Based Text*. London: Hodder Arnold, pp. 351, 358, 410, 416–417.

**Question 123 Answer: b, Heschl gyrus**
*Explanation*: Heschl's gyrus (superior temporal gyrus) contains frequency strips which correspond to the tonal frequencies of sound. An fMRI study has demonstrated an increase in the blood oxygen level–dependent (BOLD) signal in Heschl's gyrus when patients experience auditory hallucinations.

*Reference and Further Reading*: Dierks T, Linden DEJ, Jandl M (1999). Activation of Heschl's gyrus during auditory hallucinations. *Neuron*, 22: 615–621; Puri BK, Treasaden I (eds) (2010). *Psychiatry: An Evidence-Based Text*. London: Hodder Arnold, pp. 332–335.

**Question 124 Answer: d**
*Explanation*: DBT is based on Zen Buddhism. DBT promotes the use of metaphor and irreverence. Out-of-therapy telephone contact is determined by the treatment contract between the patient and the therapist but is not generally available on a 24-hour basis.

*Reference*: Palmer RL (2002). Dialectical behaviour therapy for borderline personality disorder. *Advances in Psychiatric Treatment*, 8: 10–16.

**Question 125 Answer: a, Binge eating, guilt and self-induced vomiting**
*Explanation*: IPT does not focus on the direct symptoms associated with bulimia nervosa but allows for the identification of problem areas that have contributed to the emergence of bulimia nervosa over time.

*Reference and Further Reading*: Robin AF (1999). Interpersonal therapy for bulimia nervosa. *Psychotherapy in Practice*, 55: 715–725; Puri BK, Treasaden I (eds) (2010). *Psychiatry: An Evidence-Based Text*. London: Hodder Arnold, p. 693.

# Extended Matching Items (EMIs)

## Theme: Drugs and effects on EEG
**Question 126 Answer: a, Antidepressants**
*Explanation*: The administration of antidepressant would cause an increase in delta activity.

**Question 127 Answer: c, Anxiolytics**
*Explanation*: In general, anxiolytics would cause an increased beta activity and a reduction in alpha activity.

**Question 128 Answer: b, Antipsychotics**
*Explanation*: Antipsychotics can cause an increase in beta activity and a reduction in alpha activity (at times).

**Question 129 Answer: d, Lithium**
*Explanation*: It has been noted that therapeutic levels of lithium lead to only small effects that are likely to be missed on visual analysis of routine recordings.

*Reference*: Puri BK, Hall A, Ho R (2014). *Revision Notes in Psychiatry*. London: CRC Press, p. 217

## Theme: Neurochemistry – serotonin and psychiatric disorders

### Question 130 Answer: d, Manic disorder
*Explanation*: It has been noted that the 5HT transmission from the caudal raphe nuclei and rostral raphe nuclei is increased in patients with manic disorder.

### Question 131 Answer: e, Schizophrenia
*Explanation*: There is noted to be an interesting relationship between 5-HT and DA. There are two 5-HT pathways implicated in schizophrenic patients. When excess 5-HT is produced by these two pathways, there is a corresponding reduction in the availability of DA. This could give rise to the negative symptoms of schizophrenia.

### Question 132 Answer: f, Alzheimer's dementia
*Explanation*: In this condition, the 5-HT transmission from the rostral raphe nuclei to the temporal lobe is reduced in patients.

### Question 133 Answer: c, Depressive disorder
*Explanation*: 5-HT transmission from the caudal raphe nuclei and the rostral raphe nuclei is reduced in patients with depression. It leads to insomnia and suicide ideations. Presynaptic 5HT dysfunction is a state marker in depression.

*Reference*: Puri BK, Hall A, Ho R (2014). *Revision Notes in Psychiatry*. London: CRC Press, pp. 228–229.

## Theme: Neurochemistry – neuropeptides

### Question 134 Answer: b, Somatostatin
*Explanation*: Somatostatin has inhibitory effects on growth hormone release. Its concentration in the CSF is reduced for unipolar and bipolar depression. It is also reduced in Alzheimer's dementia.

### Question 135 Answer: c, Thyrotropin-releasing factor
*Explanation*: It is indeed the smallest brain peptide that has the ability to reverse sedation caused by drugs due to the release of DA or ACH in the brain. It is noted to be of increased concentration in the CSF of depressed patients. It may be implicated in the process of learning and memory.

### Question 136 Answer: d, Cholecystokinin
*Explanation*: CCK regulates the postprandial release of bile locally in the gut and helps to control appetite in the central nervous system. The CCK receptors seemed to be involved in appetite and feeding. It is also involved in emotional behaviour.

**Question 137 Answer: e, Vasoactive intestinal peptide**
*Explanation*: This is a neuropeptide that is found in the cerebral cortex, the hypothalamus, the amygdala, the hippocampus, the autonomic ganglia, and the intestinal and respiratory tracts. It stimulates the release of ACTH, the growth hormone as well as prolactin.

**Question 138 Answer: a, Corticotrophin-releasing factor**
*Explanation*: This factor controls the release of adrenocorticotropic hormone from the anterior pituitary. Injection of CRH could lead to depressive symptoms such as reduced appetite and sex drives, weight loss and altered circadian rhythm. NA causes CRH release.

*Reference*: Puri BK, Hall A, Ho R (2014). *Revision Notes in Psychiatry*. London: CRC Press, p. 234.

## Theme: Psychotropic drugs and adverse drug reactions

**Question 139 Answer: b, Intolerance**
*Explanation*: In drug intolerance, the adverse reactions are consistent with the known pharmacological actions of the drug. These adverse drug reactions may be dose related.

**Question 140 Answer: c, Idiosyncratic reactions**
*Explanation*: Idiosyncratic adverse drug reactions are reactions that are not characteristic or predictable and are associated with an individual human difference not present in members of the general population.

**Question 141 Answer: d, Allergic reactions**
*Explanation*: Allergic reactions to drug involve the body's immune system, with the drug interacting with a protein to form an immunogen that causes sensitization and the induction of an immune response.

**Question 142 Answer: e, Pharmacokinetic interaction**
*Explanation*: Pharmacokinetic interactions between drugs include chelation, drug displacement from binding sites as well as enzyme induction or enzyme inhibition.

*Reference*: Puri BK, Hall A, Ho R (2014). *Revision Notes in Psychiatry*. London: CRC Press, p. 252.

## Theme: Genetics – gene and psychiatric disorder

**Question 143 Answer: h, Chromosome 18**
*Explanation*: Chromosome 18 is involved in Edward syndrome, which is a trisomy condition.

**Question 144 Answer: f, Chromosome 14**
*Explanation*: Presenilin 1, which is encoded on chromosome 14, is implicated in the pathogenesis of Alzheimer's disease.

**Question 145 Answer: e, Chromosome 13**
*Explanation*: Chromosome 13 is implicated in the pathogenesis of both of the conditions.

**Question 146 Answer: d, Chromosome 8**
*Explanation*: Neuregulin is encoded on chromosome 8 and involved in the pathogenesis of schizophrenia.

**Question 147 Answer: b, Chromosome 2**
*Explanation*: Chromosome 2, and in particular 2q, is involved in the pathogenesis of Autistic disorder.

*Reference*: Puri BK, Hall A, Ho R (2014). *Revision Notes in Psychiatry*. London: CRC Press, p. 260.

## Theme: Advanced psychology – dynamic therapies

**Question 148 Answer: a, Brief focal psychotherapy**
*Explanation*: The objectives of psychodynamic psychotherapy are to improve self-understanding by developing the capacity for self-reflection. In brief focal psychotherapy, the main objective is to clarify the nature of the defences and its relationship to anxiety and impulses.

**Question 149 Answer: c, Short-term dynamic psychotherapy**
*Explanation*: The focus of short-term dynamic psychotherapy is an oedipal conflict.

**Question 150 Answer: b, Time-limited psychotherapy**
*Explanation*: The focus of time-limited psychotherapy is that it focuses on the present and chronically endured pain and negative self-image.

## Theme: Genetics

**Question 151 Answer: i, Substitution**

**Question 152 Answer: j, Transition**

**Question 153 Answer: h, Silent mutation**

**Question 154 Answer: d, Missense mutation**

**Question 155 Answer: e, Nonsense mutation**

**Question 156 Answer: c, Frame shift**
*Explanation*: A mutation is a change in DNA sequence that can be transmitted from the parent cell to its daughter cells. There are two types of mutations: germline mutation refers to a mutation that originates from a gamete that is

subsequently fused with another gamete during fertilization, leading to the conception of an individual who has the mutation in every cell. A somatic mutation occurs after fertilization and is only present in a subpopulation of somatic cells.

Deletion involves loss, while insertion involves gain of genetic material. Small deletions and insertions are caused by slippage or mispairing between complementary strands due to a close homology of adjacent sequences. Large deletions and insertions account for 5% of known pathogenic mutations. Most large deletions and insertions are caused by inequal crossing-over between homologous sequences. Substitution mutations resulting in a silent, missense or nonsense mutation can be transition or transversion. A silent mutation does not alter the amino acid residue encoded. A missense mutation results in a change in the amino acid residue encoded while a nonsense muation results in the creation of a stop codon, resulting in the prematue termination of the protein. Most mutations have the effect of a loss of function. If the number of nucleotides deleted or inserted in an exon involves a multiple of three, then the sequences of codons or reading frame is preserved. If it does not, the reading frame will be disrupted, resulting in a frameshift mutation with a truncated protein product.

*Further Reading*: Puri BK, Treasaden I (eds) (2010). *Psychiatry: An Evidence-Based Text*. London: Hodder Arnold, pp. 466, 467.

## Theme: Genetics

### Question 157 Answer: c, Family studies

*Explanation*: Family studies investigate the degree of familial clustering of a disorder by comparing the frequency of a disorder in the relatives of affected index cases (such as probands) with the frequency in a representative sample drawn from the general population. First-degree relatives share 50% of their genes.

*Further Reading*: Puri BK, Treasaden I (eds) (2010). *Psychiatry: An Evidence-Based Text*. London: Hodder Arnold, p. 469.

### Question 158 Answer: e, Twin studies

*Explanation*: The main purpose of twin studies is to identify the relative contribution of genetic and environmental factors to aetiology.

*Further Reading*: Puri BK, Treasaden I (eds) (2010). *Psychiatry: An Evidence-Based Text*. London: Hodder Arnold, p. 469.

### Question 159 Answer: a, Adoption studies

*Explanation*: Twin and adoption studies can be used when genetic factors cannot be separated well from environmental factors.

*Further Reading*: Puri BK, Treasaden I (eds) (2010). *Psychiatry: An Evidence-Based Text*. London: Hodder Arnold, p. 469.

**Question 160 Answer: d, Segregation analysis**
*Explanation*: Segregation analyses use statistical methods to examine pedigrees and hypothesized modes of inheritance.

*Further Reading*: Puri BK, Treasaden I (eds) (2010). *Psychiatry: An Evidence-Based Text*. London: Hodder Arnold, p. 474.

## Theme: Genetics
**Question 161 Answer: i, Chromosome 15**
*Explanation*: This is a case of Angelman's syndrome with deletion of maternal chromosome 15.

*Further Reading*: Puri BK, Treasaden I (eds) (2010). *Psychiatry: An Evidence-Based Text*. London: Hodder Arnold, p. 471.

**Question 162 Answer: k, Chromosome 22**
*Explanation*: This is a case of DiGeorge syndrome or velcardiofacial syndrome.

**Question 163 Answer: c, Periodic stereotyped repetitive discharges at a rate of 1 per second**
*Explanation*: This is a case of cri-du-chat syndrome.

**Question 164 Answer: a, Diffuse slow activity with episodic, bilaterally synchronous and symmetrical bursts of rhythmic waves**

**Question 165 Answer: c, Periodic stereotyped repetitive discharges at a rate of 1 per second**

*Further Reading*: Puri BK, Treasaden I (eds) (2010). *Psychiatry: An Evidence-Based Text*. London: Hodder Arnold, pp. 571–573, 1101.

**Question 166 Answer: b, Unusual appearance of episodic discharges, recurring every 1–3 seconds and variable focal slow waves over the temporal areas**

*Further Reading*: Puri BK, Treasaden I (eds) (2010). *Psychiatry: An Evidence-Based Text*. London: Hodder Arnold, pp. 95, 404, 568.

**Question 167 Answer: d, High-amplitude, repetitive, bilaterally synchronous and symmetrical, polyphasic sharp-wave and slow-wave complexes, occurring every 4–15 seconds**

*Further Reading*: Puri BK, Treasaden I (eds) (2010). *Psychiatry: An Evidence-Based Text*. London: Hodder Arnold, pp. 404, 569–570.

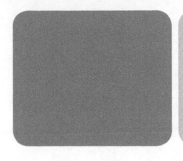

# MRCPSYCH PAPER A2 MOCK EXAMINATION 4: QUESTIONS

## GET THROUGH MRCPSYCH PAPER A2: MOCK EXAMINATION

Total number of questions: 181 (114 MCQs, 67 EMIs)
Total time provided: 180 minutes

**Question 1**
A 22-year-old male has recently sustained a head injury following a fight at his local pub. He finds that he now has great difficulties in carrying out procedural skills, and has been having difficulties working as a network technician. The most likely portion that was injured would be
  a. Medial temporal lobe
  b. Hippocampus
  c. Entorhinal cortex
  d. Amygdala
  e. Subiculum

**Question 2**
A core trainee was asked to run the memory clinic. He has just seen a 60-year-old man, whose main symptoms currently are apathy, disinhibition and reduction in speech output. Which one of the following clinical diagnosis should he be suspecting?
  a. Alzheimer's dementia
  b. Vascular dementia
  c. Mixed dementia
  d. Lewy body dementia
  e. Frontotemporal lobe dementia

**Question 3**
Which of the following is a long-acting opioid that has been helpful for patients intending to quit the use of opiates?
  a. Methadone
  b. Buprenorphine
  c. Naltrexone
  d. Dihydrocodeine
  e. Lofexidine

## Question 4
What dosage of methadone would be useful for reduction of heroin misuse?
a. 10–20 mg/day
b. 20–40 mg/day
c. 40–60 mg/day
d. 60–80 mg/day
e. More than 100 mg/day

## Question 5
A core trainee was looking at the family genogram of a patient. He notes that the mother has a particular disorder and all her sons are in turn affected. Which one of the following inheritance would account for the predominant mother to son transmission?
a. X-linked dominant
b. X-linked recessive
c. Autosomal dominant
d. Autosomal recessive
e. None of the above

## Question 6
Which of the following statements about X-linked recessive inheritance is incorrect?
a. All the male offspring who inherit the recessive abnormal allele would display the abnormal phenotypic trait.
b. Some women might manifest the phenotypic trait.
c. Male-to-male transmission usually does not take place.
d. Female heterozygotes are known to be carriers,
e. The incidence of these diseases is much higher in males than in females.

## Question 7
Which of the following biochemical disturbances have been postulated to increase the risk of suicide and aggressive behaviour?
a. Presence of low 5-Hydroxyindoleacetic acid concentration
b. Presence of high 5-Hydroxyindoleacetic acid concentration
c. Presence of high dopamine levels
d. Presence of low dopamine levels
e. Presence of low glutamate levels

## Question 8
Which of the following is incorrect with regards to the differences between bulbar palsy and pseudo-bulbar palsy?
a. The former is a lower motor neuron lesion, where the latter is an upper motor neuron lesion.
b. The tongue is noted to be flaccid and fasciculating in the former, but spastic in the latter.
c. Jaw jerk is increased for both.

d. Speech is noted to be quiet, hoarse and nasal for the former, but a characteristic Donald duck speech is noted in the latter.

e. The latter is associated with inappropriate laughter and also emotional incontinence.

## Question 9

Which of the following statements about the management of rapid cycling bipolar disorder is incorrect?

a. The current guidelines recommend an increment of the dosage of the antimanic drug or the addition of lamotrigine.

b. For long-term management, the NICE guidelines recommend a combination of lithium as first-line treatment.

c. Lithium monotherapy has been considered as the second-line next best treatment.

d. Antidepressants are to be avoided.

e. For long-term management, the NICE guidelines do not recommend the commencement of valproate in view of its potential toxicity.

## Question 10

Based on the principles of autosomal recessive inheritance, what are the chances of a child having an abnormal gene and expressing it, when both parents carry one abnormal copy of the gene?

a. 0%

b. 25%

c. 50%

d. 75%

e. 100%

## Question 11

Which of the following statements about behavioural techniques used in cognitive behavioural therapy is incorrect?

a. Rehearsal is used to help the client anticipate challenges and also to help them develop strategies to overcome difficulties.

b. Training is used to teach clients the importance of self-reliance.

c. Activity scheduling is used to increase the contact with positive activities and decrease the avoidance and withdrawal.

d. Diversion or distraction techniques are part of behavioural techniques.

e. Life skills training is part of the behavioural techniques used.

## Question 12

Dialectical behavioural therapy (DBT) is an indication for young people with repeated self-harm behaviour. Which one of the following is not an objective of DBT?

a. It helps to reduce self-harm and suicidal behaviour.

b. It helps to reduce and stop therapy-interfering behaviour.

c. It helps to reduce and stop the quality of life-interfering behaviour.

d. It helps to develop life skills.

e. It helps to develop cognitive restructuring skills.

## Question 13

Research studies have shown that a minority of cases of Alzheimer's disease are actually being inherited as an early-onset autosomal dominant disorder. The mutations that are likely to be involved to account for this include which of the following?

a. Mutations of chromosomes 1 and 14

b. Mutations of chromosomes 14 and 19

c. Mutations of chromosomes 14 and 21

d. Mutations of chromosomes 14 and 21

e. Mutations of chromosomes 19 and 22

## Question 14

In what percentage of individuals who are diagnosed with Alzheimer's dementia would the EEG be normal?

a. 2%

b. 4%

c. 6%

d. 8%

e. 10%

## Question 15

Which of the following statements about the EEG waveforms in the individual dementing condition is incorrect?

a. In Alzheimer dementia (AD), there is diffuse slowing of the EEG waveform in the early stages of the disease.

b. In Pick's disease, the EEG is less likely than in AD to be normal and would show more significant slowing of the a waves.

c. In vascular dementia, the EEG usually show asymmetry and localized slow waves, with sparing of the background activity.

d. In Creutzfeldt–Jakob disease (CJD), there is a generalized slow background rhythm with paroxysmal sharp waves.

e. In Huntington's disease, there is a low-voltage pattern which is observed.

## Question 16

Hyperreflexia, toxic psychoses and convulsions would occur when the lithium levels are greater than?

a. 0.8

b. 1.0

c. 1.2

d. 1.4

e. 2.0

**Question 17**
The process of transcription occurs in which part of a cell?
a. Nucleus
b. Ribosome
c. Smooth endoplasmic reticulum
d. Rough endoplasmic reticulum
e. Mitochondria

**Question 18**
Based on existing epidemiological studies, what has been estimated to be the prevalence of schizophrenia amongst those with learning disabilities?
a. 0.5%
b. 1%
c. 1.5%
d. 2%
e. 3%

**Question 19**
Which of the following is the main focus of brief focal psychotherapy as proposed by Malan?
a. Focusing on the nature of the defences and the relationship to anxiety and impulse
b. Focusing on the present
c. Focusing on the chronically endured pain and negative self-image
d. Focusing on the triangular conflict
e. Focusing on the awareness of defences

**Question 20**
Which of the following statements with regards to the NICE guidance on CBT and depressive disorder is correct?
a. For individuals with persistent subthreshold depressive symptoms, individual self-help based on the principles of CBT and CCBT could be offered.
b. For individuals with moderate or severe depression, individual CBT would be sufficient.
c. For individuals with moderate or severe depression, group-based CBT is not recommended.
d. Mentalization-based CBT is recommended for stable clients with two or more previous episodes of depression.
e. None of the above

**Question 21**
Who was the one who was responsible for proposing the following personality traits: neuroticism, extroversion, psychoticism and intelligence?
a. Stern
b. Kernberg
c. Cattell
d. Eysenck
e. Schneider

### Question 22
Based on neurochemistry findings, D2 receptors are coupled to which of the following?
a. Alpha subunits of G protein
b. Beta subunits of G protein
c. Acetylcholine molecules
d. Sodium channels
e. Potassium channels

### Question 23
Which of the following statements about the disease processes involving dopamine is incorrect?
a. In schizophrenia, there is reduction of the dopamine in the meso-cortical pathway that leads to anergy and loss of drive.
b. In schizophrenia, there is reduction of dopamine in the mesolimbic pathway.
c. In depression, the mesolimbic dopamine system is implicated.
d. In OCD, there is increased dopamine in the nigrostriatal pathway.
e. In bipolar disorder, there is increase in the dopamine in the nigrostriatal pathway.

### Question 24
Which of the following statements from the NICE guidelines about the use of atypical antipsychotics in schizophrenia is incorrect?
a. The atypical antipsychotic should be considered when deciding on the first-line treatment of newly diagnosed schizophrenia.
b. Atypical antipsychotic is considered the treatment of choice for managing an acute schizophrenic episode when discussion with the patient is not possible.
c. Atypical antipsychotic should be considered for an individual who is suffering from unacceptable side effects of a conventional antipsychotic.
d. Changing to an atypical antipsychotic should be considered even when a conventional antipsychotic controls the pre-existing symptoms well.
e. Clozapine should be introduced for treatment-resistant schizophrenia.

### Question 25
Almost all subjects with Down's syndrome who live beyond the age of 40 years do show evidence of Alzheimer's disease. Which particular gene has been implicated?
a. Presenilin 2 on chromosome 1
b. Presenilin 1 on chromosome 14
c. APOE gene on chromosome 19
d. Amyloid precursor protein on chromosome 21
e. Genes on the sex chromosomes

### Question 26
According to the psychoanalytic theory, borderline personality disorder frequently involves the following defence mechanism:
a. Splitting
b. Distortion

c. Intellectualization
d. Idealization
e. Rationalization

## Question 27
Studies have shown that the first manic episodes are usually precipitated by the following events, with the exception of
a. Bereavement
b. Personal separation
c. Work-related problems
d. Loss of role
e. Marital separation

## Question 28
A 4-year-old child has been referred to you for further assessment. He has gaze aversion, social avoidance and an IQ of 60. Physical examination noted that he has enlarged testes, large ears, and long face and flat feet. It is suspected that he might have fragile X disorder. The underlying defect that contributes to the condition is
a. Presence of 30 CGG repeats
b. Presence of 100 CGG repeats
c. Presence of 200 CGG repeats
d. Presence of CGG repeats on the Y chromosome
e. None of the above

## Question 29
It has been known that the long-term usage of antipsychotic medications would predispose individuals to metabolic syndrome. Based on the NICE guidelines, which one of the following recommendations is incorrect?
a. For monitoring of impaired glucose control, it is necessary to obtain a fasting glucose level at baseline.
b. It has been recommended that fasting glucose is monitored for patients at 1-month and 6-month interval after commencement of clozapine and olanzapine.
c. Antipsychotics such as clozapine, olanzapine, amisulpride and ziprasidone would contribute to impaired glucose control.
d. For dyslipidemia, it is important to monitor lipids at baseline, then at 3 monthly and then annually.
e. With regards to weight gain, it has been recommended that BMI and waist circumference are measured at baseline and at each outpatient visit.

## Question 30
Which of the following statements about dementia in Down's syndrome is true?
a. There is the presence of additional precursor protein on chromosome 21.
b. There is the loss of genetic materials from chromosome 1.
c. There is the loss of genetic materials from chromosome 14.
d. There is mutation of genetic materials on chromosome 19.
e. There is mutation of genetic materials on chromosome 14.

**Question 31**

Which of the following is the most common type of violence committed by schizophrenic patients in the outpatient?
 a. Verbal aggression
 b. Physical violence towards objects
 c. Physical violence towards others
 d. Self-directed violence
 e. Verbal and physical aggression

**Question 32**

According to the psychoanalytic theory, OCD frequently involves the following defence mechanism:
 a. Reaction formation
 b. Isolation
 c. Projection
 d. Projective identification
 e. Identification

**Question 33**

Which of the following statements about socioeconomic status in schizophrenia is incorrect?
 a. The association between schizophrenia and low social class has been attributed as one of the causative factors for schizophrenia.
 b. There tends to be a social drift in people with schizophrenia as a result of the illness.
 c. The unemployment rate of patients with schizophrenia could be as high as 70%.
 d. Low birth weight and urban birth are the known risk factors for schizophrenia.
 e. Patients who are in developing countries tend to have more acute onset and better outcomes than patients in developed countries.

**Question 34**

Which of the following is the most important postulated mode of action of buspirone?
 a. Partial agonism at 5-HT1A receptors
 b. Antagonist at 5-HT2c receptors
 c. Agonist at MT1 melatonergic receptors
 d. Agonist at MT2 melatonergic receptors
 e. Agonist at MT3 melatonergic receptors

**Question 35**

Which of the following is a characteristic EEG waveform that is commonly seen in patients diagnosed with hepatic encephalopathy?
 a. Slowing of rhythm with posterior preservation, with the presence of tri-phasic waves
 b. Low-voltage activity with posterior slowing
 c. Slowing of EEG with bursts of spike

d. Recurrent runs of 1- to 2-second waves
e. Acceleration of rhythm

## Question 36
Which of the following is a characteristic EEG finding for patients who are on antidepressants?
a. Generalized increase in EEG activity, but a reduced rhythm
b. Low-voltage activity with posterior slowing
c. Increased beta waves especially over frontal
d. Low-voltage EEG
e. Slowing with bursts of spikes

## Question 37
A 23-year-old male has been started on one of the older antidepressants, known as clomipramine, for his OCD symptoms. He has experienced weight gain. The weight gain is due to the blockage action of which one of the following?
a. Muscarinic receptor
b. Histamine receptor
c. Alpha-1 adrenergic
d. Alpha-2 adrenergic
e. Dopamine receptor

## Question 38
In order to identify the polymorphisms of the serotonin transporter gene, which one of the following methodologies could be used?
a. Northern blotting
b. Southern blotting
c. Western blotting
d. Microarray analysis
e. Linkage analysis

## Question 39
Who was the one involved in the development of self-control therapy?
a. Pavlov
b. Skinner
c. Thorndike
d. Bandura
e. Albert

## Question 40
Which of the following is not an indication for couple-based therapy?
a. The presence of interpersonal problems in a relationship
b. The presence of sexual problems in a relationship
c. The presence of grief in a couple
d. The presence of difficulties relating to a marriage
e. The presence of uncontrolled violent behaviour in a relationship

## Question 41

It is known that violence in people with schizophrenia is uncommon, but they tend to have a much higher risk than the general population. What has been the estimated prevalence of recent aggressive behaviour amongst outpatients with schizophrenia?

a. 1%
b. 2%
c. 3%
d. 4%
e. 5%

## Question 42

Based on epidemiological studies, what has been the estimated monozygotic concordance rate for Alzheimer's disease?

a. 5%
b. 10%
c. 15%
d. 20%
e. 30%

## Question 43

Which of the following statements about the intelligence of individuals with fragile X is incorrect?

a. Women with fragile X syndrome suffer from moderate learning disability.
b. Men with fragile X syndrome suffer from moderate-to-severe learning disability.
c. The verbal IQ is usually more than the performance IQ.
d. In more than 80% of male patients, the IQ has been shown to be less than 70.
e. The length of the trinucleotide repeats is inversely related to the IQ because the shorter length does not cause methylation and hence it would result in higher IQ scores.

## Question 44

Which of the following conditions is not related to either X or Y chromosomal abnormality?

a. Fragile X syndrome
b. Lesch–Nyhan syndrome
c. Klinefelter's syndrome XXY
d. Turner's syndrome
e. Patau's syndrome

## Question 45

What has been estimated to be the prevalence of childhood-onset depressive disorder?

a. 0.5%
b. 1%
c. 1.5%

d. 2%

e. 2.5%

## Question 46

What has been the estimated concordance rate for monozygotic (MZ) twins to develop schizophrenia?

a. 5%

b. 10%

c. 17%

d. 40%

e. 45%

## Question 47

A patient is questioning her need for maintenance treatment with antidepressants as she has been feeling much better in her mood for the past 6 months. Pharmacotherapy would still be needed, as studies have shown what percentage of recurrence of depression for patients with recurrent depression within 3 years that they have discontinued therapy?

a. 15%

b. 30%

c. 45%

d. 65%

e. 85%

## Question 48

Which of the following statements about antidepressant treatment is incorrect?

a. The first line treatment of depression is with antidepressants and it is important that patients receive an adequate dose for an adequate duration of 6 weeks.

b. Antidepressants should be continued for 4–6 months after the acute symptoms have settled.

c. Maintenance therapy is usually done with the same agent.

d. Lithium is effective in preventing recurrent depressive episodes and is more effective than tricyclic antidepressants.

e. Individuals who are maintained on the full effective treatment dose of antidepressants have fewer relapses as compared to those whose dose is reduced to a lower level.

## Question 49

Some patients who are on tricyclic antidepressant do complain of cognitive difficulties and sexual impairments. This is due to the blockage of which one of the following receptors?

a. Muscarinic

b. Histamine

c. Alpha-1 adrenoceptors

d. 5-HT2 receptors

e. 5-HT1c receptors

## Question 50
Which of the following is not part of a typical gene structure?
a. Upstream site that regulates transcription
b. 5' noncoding region
c. Exons
d. Intron
e. Translation initiation site

## Question 51
Which of the following is the use of oligonucleotide probes?
a. Used for detection of single base pair mutation
b. Used for detection of double base pair mutations
c. Used for identification of polymorphisms
d. Used for identification of the initiation sites
e. Used for identification of the termination sites

## Question 52
Polymorphisms of the serotonin transporter gene have been reported to be associated with all of the following conditions, with the exception of
a. OCD
b. Suicidal behaviour
c. Autism
d. Intense fear
e. Dementia

## Question 53
What is known to be approximate lifetime risk for the development of schizophrenia in siblings if one parent has had schizophrenia?
a. 3%
b. 4%
c. 6%
d. 10%
e. 17%

## Question 54
Which of the following statements about school refusal is incorrect?
a. School refusal tends to be ego-dystonic.
b. There is usually a family history of anxiety disorders and the failure of parents to separate from their own families of origin.
c. There is tendency for overprotective parenting styles.
d. There are usually two peaks to which this condition occurs, usually either at the age of 5 years, or at the age of 11 years.
e. The common symptoms include overt anxiety at the time of going to school with somatic symptoms being present.

**Question 55**

The concept of reciprocal inhibition, which is fundamental to systematic desensitization as well, was proposed by which of the following individuals?
  a. Pavlov
  b. Skinner
  c. Thorndike
  d. Wolpe
  e. Bandura

**Question 56**

Which of the following is not one of the common used behavioural techniques?
  a. Identify alternative belief
  b. Graded assignment on exposure
  c. Training to be self-reliant
  d. Activity scheduling
  e. Diversion

**Question 57**

Polymorphisms of the tryptophan hydroxylase gene have been associated with all of the following conditions, with the exception of
  a. Suicidal behaviour
  b. Bipolar disorder
  c. Early smoking commencement
  d. Alcohol abuse
  e. Heroin abuse

**Question 58**

Which of the following antidementia medications is contraindicated in people who have a history of asthma?
  a. Donepezil
  b. Rivastigmine
  c. Galantamine
  d. Memantine
  e. Rivastigmine patch

**Question 59**

The mesolimbic dopaminergic pathway has its origin from which one of the following?
  a. Substantia nigra
  b. Ventral tegmental area
  c. Limbic system
  d. Local network of dopamine (DA) in the hypothalamus
  e. Striatum

**Question 60**

The tuberoinfundibular pathway has its origin from which one of the following?
a. Substantia nigra
b. Ventral tegmental area
c. Limbic system
d. Local network of DA in the hypothalamus
e. Striatum

**Question 61**

Which of the following statements about the usage of antipsychotics in the elderly is incorrect?
a. They tend to be more sensitive to the anticholinergic side effects.
b. Parkinsonism side effects are more likely in the elderly.
c. Prevalence of tardive dyskinesia increases with age and is more common in women.
d. Acute dystonia is equally common in the young as well as in the old.
e. It has been linked with an increase in the mortality and cerebrovascular adverse events as compared to placebo.

**Question 62**

Which of the following statements with regards to linkage studies is incorrect?
a. They are able to help study the association between a disease and a genetic disorder.
b. They are able to help study the association between a specific allele and a disease.
c. They study families, instead of cases and controls.
d. Linkages are detectable over large distances >10 cM.
e. They are able to detect large relative risk (RR) of more than 2 as they are systematic in nature.

**Question 63**

Based on the psychoanalytic theory, during which one of the following psychosexual phase would boys pass through the Oedipus complex and girls the Electra complex?
a. Oral phase
b. Anal phase
c. Phallic phase
d. Latency phase
e. Genital phase

**Question 64**

Tuberous sclerosis type 3 is a genetic disorder that is caused by a translocation involving which one of the following chromosomes?
a. Chromosome 1
b. Chromosome 9
c. Chromosome 12
d. Chromosome 16
e. Chromosome 21

### Question 65
A 22-year-old male has sustained head injuries following a fight in the local pub. He needed emergency neurosurgical operation by the neurosurgeons. His mother realized that ever since the incident, he is no longer able to recall the steps of doing things right. This is likely to be due to an injury involving which part of his brain?
a. Medial temporal lobe
b. Hippocampus
c. Entorhinal cortex
d. Subiculum
e. Cerebellum

### Question 66
Working through, enactment, containment of anxiety and resolution of conflicts are part of which modality of psychotherapy?
a. Brief dynamic psychotherapy
b. Cognitive behavioural therapy
c. Cognitive analytic therapy
d. Supportive therapy
e. Interpersonal therapy

### Question 67
Which of the following statements regarding X-linked dominant inheritance is incorrect?
a. A dominant abnormal allele is carried on the X chromosome.
b. If an affected male mates with an unaffected female, all the daughters would be affected.
c. If an affected male mates with an unaffected female, all the sons would be affected.
d. If an unaffected male mates with an affected heterozygous female, half the daughters and half the sons on average are affected.
e. Male-to-male transmission does not usually take place.

### Question 68
A patient who is on lithium therapy has been admitted to the medical unit for congestive cardiac failure. The team has decided to start the patient on medications to help relieve some of the symptoms. Which of the following medication is contra-indicated as it causes an increase in the lithium levels?
a. Diltiazem
b. Propranolol
c. Thiazide diuretic
d. Sublingual glyceryl trinitrate (GTN)
e. Aspirin

## Question 69

A 60-year-old male has a 1-year history of memory impairments, associated with apathy, depression, hallucinations and delusions. On physical examination, it is noted that he has Parkinsonism-like features. Which one of the following neurochemicals had been implicated in this condition?
a. Lack of serotonin
b. Lack of dopamine
c. Lack of acetylcholine
d. Lack of neuropeptides
e. Lack of GABA

## Question 70

Which of the following with regards to the pharmacokinetics in old age is incorrect?
a. There is decreased first-pass availability.
b. There is a decrease in the rate of gastric emptying.
c. There is a reduction in the hepatic mass and blood flow.
d. There is reduction in renal blood flow.
e. There is a reduction in the glomerular filtration rate and the rate of elimination.

## Question 71

Approximately what proportion of individuals with mild mental retardation is expected to have a comorbid diagnosis of epilepsy?
a. 5%
b. 8%
c. 10%
d. 15%
e. 20%

## Question 72

Which of the following is not an X-linked dominant disorder?
a. Ornithine transcarbamylase
b. Aicardi syndrome
c. Coffin–Lowry syndrome
d. Rett syndrome
e. Hunter syndrome

## Question 73

One of the common side effects upon commencement of clozapine is hypersalivation. This is caused by the agonist of which one of the following receptors?
a. Dopamine D2
b. Serotonin 5-HT2
c. Serotonin 5-HT3
d. Muscarinic M3
e. Muscarinic M4

**Question 74**
What has been known to be the commonest non-cognitive feature in patients with dementia with Lewy bodies?
a. Apathy
b. Depression
c. Complex visual hallucinations
d. Complex auditory hallucinations
e. Paranoid delusions

**Question 75**
Which of the following statements about bipolar disorder is true?
a. There is an unequal male to female ratio for the disorder
b. The age of onset of bipolar disorder is earlier than that of unipolar disorder.
c. Bipolar disorder usually affects those in the lower socioeconomic classes.
d. Bipolar patients with only manic episodes have worst outcomes as compared to patients with depressive episodes.
e. Patients with mixed episodes do have a better prognosis.

**Question 76**
What has been estimated to be the prevalence of depressive disorder in patients who have suffered from a cerebrovascular accident?
a. 2%
b. 4%
c. 6%
d. 10%
e. 30%

**Question 77**
Which of the following is not postulated to be the effect of electroconvulsive therapy (ECT)?
a. Increased cerebral noradrenaline activity
b. Increased cerebral tyrosine hydroxylase activity
c. Increased plasma catecholamines, particularly adrenaline
d. Reduced beta-adrenergic receptor density
e. Increased alpha-adrenergic receptor density

**Question 78**
Based on epidemiological studies, the estimated incidence per 100,000 for men who have committed suicide in the United Kingdom is
a. 2
b. 4
c. 5
d. 7
e. 11

**Question 79**
Based on epidemiological studies, the estimated incidence per 100,000 for females
who have committed suicide in the United Kingdom is
a. 1
b. 2
c. 3
d. 5
e. 7

**Question 80**
Which of the following statements about agomelatine is incorrect?
a. It is classified as one of the recently introduced antidepressants.
b. It is an agonist at the MT1 melatonergic receptors.
c. It is an agonist at the MT2 melatonergic receptors.
d. It is an antagonist at the 5-HT2C receptors.
e. It is a partial agonist at the MT2 melatonergic receptors.

**Question 81**
Which of the following benzodiazepines has been recommended for use for
women who are breastfeeding?
a. Alprazolam
b. Lorazepam
c. Clonazepam
d. Diazepam
e. None of the above

**Question 82**
What is the estimated prevalence of dementia amongst individuals who are
between the ages of 75 and 79 years, given that there is a doubling of the prevalence
every 5 years?
a. 1.5%
b. 3%
c. 6%
d. 12%
e. 24%

**Question 83**
In facilitating neurotransmission, which one of the following receptors acts as a
fast-acting ion channel?
a. Serotonin receptor
b. Dopamine receptor
c. Muscarinic acetylcholine receptor
d. Nicotinic acetylcholine receptor
e. None of the above

## Question 84

A 22-year-old male was involved in a fight and sustained a head injury, for which he was treated. Months later, it was noted that he had personality changes characterized by the following: disinhibition, reduced social and ethical control, sexual indiscretions, poor judgements, elevated mood and lack of concern for the feelings of other people. What is the most likely injury that he has sustained?
a. Hematoma in the frontal lobe
b. Bilateral parietal contusions
c. Right occipital damage
d. Left occipital damage
e. Contrecoup injury to the temporal lobe

## Question 85

Based on epidemiological studies, what has been estimated to be the prevalence of mental abnormalities in those in prison in the United Kingdom?
a. 5%
b. 10%
c. 15%
d. 20%
e. 30%

## Question 86

All of the following disorders are correctly paired with their genetic abnormalities, with the exception of
a. Down's syndrome: fusion between chromosomes 21 and 14
b. Fragile X: presence of multiple trinucleotide repeats of CGG
c. Turner's syndrome: presence of an extra pair of Y chromosome
d. Klinefelter's syndrome: presence of a 47XXY karyotype
e. Duchenne muscular dystrophy: abnormalities at Xp21

## Question 87

Approximately what percentage of individuals with prodromal symptoms will convert to schizophrenia?
a. 5%
b. 10%
c. 20%
d. 25%
e. 35%

## Question 88

Juvenile delinquency has been defined as the law-breaking behaviour in 10-to 21-year-olds, which might predispose individuals to re-offence when they are adults. Based on existing epidemiological studies, approximately what percentage of them would have stopped their behaviours by the age of 19?
a. 10%
b. 20%
c. 30%

d. 40%

e. 50%

## Question 89

Which of the following medications would not account for a patient turning delirious in the psychiatric ward?

a. Phenothiazines

b. Antidepressants

c. Benzodiazepines

d. Lithium

e. Anti-hypertensives

## Question 90

What has been estimated to be the prevalence of epilepsy amongst patients with severe mental retardation?

a. 5%

b. 10%

c. 15%

d. 20%

e. 35%

## Question 91

Which of the following statements about the findings from epidemiological studies of depression is incorrect?

a. The prevalence in the general population has been around 2%–5%.

b. It has been estimated that at least 1 in 4 women and 1 in 10 men have depressive disorder in their lifetime.

c. People living in deprived industrial area are more unlikely to be treated for depression than people living in other areas.

d. The peak age of onset of depression is 30 years.

e. People younger than 40 years are three times more likely to develop depression than older people.

## Question 92

Which of the following antidepressants is recommended for use for women who are breastfeeding their infants?

a. Paroxetine

b. Fluoxetine

c. Citalopram

d. Fluvoxamine

e. None of the above

## Question 93

A 25-year-old woman suffers from depression and has taken fluoxetine for 2 weeks. She complains of insomnia at night. Her GP wants to find out the receptor involved in causing the insomnia. Your answer is

a. Agonism of $5\text{-}HT_1$ receptors

b. Agonism of $5\text{-}HT_2$ receptors

c. Agonism of 5-HT$_3$ receptors

d. Agonism of 5-HT$_4$ receptors

e. Agonism of 5-HT$_6$ receptors

**Question 94**

A 35-year-old middle-class man has been dependent on heroin and is highly motivated to remain abstinent. He wants to take an opioid antagonist with a relatively long half-life. Your recommendation is

a. Buprenorphine

b. Dihydrocodeine

c. Methadone

d. Naloxone

e. Naltrexone

**Question 95**

A 13-year-old obese white Caucasian boy with learning disability is referred. He presents with an irresistible hunger drive and incessant skin picking with compulsion and anxiety. His mother reports that he tends to talk to himself. On physical examination, he has almond-shaped eyes, a fish-shaped mouth, micro-orchidism and truncal obesity. Which of the following is the most likely finding by molecular genetic testing?

a. Microdeletion of chromosome 15q 11-13 of maternal origin

b. Microdeletion of chromosome 15q 11-13 of paternal origin

c. Microdeletion of chromosome 16p 13.3

d. Microdeletion of chromosome 17q 21-31 of maternal origin

e. Microdeletion of chromosome 17q 21-31 of paternal origin

**Question 96**

The Royal College of Psychiatrists wants to assess the quality of the MRCPsych Paper 2. The Royal College selected the Paper 2 used in spring 2008. The items in the examination paper were split into two tests equivalent in content and difficulty. The two tests were administered to a group of 100 volunteer candidates. The correlation of two separate tests was assessed with an adjustment for the test length by the Kuder–Richardson formula. What is the Royal College trying to measure?

a. The degree of agreement amongst the same candidates at different times

b. The degree of agreement amongst different candidates within the same time frame

c. The internal consistency of the MRCPsych Paper 2 used in spring 2008

d. The stability of the MRCPsych Paper 2 used in spring 2008 under identical conditions at different times

e. The validity of the MRCPsych Paper 2 in measuring the competency of trainees

**Question 97**

A 13-year-old adolescent suffering from depressive disorder was referred to a psychologist for psychotherapy. She missed three psychotherapy sessions and her father finds her missing. Today, her father informs the psychologist that the patient has committed suicide. Which of the following parental factors is not associated with suicide in this young person?

   a. Divorce of parents when she was 6
   b. Early death of mother owing to kidney disease
   c. Poor education level of both parents
   d. Her father also suffers from depressive disorder
   e. Upper social class and high expectation of children

**Question 98**

A 40-year-old man presented with depression, anxiety, aggression and sensory pain. He showed cerebellar ataxia on physical examination and severe deficits on cognitive assessment. He passed away shortly after admission. He worked as a food factory worker and processed meat products made from cows infected with bovine spongiform encephalopathy (BSE). Following the death of the patient, a post-mortem examination was performed. In which of the following neuroanatomical areas were florid plaques and spongiform changes most likely to be found?

   a. Brainstem
   b. Occipital cortex
   c. Parietal cortex
   d. Prefrontal cortex
   e. Temporal cortex

**Question 99**

What is the lifetime prevalence of non-suicidal self-injury amongst adolescents?

   a. 2%–12%
   b. 13%–23%
   c. 24%–34%
   d. 3%–45%
   e. 56%–66%

**Question 100**

A 60-year-old woman suffering from bipolar disorder has developed acute renal failure. You were given a list of psychotropic medications which the patient has taken (see the following options). The renal consultant wants to find out which medication has the highest percentage of excretion unchanged in urine. Your response is

   a. Amisulpride
   b. Lithium
   c. Lamotrigine
   d. Mirtazapine
   e. Olanzapine

**Question 101**

The son of a 75-year-old man with Alzheimer's disease wants to consult you on the predicted risk of developing Alzheimer's disease amongst the first-degree relatives like himself. Your response is

a. 5%–9%

b. 10%–14%

c. 15%–19%

d. 20%–24%

e. 25%–29%

**Question 102**

A 45-year-old man had a motor vehicle accident and sustained a head injury involving the frontal part of his brain. He was subsequently noted by family to be easily irritable, callous and impatient. He was also amotivational and non-empathic towards others. Which part of the frontal lobe is most likely to be affected?

a. Anterior cingulate

b. Distal prefrontal cortex

c. M1

d. Orbitofrontal cortex

e. Supplementary motor area

**Question 103**

A rescarcher has conducted the following experiments on 10 people with schizophrenia and 10 people without schizophrenia. Each participant is presented with a sequence of letters, and the task consists of indicating when the current letter matches the one from five steps earlier in the sequence while undergoing functional magnetic resonance imaging. Which of the following neuroanatomical areas shows less activation in people with schizophrenia compared with controls?

a. Dorsolateral prefrontal cortex

b. Frontal eye fields

c. Orbitofrontal cortex

d. Primary motor cortex

e. Ventromedial prefrontal cortex

**Question 104**

A 20-year-old motorcyclist complains that he has forgotten the way to ride a motorcycle. Damage in which of the following neuroanatomical areas accounts for his symptom?

a. Amygdala

b. Dentate gyrus

c. Entorhinal cortex

d. Dorsal striatum

e. Hippocampus

### Question 105
A 25-year-old man with bipolar disorder has tried different types of mood stabilizers and antipsychotics without much success in controlling his manic symptoms. The consultant psychiatrist has read an article stating that the calcium channel blocker verapamil has been extensively studied for the treatment of mania. This article also suggests that psychiatrists faced with patients with mania who do not respond to other antimanic agents may consider using verapamil as adjunctive therapy. The consultant is very keen to add verapamil to the following list of medications (see the following options). Which of the following drugs has the highest risk of causing toxicity when combined with verapamil?
a. Amitriptyline
b. Lamotrigine
c. Lithium
d. Valproate
e. Risperidone

### Question 106
What are the classical EEG changes seen in hepatic encephalopathy?
a. Alpha waves
b. Alpha and theta waves
c. Delta waves
d. Low voltage
e. Triphasic waves

### Question 107
The Department of Health announces that there were 8.4 stillbirths for every 1000 live births from 2009 to 2010. This figure refers to the
a. Age-specific mortality rate
b. Infant mortality rate
c. Neonatal mortality rate
d. Perinatal mortality rate
e. Stillbirth mortality rate

### Question 108
A 60-year-old man is brought in by his partner as he has been aggressive and disinhibited.

He suffers a severe contrecoup head injury from a fall in the bathtub. The magnetic resonance imaging (MRI) scan reveals a brighter area that represents contusions resulting from the contrecoup injury. Which of the following neuroanatomical areas is the most likely to be involved?
a. Contrecoup in occipital lobe
b. Contrecoup in orbitofrontal lobe
c. Contrecoup in parietal lobe

d. Contrecoup in primary motor cortex
e. Contrecoup in temporal lobe

## Question 109
'The heritability of autism is 0.6'. What does this statement mean?
a. Sixty percent of people with autism have specific alleles in coupling at linked loci more or less often than would be expected by chance.
b. Sixty percent of people with autism have two or more loci at which alleles show linkage.
c. Sixty percent of total phenotypic variance of autism in a population results from genetic factors.
d. The constant proportion of different genotypes of autism in a population is 60%.
e. The proportion of autism resulting from mutation in an allele is 60%.

## Question 110
Which of the following is the mechanism of action of acamprosate?
a. GABA antagonist
b. Glutamate antagonist
c. Inhibition of alcohol dehydrogenase
d. Inhibition of alcohol aldehyde dehydrogenase
e. Opioid antagonist

## Question 111
Lofexidine is used in the treatment of opioid withdrawal. Its mechanism of action involves
a. $\alpha_1$ adrenergic receptor agonist
b. $\alpha_1$ adrenergic receptor antagonist
c. $\alpha_2$ adrenergic receptor agonist
d. $\alpha_2$ adrenergic receptor antagonist
e. $\beta_1$ receptor agonist

## Question 112
A developing country is in a very poor financial condition and the government can only purchase one type of antipsychotics. The government administered a survey to 800 patients with schizophrenia and they were given two drugs from which to choose. The government informed the patients that Drug A could cure 300 people and make them free of psychotic symptoms. Drug B had a 60% chance of failure. Both drugs had the same expected benefits of curing around 300 patients; 90% of respondents chose drug A but only 10% chose drug B. This phenomenon is known as
a. Cognitive bias
b. Cognitive dissonance
c. Cognitive distortion
d. Cognitive framing
e. Cognitive representation

**Question 113**

Which of the following has the least impact on the cognitive representation of disease amongst people with chronic schizophrenia?

a. Aetiology of schizophrenia
b. Impact of schizophrenia on patients' lives
c. Measures and strategies available to control schizophrenia
d. Positive symptoms
e. Prevalence of schizophrenia

**Question 114**

A 40-year-old woman suffering from treatment-resistant schizophrenia has taken clozapine 450 mg per day for 2 months. Which of the following side effects would not improve even the dose is reduced?

a. Hypotension
b. Neutropenia
c. Sedation
d. Seizure
e. Weight gain

# Extended Matching Items (EMIs)

## Theme: Major psychiatric disorders and findings in association studies

**Options:**

a. Schizophrenia
b. Depressive disorder
c. Bipolar disorder
d. Post-traumatic stress disorder
e. Autism
f. Hyperkinetic disorder

**Lead in:** Select the most appropriate answer for each of the following. Each option may be used once, more than once or not at all.

**Question 115**

Association studies found inconsistent results.

**Question 116**

Association studies found the involvement of dopamine D3 receptor genes and 5-HT2A receptor genes.

**Question 117**

Association studies have found the involvement of genes encoding for tyrosine hydroxylase, serotonin transporter and catechol-$O$-methyltransferase (COMT).

**Question 118**

Association studies have found the involvement of serotonin transporter gene in this condition.

**Question 119**

Association studies have found the involvement of the dopamine D4 receptor gene in this condition.

## Theme: Transmission of genetic disorders

**Options:**

a. Autosomal dominant inheritance
b. Autosomal recessive inheritance
c. X-linked dominant inheritance
d. X-linked recessive inheritance
e. Disorders of carbohydrate metabolism and lysosomal storage

**Lead in:** Select the most appropriate answer for each of the following. Each option may be used once, more than once or not at all.

**Question 120**

Rett's syndrome is inherited in this form of inheritance.

**Question 121**

Gaucher's disease is inherited in this form of inheritance.

**Question 122**

Phenylketonuria is inherited in this form of inheritance.

**Question 123**

Early-onset Alzheimer's dementia is an example of this.

## Theme: Advanced psychology

**Options:**

a. Couple therapy
b. Motivational interviewing
c. Eye movement and desensitization reprocessing
d. Grief counselling
e. Brief insight-oriented therapy
f. Art therapies

**Lead in:** Select the most appropriate answer for each of the following. Each option may be used once, more than once or not at all.

**Question 124**

This particular form of therapy deals with grief in a couple as well as sex-related problems. Which form of therapy is this?

**Question 125**

This form of therapy is useful for patients who are non-concordant to psychotropic medications.

**Question 126**
This form of therapy focuses much on traumatic events, negative cognitions and affective responses.

**Question 127**
This form of therapy is largely counselling work that allows the client to gradually accept the loss.

**Question 128**
This particular form of therapy has its basis on the psychoanalytical therapy, but with different techniques and time frames.

## Theme: Genetics
**Options:**
   a. <1%
   b. 2%
   c. 5%
   d. 10%

**Lead in:** A couple has adopted a child with Down's syndrome. They want to find out the chances of developing psychiatric disorder when their adopted child becomes an adult. Match the correct number to the each of the following psychiatric comorbidities. Each option might be used once, more than once or not at all.

**Question 129**
Anxiety disorders. (Choose one option.)

**Question 130**
Depressive disorder. (Choose one option.)

**Question 131**
Dementia. (Choose one option.)

**Question 132**
OCD. (Choose one option.)

**Question 133**
Schizophrenia. (Choose one option.)

**Question 134**
Self-injury. (Choose one option.)

## Theme: Genetics
**Options:**
   a. 5%
   b. 9%
   c. 13%
   d. 45%

**Lead in:** A 28-year-old man suffers from a first episode of schizophrenia. His family members want to find out their risk of developing schizophrenia. Match the correct number to the following psychiatric comorbidity. Each option might be used once, more than once or not at all.

**Question 135**
The risk for his brother to develop schizophrenia. (Choose one option.)

**Question 136**
The risk of his son to develop schizophrenia. (Choose one option.)

**Question 137**
The risk of his father to develop late-onset schizophrenia. (Choose one option.)

## Theme: Psycho-pharmacology and neurology
**Options:**
   a. Absent P waves
   b. Biphasic P waves
   c. PR interval = 100 ms
   d. PR interval = 300 ms
   e. QRS complex = 200 ms
   f. QTc = 500 ms
   g. RR interval 450 ms
   h. RR interval = 1500 ms
   i. R wave in $V_6$ = 30 mm
   j. ST segment depression
   k. ST segment elevation
   l. Diffuse ST segment elevation
   m. ST segment elevation with saddle
   n. Absent T wave
   o. Diffuse T wave inversion
   p. Tall T waves
   q. Q wave
   r. Heart rate: 120 per minute
   s. Heart rate: 30 per minute

**Lead in:** Match the aforementioned electrocardiogram (ECG) findings to the most typical ECG features found in the following scenarios. Each option might be used once, more than once or not at all.

**Question 138**
A 40-year-old married woman with major depression checked into a hotel and took 100 amitriptyline tablets (100 mg each). She remains obtunded at the Accident and Emergency Department and is about to be transferred to an intensive care unit. (Choose three options.)

### Question 139

A 40-year-old man suffering from treatment-resistant schizophrenia has been taking clozapine for the past 5 years. He experiences tiredness, shallow and difficult breathing and chest pain. The temperature is 39 degrees Celsius. (Choose three options.)

### Question 140

A 55-year-old man suffering from depression does not respond to various types of antidepressants. His antidepressant treatment is augmented with thyroxine. He presents to the Accident and Emergency Department with a 2-hour history of chest pain, nausea and sweatiness. (Choose four options.)

### Question 141

A 35-year-old woman complains of a 3-month history of ankle swelling, together with increased abdominal distension and breathlessness over the past week. She admits to having taken amphetamines on a daily basis for the last 5 years. (Choose four options.)

### Question 142

A 70-year-old man with Alzheimer's disease is admitted because of a blackout. He has taken donepezil on a daily basis for the past year. (Choose two options.)

## Theme: Neuropathology

**Options:**
  a. Alzheimer's disease
  b. Bipolar disorder
  c. Chronic depression
  d. Huntington's disease
  e. Lewy body dementia
  f. Obsessive-compulsive disorder
  g. Progressive supranuclear palsy
  h. Schizophrenia
  i. Variant Creutzfeldt–Jakob disease
  j. Wernicke's encephalopathy
  k. Wilson's disease

**Lead in:** Match the aforementioned neuropsychiatric conditions to the following MRI changes. Each option might be used once, more than once or not at all.

### Question 143

Atrophy of the head of caudate nucleus. (Choose one option.)

### Question 144

Hockey-stick sign. (Choose one option.)

**Question 145**
Hyperintensities in bilateral mammillary bodies. (Choose one option.)

**Question 146**
Pulvinar sign. (Choose one option.)

## Theme: Neuroanatomy

**Options:**
a. Broca's area
b. Superior mesial region
c. Inferior mesial region
d. Orbital cortex
e. Basal forebrain

**Lead in:** Please select the most appropriate options from the aforementioned for each of the following questions.

**Question 147**
A lesion of this particular area can lead to motor aphasia.

**Question 148**
A lesion of this area would lead to sociopathy.

**Question 149**
A lesion of this area would lead to akinetic mutism.

**Question 150**
An injury to this area of the central nervous system would lead to both anterograde and retrograde amnesia.

## Theme: Neuropathology

**Options:**
a. Gliomas
b. Metastases
c. Meningeal tumours
d. Pituitary adenomas
e. Neuilemmomas
f. Haemangioblastomas
g. Medulloblastoma

**Lead in:** Please select the most appropriate options from the aforementioned for each of the following questions.

**Question 151**
Which of the aforementioned is the most common cerebral tumour?

**Question 152**
Null cell adenoma is the third most common type of which of the aforementioned.

**Question 153**
These tumours are derived from blood vessels.

**Question 154**
These are considered to be embryonal tumours.

## Theme: Advanced psychological process and treatment – group therapy

**Options:**
  a. Open-group therapy
  b. Closed-group therapy
  c. Heterogeneous group therapy
  d. Homogenous group therapy
  e. Continuous group therapy
  f. Brief group therapy
  g. Leadership

**Lead in:** Select the most appropriate option for each of the following questions.

**Question 155**
In this particular form of group therapy, there is no particular end date of the therapy.

**Question 156**
In this form of group therapy, replacement of group members is allowed.

**Question 157**
This particular form of group therapy allows the mixture of clients from differing backgrounds.

## Theme: Psychiatric epidemiology

**Options:**
  a. Relative risk
  b. Attributable risk
  c. Relative risk increased
  d. Absolute risk reduction
  e. Relative risk reduction
  f. Number needed to treat
  g. Odds ratio

**Lead in:** Based on your understanding of epidemiology, please select the most appropriate option for each of the following questions.

**Question 158**
This helps to summarize the results of a trial and also in individualized decision making.

**Question 159**
This is a ratio of the subjects in the disease group who have been exposed to the subjects in the control group who have not been exposed.

**Question 160**
This refers to a measure of the difference in the risk between the two groups being studied but this time indexing the risk reduction following exposure to the index factor.

**Question 161**
This is also known as the risk difference or the absolute excess risk.

**Question 162**
This refers to the ratio of the incidence of the disease in people who are exposed to the risk factor to the incidence of the disease in people who are not exposed to the same risk factor.

## Theme: Genetics and morbid risks in first-degree relatives

**Options:**
  a. 3%
  b. 3.5%
  c. 5%
  d. 10%
  e. 18%
  f. 24.6%
  g. 15%

**Lead in:** Morbid risk (MR) (also known as lifetime incidence) is used to express the rates of illness in relatives. Based on your understanding of morbid risk, please match the MR in first-degree relatives for each of the following disorders.

**Question 163**
Schizophrenia amongst White populations

**Question 164**
Schizophrenia amongst Afro-Caribbeans

**Question 165**
Bipolar disorder

**Question 166**
Obsessive-compulsive disorder

**Question 167**
Alzheimer's disease

**Question 168**
Autism

## Theme: Neurochemistry of neuropeptides
**Options:**
  a. Corticotropin-releasing factor (CRF)
  b. Somatostatin
  c. Thyrotropin-releasing hormone (TRH)
  d. Cholecystokinin (CCK)
  e. Vasoactive intestinal peptide (VIP)

**Lead in:** Please select the appropriate neuropeptides for each of the following questions.

**Question 169**
In depressive disorder, the concentrations of these two neuropeptides are increased in the cerebrospinal fluid.

**Question 170**
Overactivity of this neuropeptide leads to excessive noradrenaline release.

**Question 171**
The amount of this neuropeptide is reduced in Alzheimer's disease.

**Question 172**
This particular neuropeptide is involved in appetite and feeding, as well as in emotional behaviour.

**Question 173**
This is a neuropeptide that inhibits the release of somatostatin.

## Theme: Neuropathology
**Options:**
  a. Schizophrenia
  b. Autism
  c. Parkinson's disease
  d. Huntington's disease

**Lead in:** Please select the most appropriate option from the aforementioned options for each of the following questions.

**Question 174**
Hypoplasia of the cerebellar vermis is the characteristic feature of this condition.

**Question 175**
In this condition, there is characteristic neuronal loss, as well as reactive astrocytosis and presence of Lewy bodies in the substantia nigra.

**Question 176**
In this condition, there is the dilatation of the lateral and the third ventricles, along with marked atrophy of the cerebral cortex.

## Theme: Neurochemistry of serotonin

**Options:**
  a. 5-HT1A
  b. 5-HT1B
  c. 5-HT1D
  d. 5-HT2
  e. 5-HT2c
  f. 5-HT3
  g. 5-HT4
  h. 5-HT6
  i. 5-HT7

**Lead in:** Select the serotonin receptor type for each of the following questions.

**Question 177**
Buspirone exerts its clinical effects through the partial agonism of which of the aforementioned receptors?

**Question 178**
This particular receptor type is implicated in Cloninger's type II alcoholism.

**Question 179**
This receptor is involved in the contraction of the colon and bladder.

**Question 180**
Antagonism of this receptor helps to improve cognition.

**Question 181**
This particular receptor is involved in the circadian rhythm.

## GET THROUGH MRCPSYCH PAPER A2: MOCK EXAMINATION

**Question 1 Answer: d, Amygdala**
*Explanation*: The storage of implicit memories or procedural memories would be dependent on the functioning of the cerebellum, the amygdala, and specific sensory and motor systems that are typically used in learned task.

*Reference*: Puri BK, Hall A, Ho R (2014). *Revision Notes in Psychiatry*. London: CRC Press, p. 103.

**Question 2 Answer: e, Frontotemporal lobe dementia**
*Explanation*: The most likely clinical diagnosis would be frontotemporal lobe dementia. Patients with this particular form of dementia usually have a much younger age of onset, and have more severe apathy, disinhibitions, reduction in speech output as well as loss of insight and coarsening of social behaviour.

*Reference*: Puri BK, Hall A, Ho R (2014). *Revision Notes in Psychiatry*. London: CRC Press, p. 696.

**Question 3 Answer: a, Methadone**
*Explanation*: Methadone is a synthetic opiate that could be taken either orally or intravenously. It is considered to be a long-acting opioid agonist, with half-life of between 24 to 36 hours and this would allow for once daily oral prescription.

*Reference*: Puri BK, Hall A, Ho R (2014). *Revision Notes in Psychiatry*. London: CRC Press, p. 535.

**Question 4 Answer: d, 60–80 mg/day**
*Explanation*: Methadone at the dose of 60–100mg/day is actually more effective than lower dosages in reduction of heroin misuse. At the dose of 20–40 mg/day, it would help for withdrawal symptoms. The starting dose of the medication is usually 10–30 mg per day and then a gradual increment by 5–10 mg per week to reach the therapeutic dosage.

*Reference*: Puri BK, Hall A, Ho R (2014). *Revision Notes in Psychiatry*. London: CRC Press, p.535.

**Question 5 Answer: b, X-linked recessive inheritance**
*Explanation*: In X-linked recessive inheritance, a recessive abnormal allele is carried on the X chromosome. All the males which carry the genotype XY would inherit the allele and hence manifest the abnormal phenotypic trait.

*Reference*: Puri BK, Hall A, Ho R (2014). *Revision Notes in Psychiatry*. London: CRC Press, p. 267.

**Question 6 Answer: b, Some women might manifest the phenotypic trait.**
*Explanation*: Women are not likely to display the trait. This is because the single recessive mutation for a gene on the X chromosome in women is compensated for by the normal allele on the other X chromosome so that the disease does not occur.

*Reference*: Puri BK, Hall A, Ho R (2014). *Revision Notes in Psychiatry*. London: CRC Press, p. 267.

**Question 7 Answer: a, Presence of low 5-HIAA concentration**
*Explanation*: Low 5-HIAA concentration in the cerebral spinal fluid has been associated with increased suicidal behaviour and aggression. This is irrespective of the clinical diagnosis that the patient already has. Hence, it has been concluded that serotonin has played an important role in the biology of aggression as well as the control of impulsive behaviour.

*Reference*: Puri BK, Hall A, Ho R (2014). *Revision Notes in Psychiatry*. London: CRC Press, p. 397.

**Question 8 Answer: c, Jaw jerk is increased for both.**
*Explanation*: Jaw jerk is considered to be normal for bulbar palsy but increased for pseudobulbar palsy.

*Reference*: Puri BK, Hall A, Ho R (2014). *Revision Notes in Psychiatry*. London: CRC Press, p. 167.

**Question 9 Answer: e, For long-term management, the NICE guidelines do not recommend the commencement of valproate in view of its potential toxicity.**
*Explanation*: All of the aforementioned are true, with the exception of (e), as valproate is actually commonly used as part of long-term treatment. In addition, the guidelines also recommend that thyroid function tests are to be rechecked every 6-months.

*Reference*: Puri BK, Hall A, Ho R (2014). *Revision Notes in Psychiatry*. London: CRC Press, p. 397.

**Question 10 Answer: b, 25%**
*Explanation*: When both the parents carry one abnormal copy of the gene, there is a 25% chance of the child inheriting the mutation, and hence expressing the disease.

*Reference*: Puri BK, Hall A, Ho R (2014). *Revision Notes in Psychiatry*. London: CRC Press, p. 267.

**Question 11 Answer: e, Life skills training is part of the behavioural techniques used.**
*Explanation*: All of the aforementioned statements about behavioural techniques in CBT are correct, with the exception of (e), which is a technique used in dialectical behavioural therapy. Assignment is another of the behavioural techniques and tasks being used.

*Reference*: Puri BK, Hall A, Ho R (2014). *Revision Notes in Psychiatry*. London: CRC Press, p. 336.

**Question 12 Answer: e, It helps to develop cognitive restructuring skills**.
*Explanation*: DBT is usually indicated as a form of psychotherapy for borderline personality disorder. This disorder develops due to the interaction between an emotionally vulnerable person and an invalidating environment. DBT helps the person to build a life that is worth living. It does not help them to develop cognitive skills.

*Reference*: Puri BK, Hall A, Ho R (2014). *Revision Notes in Psychiatry*. London: CRC Press, p. 336.

**Question 13 Answer: c, Mutations of chromosomes 14 and 21**
*Explanation*: A small minority of cases of Alzheimer's disease are inherited as early-onset autosomal dominant disorder. The mutations concerned tend to be found on chromosomes 14 and 21.

*Reference*: Puri BK, Hall A, Ho R (2014). *Revision Notes in Psychiatry*. London: CRC Press, p. 267.

**Question 14 Answer: c, 6%**
*Explanation*: In around 6% of the individuals, the EEG will be normal. The following changes are usually observed in the EEG of patients with AD, which include diffuse slowing in early stages and reduced alpha and beta activities. There are also more paroxysmal bi-frontal waves.

*Reference*: Puri BK, Hall A, Ho R (2014). *Revision Notes in Psychiatry*. London: CRC Press, p. 686.

**Question 15 Answer: b, In Pick's disease, the EEG is less likely than in AD to be normal and would show more significant slowing of the a waves.**
*Explanation*: This is incorrect. In Pick's disease, it has been observed that the EEG is more likely to be normal in AD and there would be less slowing of the a waves.

*Reference*: Puri BK, Hall A, Ho R (2014). *Revision Notes in Psychiatry*. London: CRC Press, p. 686.

**Question 16 Answer: e, 2.0**
*Explanation*: At levels greater than 2.0 mM, the aforementioned are seen. There might also be syncope, oliguria, circulatory failure, coma and even death.

*Reference*: Puri BK, Hall A, Ho R (2014). *Revision Notes in Psychiatry*. London: CRC Press, p. 252.

**Question 17 Answer: a, Nucleus**
*Explanation*: Transcription is a step in gene expression in which the information from the DNA is transcribed onto a mRNA transcript. Euchromatin is transcriptionally active. This process occurs in the nucleus.

*Reference*: Puri BK, Hall A, Ho R (2014). *Revision Notes in Psychiatry*. London: CRC Press, p. 260.

**Question 18 Answer: e, 3%**
*Explanation*: The prevalence of people with learning disabilities who also have schizophrenia has been estimated to be around 3%. This is much higher than the average prevalence in the general population. It has been noted that the prevalence of schizophrenia is inversely related to the Intelligence Quotient (IQ). More importantly, a diagnosis of schizophrenia cannot be made if the IQ is considered to be less than 45.

*Reference*: Puri BK, Hall A, Ho R (2014). *Revision Notes in Psychiatry*. London: CRC Press, p. 670.

**Question 19 Answer: a, Focusing on the nature of the defences and the relationship to anxiety and impulse**
*Explanation*: Brief focal psychotherapy was proposed by Malan and it is a subtype of brief dynamic psychotherapy. It helps to clarify the nature of the defences and its relationship to anxiety and impulse.

*Reference*: Puri BK, Hall A, Ho R (2014). *Revision Notes in Psychiatry*. London: CRC Press, p. 331.

**Question 20 Answer: a, For individuals with persistent subthreshold depressive symptoms, individual self-help based on the principles of CBT and CCBT could be offered.**
*Explanation*: The aforementioned is true. For patient with moderate or severe depression, a combination of individual CBT or group-based CBT with antidepressants is recommended. For relapse prevention, CBT is recommended for clients who have received antidepressant treatment, and mentalization-based CBT is recommended for stable clients with three or more previous episodes of depression.

*Reference*: Puri BK, Hall A, Ho R (2014). *Revision Notes in Psychiatry*. London: CRC Press, p. 393.

**Question 21 Answer: d, Eysenck**
*Explanation*: Eysenck was the one who did factor analysis and proposed all of the aforementioned personality traits.

*Reference*: Puri BK, Hall A, Ho R (2014). *Revision Notes in Psychiatry*. London: CRC Press, p. 433.

**Question 22 Answer: a, Alpha subunits of the G proteins**
*Explanation*: The D2 dopaminergic receptors are coupled to G proteins, to produce their physiological effects. The main dopaminergic receptors and their main effectors are via the G protein alpha-subunits.

*Reference*: Puri BK, Hall A, Ho R (2014). *Revision Notes in Psychiatry*. London: CRC Press, p. 224.

**Question 23 Answer: b, In schizophrenia, there is a reduction of dopamine in the mesolimbic pathway.**
*Explanation*: (a) is true whereas (b) is incorrect. There is an increase in the pathway. The dopamine hypothesis proposes that there are increased levels of dopamine or dopamine receptors that cause schizophrenia.

*Reference*: Puri BK, Hall A, Ho R (2014). *Revision Notes in Psychiatry*. London: CRC Press, p. 223.

**Question 24 Answer: d, Changing to an atypical antipsychotic should be considered even when a conventional antipsychotic controls the pre-existing symptoms well.**
*Explanation*: There is no acute indication for a change if the conventional antipsychotics control symptoms well and the individual has not suffered from unacceptable side effects.

*Reference*: Puri BK, Hall A, Ho R (2014). *Revision Notes in Psychiatry*. London: CRC Press, p. 364.

**Question 25 Answer: d, Amyloid precursor protein on chromosome 21**
*Explanation*: This has been linked with the early-onset symptoms of dementia in Down's syndrome.

*Reference*: Puri BK, Hall A, Ho R (2014). *Revision Notes in Psychiatry*. London: CRC Press, p. 258.

**Question 26 Answer: a, Splitting**
*Explanation*: Splitting is often seen in patients with borderline personality disorder. They tend to divide good objects, affects and memories from bad ones.

*Reference*: Puri BK, Hall A, Ho R (2014). *Revision Notes in Psychiatry*. London: CRC Press, p. 137.

**Question 27 Answer: e, Martial separation**
*Explanation*: All of the aforementioned are factors that could potentially precipitate a manic episode, with the exception of martial separation, which most commonly would cause a depressive episode. In addition, highly expressed emotions and sleep deprivation are also other relevant precipitating factors.

*Reference*: Puri BK, Hall A, Ho R (2014). *Revision Notes in Psychiatry*. London: CRC Press, p. 383.

**Question 28 Answer: c, Presence of 200 CGG repeats**
*Explanation*: Fragile X is an X-linked dominant genetic disorder with low penetrance. The fragile site is located at band q27.3 on the X chromosome. The trinucleotide repeats of CGG are found on the long arm of the X chromosome. Normal number of repeats is 30, and the repeats for carriers range from 55 to 200. Full mutation with more than 200 repeats would lead to hypermethylation at the fragile X mental retardation gene (FMR) gene.

*Reference*: Puri BK, Hall A, Ho R (2014). *Revision Notes in Psychiatry*. London: CRC Press, p. 666.

**Question 29 Answer: c, Antipsychotic such as clozapine, olanzapine, amisulpride and ziprasidone would contribute to impaired glucose control.**
*Explanation*: Impaired glucose control is more common for antipsychotics such as clozapine and olanzapine. Antipsychotics such as amisulpride, asenapine and ziprasidone contribute minimally.

*Reference*: Puri BK, Hall A, Ho R (2014). *Revision Notes in Psychiatry*. London: CRC Press, p. 584.

**Question 30 Answer: a, There is the presence of additional precursor protein on chromosome 21.**
*Explanation*: Previous research has shown that almost all subjects with Down's syndrome who live beyond the age of 40 years do show evidence of Alzheimer's disease. This is due to the presence of additional precursor protein on chromosome 21.

*Reference*: Puri BK, Hall A, Ho R (2014). *Revision Notes in Psychiatry*. London: CRC Press, p. 258.

**Question 31 Answer: a, Verbal aggression**
*Explanation*: Verbal aggression is the most common form of violence displayed by outpatients with schizophrenia.

*Reference*: Puri BK, Hall A, Ho R (2014). *Revision Notes in Psychiatry*. London: CRC Press, p. 370.

### Question 32 Answer: b, Isolation

*Explanation*: In isolation, thoughts, affects and behaviours are isolated so that their links with other thoughts or memories are broken. In addition to isolation, patients also tend to make use of undoing. This refers to an attempt to negate or atone for forbidden thoughts, affects or memories.

*Reference*: Puri BK, Hall A, Ho R (2014). *Revision Notes in Psychiatry*. London: CRC Press, p. 136.

### Question 33 Answer: a, The association between schizophrenia and low social class has been attributed as one of the causative factors for schizophrenia.

*Explanation*: Current research has shown that this is now being perceived as a consequence rather than an aetiology of schizophrenia.

*Reference*: Puri BK, Hall A, Ho R (2014). *Revision Notes in Psychiatry*. London: CRC Press, p. 281.

### Question 34 Answer: a, Partial agonism at 5-HT1A receptors

*Explanation*: The aforementioned is true with regards to the mechanism of action for the above-mentioned drug.

*Reference*: Puri BK, Hall A, Ho R (2014). *Revision Notes in Psychiatry*. London: CRC Press, p. 246.

### Question 35 Answer: a, Slowing of rhythm with posterior preservation, with the presence of tri-phasic waves

*Explanation*: This is the characteristic EEG waveform finding in patients diagnosed with hepatic encephalopathy.

*Reference*: Puri BK, Hall A, Ho R (2014). *Revision Notes in Psychiatry*. London: CRC Press, p. 691.

### Question 36 Answer: a, Generalized increase in EEG activity, but a reduced rhythm

*Explanation*: Antidepressants would cause a generalized increase in EEG activity, but a reduced rhythm; in overdose, a widespread activity and spikes would be present.

*Reference*: Puri BK, Hall A, Ho R (2014). *Revision Notes in Psychiatry*. London: CRC Press, p. 691.

### Question 37 Answer: b, Histamine receptors

*Explanation*: The weight gain induced by tricyclic antidepressants is due to the blockage of the histamine receptors, as well as the serotonin receptors.

*Reference*: Puri BK, Hall A, Ho R (2014). *Revision Notes in Psychiatry*. London: CRC Press, p. 254.

**Question 38 Answer: b, Southern blotting**
*Explanation*: Southern blotting is a technique which allows for the transfer of DNA fragments from the gel, where electrophoresis and DNA denaturation have taken place to a filter. It would enable identification of the polymorphisms of the relevant genes.

*Reference*: Puri BK, Hall A, Ho R (2014). *Revision Notes in Psychiatry*. London: CRC Press, p. 263.

**Question 39 Answer: d, Bandura**
*Explanation*: Bandura helped to develop the therapeutic technique of self-control therapy, based on the concepts of self-regulation. It could be used as part of a treatment package for the cessation of smoking, as well as to counter overeating and in helping students to improve their ability to study.

*Reference*: Puri BK, Hall A, Ho R (2014). *Revision Notes in Psychiatry*. London: CRC Press, p. 30.

**Question 40 Answer: e, The presence of uncontrolled violent behaviour in a relationship**
*Explanation*: This is actually a contraindication to couple-based therapy. The other contraindication would include the presence of clear evidence that one partner is making use of the couple therapy to terminate an existing relationship.

*Reference*: Puri BK, Hall A, Ho R (2014). *Revision Notes in Psychiatry*. London: CRC Press, p. 345.

**Question 41 Answer: e, 5%**
*Explanation*: Based on recent studies, the prevalence of recent aggressive behaviours amongst outpatients with schizophrenia has been estimated to be around 5%.

*Reference*: Puri BK, Hall A, Ho R (2014). *Revision Notes in Psychiatry*. London: CRC Press, p. 370.

**Question 42 Answer: e, 30%**
*Explanation*: The estimated monozygotic concordance rate for Alzheimer's dementia has been estimated to be around 31%.

*Reference*: Puri BK, Hall A, Ho R (2014). *Revision Notes in Psychiatry*. London: CRC Press, p. 273.

**Question 43 Answer: a, Women with fragile X syndrome suffer from moderate learning disability.**
*Explanation*: Women with fragile X syndrome tend to suffer only from mild learning disability.

*Reference*: Puri BK, Hall A, Ho R (2014). *Revision Notes in Psychiatry*. London: CRC Press, p. 666.

**Question 44 Answer: e, Patau's syndrome**
*Explanation*: The aforementioned are conditions that are related to abnormalities involving either the X or Y chromosome.

*Reference*: Puri BK, Hall A, Ho R (2014). *Revision Notes in Psychiatry*. London: CRC Press, p. 258.

**Question 45 Answer: b, 1%**
*Explanation*: The prevalence of childhood-onset depressive disorder has been estimated to be 1%. It is rare in childhood. The frequency for boys and girls has been noted to be equal until the age of 14 years. Childhood depression is less common than childhood dysthymia.

*Reference*: Puri BK, Hall A, Ho R (2014). *Revision Notes in Psychiatry*. London: CRC Press, p. 648.

**Question 46 Answer: e, 45%**
*Explanation*: The estimated concordance rate for monozygotic twins is 45% whereas that for dizygotic twins is approximately 10%.

*Reference*: Puri BK, Hall A, Ho R (2014). *Revision Notes in Psychiatry*. London: CRC Press, p. 358.

**Question 47 Answer: e, 85%**
*Explanation*: Following the discontinuation of pharmacotherapy, it has been shown that there is a recurrence rate of 85% in patients with recurrent depression within 3 years of stopping the medications.

*Reference*: Puri BK, Hall A, Ho R (2014). *Revision Notes in Psychiatry*. London: CRC Press, p. 389.

**Question 48 Answer: d, Lithium is effective in preventing recurrent depressive episodes and is more effective than tricyclic antidepressants.**
*Explanation*: Lithium is effective in prevention of recurrent depressive episodes, but studies have shown that it is actually less effective as compared to tricyclic antidepressant.

*Reference*: Puri BK, Hall A, Ho R (2014). *Revision Notes in Psychiatry*. London: CRC Press, p. 389.

**Question 49 Answer: c, Alpha-1 adrenoceptors**
*Explanation*: The blockage of the aforementioned receptors would lead to drowsiness, postural hypotension, sexual dysfunction and also cognitive impairment.

*Reference*: Puri BK, Hall A, Ho R (2014). *Revision Notes in Psychiatry*. London: CRC Press, p. 252.

**Question 50 Answer: e, Translation initiation site**
*Explanation*: A transcription initiation site is present, but not a translation initiation site. In addition, other gene structures would include a promoter site (TATA) as well as a 3' noncoding region, which usually contain a poly-A addition site.

*Reference*: Puri BK, Hall A, Ho R (2014). *Revision Notes in Psychiatry*. London: CRC Press, p. 259.

**Question 51 Answer: a, Used for detection of single based pair mutations**
*Explanation*: These are considered to be small gene probes that could be used to help detect single based pair mutations.

*Reference*: Puri BK, Hall A, Ho R (2014). *Revision Notes in Psychiatry*. London: CRC Press, p. 262.

**Question 52 Answer: e, Dementia**
*Explanation*: Polymorphisms of the serotonin transporter gene have been associated with all of the aforementioned conditions, with the exception of (e) dementia.

*Reference*: Puri BK, Hall A, Ho R (2014). *Revision Notes in Psychiatry*. London: CRC Press, p. 263.

**Question 53 Answer: e, 17%**
*Explanation*: The approximate lifetime risks for the development of schizophrenia amongst siblings if one parent has schizophrenia would be estimated to be 17%.

*Reference*: Puri BK, Hall A, Ho R (2014). *Revision Notes in Psychiatry*. London: CRC Press, p. 358.

**Question 54 Answer: d, There are usually two peaks at which this condition occurs, usually either at the age of 5 years, or at the age of 11 years.**
*Explanation*: There are three peaks of age at which school refusal occurs. It could occur at the age of 5, 11 and between 14 to 16 years.

*Reference*: Puri BK, Hall A, Ho R (2014). *Revision Notes in Psychiatry*. London: CRC Press, p. 645.

**Question 55 Answer: d, Wolpe**
*Explanation*: Wolpe proposed that relaxation inhibits anxiety and hence the two are considered to be mutually exclusive.

*Reference*: Puri BK, Hall A, Ho R (2014). *Revision Notes in Psychiatry*. London: CRC Press, p. 28.

**Question 56 Answer: a, Identification of the alternative belief**
*Explanation*: The common behavioural techniques include rehearsal, assignment, training to be self-reliant, pleasure and mastery and activity scheduling, as well as diversion or distraction techniques.

*Reference*: Puri BK, Hall A, Ho R (2014). *Revision Notes in Psychiatry*. London: CRC Press, p. 335.

**Question 57 Answer: e, Heroin abuse**
*Explanation*: Polymorphisms of the tryptophan hydroxylase gene has been associated with all of the aforementioned conditions, with the exception of (e).

*Reference*: Puri BK, Hall A, Ho R (2014). *Revision Notes in Psychiatry*. London: CRC Press, p. 263.

**Question 58 Answer: a, Donepezil**
*Explanation*: Donepezil is contraindicated in people who are suffering from asthma. Common side effects of the medications include excessive cholinergic effects such as nausea, diarrhoea, dizziness, urinary incontinence and insomnia.

*Reference*: Puri BK, Hall A, Ho R (2014). *Revision Notes in Psychiatry*. London: CRC Press, p. 693.

**Question 59 Answer: b, Ventral tegmental area**
*Explanation*: The mesolimbic dopaminergic pathway has its origin from the ventral tegmental area to the limbic system.

*Reference*: Puri BK, Hall A, Ho R (2014). *Revision Notes in Psychiatry*. London: CRC Press, p. 222.

**Question 60 Answer: d, Local network of DA in the hypothalamus**
*Explanation*: The tuberoinfundibular pathway has its origin from the local network of the DA in the hypothalamus.

*Reference*: Puri BK, Hall A, Ho R (2014). *Revision Notes in Psychiatry*. London: CRC Press, p. 222.

**Question 61 Answer: d, Acute dystonia are equally common in the young as well as in the old.**
*Explanation*: Acute dystonia are usually more common in the young and are rare in the elderly.

*Reference*: Puri BK, Hall A, Ho R (2014). *Revision Notes in Psychiatry*. London: CRC Press, p. 682.

**Question 62 Answer: b, They are able to help study the association between a specific allele and a disease.**
*Explanation*: Only association studies are able to help study the aforementioned. Linkage studies differ from association studies as association studies look into both cases and controls.

*Reference*: Puri BK, Hall A, Ho R (2014). *Revision Notes in Psychiatry*. London: CRC Press, p. 265.

**Question 63 Answer: c, Phallic phase**
*Explanation*: At around the age of 3 years to the end of 5 years, boys and girls pass through the aforementioned phases.

*Reference*: Puri BK, Hall A, Ho R (2014). *Revision Notes in Psychiatry*. London: CRC Press, p. 133.

**Question 64 Answer: c, Chromosome 12**
*Explanation*: Tuberous sclerosis 1 is usually caused by a gene on chromosome 9. Tuberous sclerosis 2 is caused by a gene on chromosome 16. Tuberous sclerosis 3 is caused by a translation that involves chromosome 12.

*Reference*: Puri BK, Hall A, Ho R (2014). *Revision Notes in Psychiatry*. London: CRC Press, p. 267.

**Question 65 Answer: e, Cerebellum**
*Explanation*: Procedural knowledge refers to knowing how to perform a specific set of tasks. Its storage would require the functioning of the cerebellum, the amygdala and other specific sensory and motor systems.

*Reference*: Puri BK, Hall A, Ho R (2014). *Revision Notes in Psychiatry*. London: CRC Press, p. 103.

**Question 66 Answer: a, Brief dynamic therapy**
*Explanation*: These are part of brief dynamic therapy. In brief dynamic therapy, it is important to establish a therapeutic alliance, and then set goals, and allow free association by the client. There is a need to focus on internal conflicts and interpretation of transference. Confrontation, working through, and enactment could be used. Eventually, it is hoped that there will be resolution of conflicts and the client would be able to link the past, present and the transference.

*Reference*: Puri BK, Hall A, Ho R (2014). *Revision Notes in Psychiatry*. London: CRC Press, p. 331.

**Question 67 Answer: c, If an affected male mates with an unaffected female, all the sons would be affected.**
*Explanation*: In X-linked dominant inheritance, usually when an affected male mates with an unaffected female, all the sons would not be affected.

Reference: Puri BK, Hall A, Ho R (2014). *Revision Notes in Psychiatry*. London: CRC Press, p. 269.

### Question 68 Answer: c, Thiazide diuretic
*Explanation*: The team should reconsider the usage of thiazide diuretics in the treatment of the underlying medical condition. The reason is that it could reduce the amount of lithium excretion and hence cause acute lithium intoxication.

Reference: Puri BK, Hall A, Ho R (2014). *Revision Notes in Psychiatry*. London: CRC Press, p. 252.

### Question 69 Answer: c, Lack of acetylcholine
*Explanation*: It has been shown that the cholinergic deficits are more pronounced in dementia with Lewy body.

Reference: Puri BK, Hall A, Ho R (2014). *Revision Notes in Psychiatry*. London: CRC Press, p. 702.

### Question 70 Answer: a, There is decreased first-pass availability.
*Explanation*: As an individual ages, there is expected to be an increase in the first-pass availability.

Reference: Puri BK, Hall A, Ho R (2014). *Revision Notes in Psychiatry*. London: CRC Press, p. 681.

### Question 71 Answer: d, 15%
*Explanation*: The prevalence of epilepsy amongst those with mild mental retardation has been estimated to be around 12%–18%.

Reference: Puri BK, Hall A, Ho R (2014). *Revision Notes in Psychiatry*. London: CRC Press, p. 664.

### Question 72 Answer: e, Hunter syndrome
*Explanation*: All of the aforementioned are X-linked dominant disorders, with the exception of Hunter syndrome, which is an X-linked recessive disorder.

Reference: Puri BK, Hall A, Ho R (2014). *Revision Notes in Psychiatry*. London: CRC Press, p. 269.

### Question 73 Answer: e, Muscarinic M4 agonism
*Explanation*: Clozapine has been known to cause neutropenia and potentially fatal agranulocytosis. Other side effects would include hypersalivation and side effects common to those of chlorpromazine, including the extrapyramidal symptoms.

Reference: Puri BK, Hall A, Ho R (2014). *Revision Notes in Psychiatry*. London: CRC Press, p. 251.

**Question 74 Answer: c, Complex visual hallucinations**

*Explanation*: The most common noncognitive feature in patients with dementia with Lewy bodies might be complex visual hallucinations. Complex visual hallucinations have been known to affect at least 80% of the individuals.

*Reference*: Puri BK, Hall A, Ho R (2014). *Revision Notes in Psychiatry*. London: CRC Press, p. 702.

**Question 75 Answer: b, The age of onset of bipolar disorder is earlier than that of unipolar disorder.**

*Explanation*: (b) is correct. There is an equal female-to-male ratio. The age of onset of bipolar disorder is noted to be much earlier than that of unipolar disorder. Bipolar disorder is usually found in occupations that require creativity such as artists and writers. Bipolar disorder patients with only manic episodes have better outcomes than patients with severe depressive episodes. Patients with mixed episodes have the worse prognosis.

*Reference*: Puri BK, Hall A, Ho R (2014). *Revision Notes in Psychiatry*. London: CRC Press, p. 286.

**Question 76 Answer: e, 30%**

*Explanation*: The prevalence of post-stroke depression amongst patients suffering from cerebrovascular accident has been estimated to be around 30%. It has been noted that the incidence of depression is lower amongst patients suffering from an occlusion of the posterior cerebral arteries as compared to those with occlusions in the anterior and middle cerebral arteries.

*Reference*: Puri BK, Hall A, Ho R (2014). *Revision Notes in Psychiatry*. London: CRC Press, p. 491.

**Question 77 Answer: e, Increased alpha-adrenergic receptor density**

*Explanation*: All of the aforementioned are postulated to the effects of ECT. Option (d) has been believed to be due to receptor down-regulation.

*Reference*: Puri BK, Hall A, Ho R (2014). *Revision Notes in Psychiatry*. London: CRC Press, p. 248.

**Question 78 Answer: e, 11**

*Explanation*: 11/100,000 men have committed suicide in the United Kingdom and this accounts for around 2% of all male deaths. Suicide, according to a study by Power (1997), accounts for 1% of all deaths in the United Kingdom.

*Reference*: Puri BK, Hall A, Ho R (2014). *Revision Notes in Psychiatry*. London: CRC Press, p. 288.

**Question 79 Answer: c, 3**
*Explanation*: 3/100,000 women have committed suicide in the United Kingdom. This accounts for approximately 1% of all female deaths in the United Kingdom.

*Reference*: Puri BK, Hall A, Ho R (2014). *Revision Notes in Psychiatry*. London: CRC Press, p. 288.

**Question 80 Answer: e, It is a partial agonist at the MT2 melatonergic receptors.**
*Explanation*: All of the following are true with regards to the clinical profile of agomelatine, with the exception of (e).

*Reference*: Puri BK, Hall A, Ho R (2014). *Revision Notes in Psychiatry*. London: CRC Press, p. 246.

**Question 81 Answer: b, Lorazepam**
*Explanation*: For breast-feeding females who have anxiety and insomnia, the benzodiazepines that are recommended for usage are lorazepam and zolpidem. It would be advisable to ask the mother not to sleep with her baby in order to avoid suffocation accident inflicted on the newborn.

*Reference*: Puri BK, Hall A, Ho R (2014). *Revision Notes in Psychiatry*. London: CRC Press, p. 570.

**Question 82 Answer: c, 6%**
*Explanation*: The prevalence of dementia for individuals who are aged between 75 and 79 years would be around 6%.

*Reference*: Puri BK, Hall A, Ho R (2014). *Revision Notes in Psychiatry*. London: CRC Press, p. 678.

**Question 83 Answer: d, Nicotinic acetylcholine receptor**
*Explanation*: Nicotinic acetylcholine receptor is classified as an ion channel.

*Reference*: Puri BK, Hall A, Ho R (2014). *Revision Notes in Psychiatry*. London: CRC Press, p. 220.

**Question 84 Answer: a, Hematoma in the frontal lobe**
*Explanation*: The personality changes are characteristic of a frontal lobe lesion.

*Reference*: Puri BK, Hall A, Ho R (2014). *Revision Notes in Psychiatry*. London: CRC Press, p. 110.

**Question 85 Answer: e, 30%**
*Explanation*: The prevalence of mental abnormalities in those in prison in the United Kingdom has been estimated to be 33%.

*Reference*: Puri BK, Hall A, Ho R (2014). *Revision Notes in Psychiatry*. London: CRC Press, p. 719.

**Question 86 Answer: c, Turner's syndrome: presence of an extra pair of Y chromosome**
*Explanation*: For Turner's syndrome, the mode of inheritance is due to the nondisjunction of the paternal XY chromosome that results in sex chromosomal abnormalities; 50% of the patients have a karyotype consisting of 45X or 46XX mosaicism.

*Reference*: Puri BK, Hall A, Ho R (2014). *Revision Notes in Psychiatry*. London: CRC Press, p. 662.

**Question 87 Answer: e, 35%**
*Explanation*: The conversion rate to schizophrenia has been estimated to be around 35%. Around 70% would achieve full remission within a course of 3–4 months; 80% are able to achieve stable remission within a year.

*Reference*: Puri BK, Hall A, Ho R (2014). *Revision Notes in Psychiatry*. London: CRC Press, p. 369.

**Question 88 Answer: e, 50%**
*Explanation*: Approximately 50% of individuals have stopped their delinquent behaviour by the age of 19 years.

*Reference*: Puri BK, Hall A, Ho R (2014). *Revision Notes in Psychiatry*. London: CRC Press, p. 719.

**Question 89 Answer: e, Anti-hypertensives**
*Explanation*: All of the aforementioned medications could result in delirium, with the exception of (e). In addition, all of the aforementioned medications are also associated with changes in the EEG waveform seen in patients with delirium.

*Reference*: Puri BK, Hall A, Ho R (2014). *Revision Notes in Psychiatry*. London: CRC Press, p. 691.

**Question 90 Answer: e, 35%**
*Explanation*: The prevalence of epilepsy amongst patients with severe mental retardation has been estimated to be around 30%–37%.

*Reference*: Puri BK, Hall A, Ho R (2014). *Revision Notes in Psychiatry*. London: CRC Press, p. 664.

**Question 91 Answer: c, People living in deprived industrial areas are more unlikely to be treated for depression than people living in other areas.**
*Explanation*: This is incorrect. They are more likely to be treated for depression.

*Reference*: Puri BK, Hall A, Ho R (2014). *Revision Notes in Psychiatry*. London: CRC Press, p. 286.

### Question 92 Answer: a, Paroxetine

*Explanation*: For women who are breast-feeding, paroxetine and sertraline have been recommended as the antidepressant of choice.

*Reference*: Puri BK, Hall A, Ho R (2014). *Revision Notes in Psychiatry*. London: CRC Press, p. 566.

### Question 93 Answer: b, Agonism of 5-HT$_2$ receptors

*Explanation*: The receptor is involved in the regulation of slow wave sleep. It is also implicated in anxiety-related disorders.

*Further Reading*: Puri BK, Treasaden I (eds) (2010). *Psychiatry: An Evidence-Based Text*. London: Hodder Arnold, pp. 698, 708, 724, 762.

### Question 94 Answer: e

*Explanation*: Both naloxone and naltrexone are opioid antagonists. Naltrexone has a longer half-life (4 hours) compared with naloxone (less than one hour).

*Further Reading*: Puri BK, Treasaden I (eds) (2010). *Psychiatry: An Evidence-Based Text*. London: Hodder Arnold, p. 913.

### Question 95 Answer: b, Microdeletion of chromosome 15q 11-13 of paternal origin

*Explanation*: This person suffers from Prader-Willi syndrome.

Option (a) refers to Angelman syndrome.

*Further Reading*: Puri BK, Treasaden I (eds) (2010). *Psychiatry: An Evidence-Based Text*. London: Hodder Arnold, pp. 471, 1086, 1091.

### Question 96 Answer: c, The internal consistency of the MRCPsych Paper 2 used in spring 2008

*Explanation*: Here, the Royal College of Psychiatrists is trying to measure the split-half reliability of the MRCPsych Paper 2 used in spring 2008.

Option (a) refers to intra-rater reliability.

Option (b) refers to inter-rater reliability.

Option (d) refers to test-retest reliability.

### Question 97 Answer: e, Upper social class and high expectation of children

*Explanation*: The parental risk factors should be low social class but not high social class. Parental factors associated with an increased risk of suicide in young people include suicide or early death, admission to hospital for a mental illness, unemployment, low income, poor schooling, divorce as well as mental illness in siblings and mental illness and short duration of schooling in the young people themselves. The strongest risk factor is mental illness in the young people.

*Reference and Further Reading*: Agerbo E, Nordentoft M, Mortensen PB (2002). Familial, psychiatric, and socioeconomic risk factors for suicide in young people: Nested case-control study. *BMJ*, 325: 74; Puri BK, Treasaden I (eds) (2010). *Psychiatry: An Evidence-Based Text*. London: Hodder Arnold, pp. 855–856.

**Question 98 Answer: b, Occipital cortex**
*Explanation*: This man suffers from variant Creutzfeldt–Jakob disease (vCJD) where immunohistochemistry for prion protein often shows strong staining of plaques in the occipital cortex. In contrast, conventional CJD and kuru-type plaques are commonly found in the cerebellar cortex.

*Reference and Further Reading*: Sánchez-Juan P, Houben J, Hoff I, Jansen C, et al. (2007). The first case of variant Creutzfeldt–Jakob disease in the Netherlands. *Journal of Neurology*, 254: 958–960; Puri BK, Treasaden I (eds) (2010). *Psychiatry: An Evidence-Based Text*. London: Hodder Arnold, pp. 572–573.

**Question 99 Answer: b, 13%–23%**

*Reference*: Jacobson CM, Gould M (2007). The epidemiology and phenomenology of non-suicidal self-injurious behaviour among adolescents: A critical review of the literature. *Achieve of Suicide Research*, 11: 129–147.

**Question 100 Answer: b, Lithium**
*Explanation*: Only lithium and sulpiride are 95% excreted unchanged in urine. The percentages for the other options are as follows: mirtazapine (75%) olanzapine (57%), amisulpride (50%) and lamotrigine (<10%).

*Reference*: Taylor D, Paton C, Kapur S (2009). *The Maudsley Prescribing Guidelines*. London: Informa Healthcare.

**Question 101 Answer: b, 10%–14%**
*Explanation*: The risk for the general population is 5%.

*Reference and Further Reading*: Liddel MB (2001). Genetic risk of Alzheimer's disease: Advising relatives. *British Journal of Psychiatry*, 178: 7–11; Puri BK, Treasaden I (eds) (2010). *Psychiatry: An Evidence-Based Text*. London: Hodder Arnold, pp. 1103–1104.

**Question 102 Answer: d, Orbitofrontal cortex**
*Explanation*: The orbitofrontal cortex is associated with the control of behaviour, especially social behaviour and guided by emotion, empathy and theory of the mind.

*Reference*: Puri BK, Treasaden I (eds) (2010). *Psychiatry: An Evidence-Based Text*. London: Hodder Arnold, pp. 509–510.

**Question 103 Answer: a, Dorsolateral prefrontal cortex**
*Explanation*: The task described here is known as the 'n-back' task which is a continuous performance task which assesses working memory. Lesions in dorsolateral prefrontal cortex cause negative symptoms and working memory impairment in people with schizophrenia.

*Reference and Further Reading*: Tan HY, Choo WC, Fones CS, Chee MW (2005). fMRI study of maintenance and manipulation processes within working memory in first-episode schizophrenia. *American Journal of Psychiatry*, 162: 1849–1858; Puri BK,Treasaden I (eds) (2010). *Psychiatry: An Evidence-Based Text*. London: Hodder Arnold, pp. 332–333, 340.

**Question 104 Answer: d, Dorsal striatum**
*Explanation*: This motorcyclist has lost his procedural memory. Procedural memory is formed by the cerebellum, basal ganglia and motor cortex. The dorsal striatum is part of the basal ganglia and damage in this area would affect procedural memory. Procedural memory is not affected by damage to the amygdala, dentate gyrus, entorhinal cortex or hippocampus.

*Further Reading*: Puri BK,Treasaden I (eds) (2010). *Psychiatry: An Evidence-Based Text*. London: Hodder Arnold, pp. 335, 339–341, 352, 509, 803.

**Question 105 Answer: c, Lithium**
*Explanation*: Multiple cases of toxicity when combining lithium and verapamil, particularly neurotoxicity, have been reported.

*Reference*: Singh GP, Sidana A, Sharma RP (2004). Renewed interest in calcium channel blockers as antimania agents in the third millennium. *Hong Kong Journal of Psychiatry*, 14: 12–15; Freeman MP, Stoll AL (1998). Mood stabilizer combinations: A review of safety and efficacy. *American Journal of Psychiatry*, 155: 12–21.

**Question 106 Answer: e, Triphasic waves**
*Explanation*: The classical EEG changes of hepatic encephalopathy are high-amplitude, low-frequency waves of 1.5–3 Hz, which are known as 'triphasic waves' (occurring in 25% of cases).

*Reference*: Sadock BJ, Sadock VA, (eds) (2009). *Kaplan & Sadock's. Comprehensive Textbook of Psychiatry* (9th edition). Philadelphia, PA: Lippincott Williams & Wilkins.

**Question 107 Answer: d, Perinatal mortality rate**
*Explanation*: Perinatal mortality rate is the number of stillbirths and deaths (of less than 7 days) over the total number of live births and stillbirths in a one-year period.

*Reference*: Puri BK, Hall A, Ho R (2014). *Revision Notes in Psychiatry*. London: CRC Press, p. 280.

**Question 108 Answer: b, Contrecoup in orbitofrontal lobe**
*Explanation*: Orbitofrontal damage is usually associated with personality changes, impaired social judgement, impulsiveness, hyperactivity, disinhibition, lability of mood, excitability and childishness.

*Further Reading*: Puri BK, Treasaden I (eds) (2010). *Psychiatry: An Evidence-Based Text*. London: Hodder Arnold, pp. 557–559.

**Question 109 Answer: c, Sixty percent of total phenotypic variance of autism in a population results from genetic factors.**
*Explanation*: Autism is a disorder with high heritability. The monozygotic to dizygotic ratio has been estimated to be 36:0. The recurrence rate in siblings is roughly 3% for narrowly defined autism but is about 10%–20% for milder variants. The loci may involve chromosomes 2q and 7q. Family history of schizophrenia-like psychosis or affective disorder has been found to be associated.

*Further Reading*: Puri BK, Treasaden I (eds) (2010). *Psychiatry: An Evidence-Based Text*. London: Hodder Arnold, p. 468.

**Question 110 Answer: b, Glutamate antagonist**
*Explanation*: Acamprosate is a GABA agonist and glutamate antagonist.

*Further Reading*: Puri BK, Treasaden I (eds) (2010). *Psychiatry: An Evidence-Based Text*. London: Hodder Arnold, p. 913.

**Question 111 Answer: c, $\alpha_2$ adrenergic receptor agonist**
*Explanation*: This is an alpha-2 agonist, which acts centrally to reduce sympathetic tone. In addition, it helps to counteract the adrenergic hyperactivity during opioid withdrawal. It is indicated for detoxification within a short period of time as well as dependence in young people. The starting dose is 800 mcg daily, with an increment of 2.4 mg in divided daily doses over 3 days, and then a reduction in 4 days.

*Further Reading*: Puri BK, Treasaden I (eds) (2010). *Psychiatry: An Evidence-Based Text*. London: Hodder Arnold, p. 1040.

**Question 112 Answer: d, Cognitive framing**
*Explanation*: Cognitive framing is a concept used in psychology and social science. Cognitive frames are formed based on our life experiences. Drug A is associated with the word 'cure' and evokes a positive frame in which it offers hope of cure, although it benefits only around 40% of patients. Drug B is associated with the word 'failure' and evokes a negative frame. The choices which patients made in this survey were influenced by the positive and negative frames.

*Reference*: Puri BK, Hall A, Ho R (2014). *Revision Notes in Psychiatry*. London: CRC Press, p. 387.

**Question 113 Answer: e, Prevalence of schizophrenia**
*Explanation*: The cognitive representation of a disease is the belief that patients have in relation to their illness at a given time. Cognitive representation is determined by five factors: aetiology, symptoms, impact of the disease on patients' lives, measures for controlling the disease and progress of the disease.

*Reference*: Puri BK, Hall A, Ho R (2014). *Revision Notes in Psychiatry*. London: CRC Press, p. 363.

**Question 114 Answer: b, Neutropenia**
*Explanation*: Neutropenia is not dose related.

*Further Reading*: Puri BK,Treasaden I (eds) (2010). *Psychiatry: An Evidence-Based Text*. London: Hodder Arnold, pp. 425–427, 603.

# Extended Matching Items (EMIs)

## Theme: Major psychiatric disorders and findings in association studies

**Question 115 Answer: b, Depressive disorder**
*Explanation*: Findings for depressive disorder in association studies yield inconsistent results.

**Question 116 Answer: a, Schizophrenia**
*Explanation*: Association studies found an association between schizophrenia and the dopamine D3 receptor gene and 5 HT2A receptor genes. Schizophrenia is associated with the COMT gene as well.

**Question 117 Answer: c, Bipolar disorder**
*Explanation*: Association studies have found an association with the genes encoding for tyrosine hydroxylase, serotonin transporter and COMT. Anticipation (which refers to the phenomenon whereby a disease has an earlier age of onset and increased severity in succeeding generations) has been described in bipolar disorder.

**Question 118 Answer: d, Post-traumatic stress disorder**
*Explanation*: There has been an association between serotonin transporter promoter gene and post-traumatic stress disorder.

**Question 119 Answer: f, Hyperkinetic disorder**
*Explanation*: In hyperkinetic disorder, there is an association between the dopamine D4 gene and the disorder.

*Reference*: Puri BK, Hall A, Ho R (2014). *Revision Notes in Psychiatry*. London: CRC Press, p. 268.

## Theme: Transmission of genetic disorders

**Question 120 Answer: c, X-linked dominant inheritance**
*Explanation*: In X-linked dominant disorders, a dominant abnormal allele is carried on the X chromosome. If an affected male mates with an unaffected female, all the daughters and none of the sons are affected. If an unaffected male mates with an affected heterozygous female, half the daughters and half the sons, on average, are affected. Again, male-to-male transmission does not take place.

**Question 121 Answer: e, Disorders of carbohydrate metabolism and lysosomal storage**
*Explanation*: The incidence rate of type I disease is between 1 in 600 and 1 in 2400 in Jewish populations. There is a reduction in lysosomal cerebroside-beta-glucosidase, thus causing an abnormal accumulation of glucosylceramide.

**Question 122 Answer: b, Autosomal recessive inheritance**
*Explanation*: Autosomal recessive disorders result from the presence of two abnormal recessive alleles causing the individual to manifest the abnormal phenotypic trait. Features of autosomal transmission include the following: heterozygous individuals are generally carriers who do not manifest the abnormal phenotypic trait; the rarer the disorder, the more likely it is that the parents are related and the disorder tends to miss generations but the affected individuals in a family tend to be found among siblings: horizontal transmission takes place.

**Question 123 Answer: a, Autosomal dominant disorder**
*Explanation*: A minority of cases of Alzheimer's disease is inherited as early-onset autosomal dominant disorder. The mutations concerned tend to be found on chromosome 14 or chromosome 21. Autosomal dominant disorder results from the presence of an abnormal dominant allele, causing the individual to manifest the abnormal phenotypic trait.

## Theme: Advanced psychology

**Question 124 Answer: a, Couple therapy**
*Explanation*: Couple therapy involves the therapist seeing two clients who are in a relationship, but not necessarily in a marriage. The indications include interpersonal problems in a relationship, issues or difficulties related to a marriage or partnership, grief in a couple (for example the sudden loss of a child) as well as sexual problems.

**Question 125 Answer: b, Motivational interviewing**
*Explanation*: Motivating interviewing is helpful for patients with substance misuse as well as nonconcordance to psychotropic medications.

**Question 126 Answer: c, Eye movement and desensitization reprocessing**
*Explanation*: EDMR focuses on the aforementioned. The aim is to desensitize the individual to the affective responses. This is accompanied by bilateral stimulation

and rapid eye movement when the client is asked to follow the regular movement of the therapist's forefinger.

**Question 127 Answer: d, Grief counselling**
*Explanation*: Grief counselling allows the client to talk about the loss, to express feelings of sadness, guilt, or anger and to understand the course of the grieving process. This therapy also allows the client to accept the loss, working through the grief process and adjusting one's life without the deceased.

**Question 128 Answer: e, Brief insight-oriented therapy**
*Explanation*: Insight refers to the person's understanding of his or her psychological function and personality. Treatment framework involves the therapist assisting the client to gain new and better insight into possible explanations for his or her feelings, responses, behaviours and interpersonal relationship. It also expects the client to develop insight into his or her responses to the therapist and other significant relationship in the past.

*Reference*: Puri BK, Hall A, Ho R (2014). *Revision Notes in Psychiatry*. London: CRC Press, pp. 346–348.

**Question 129 Answer: a, <1%**
*Explanation*: Anxiety disorders are uncommon among people with Down's syndrome. The prevalence is around 0.3%.

**Question 130 Answer: d, 10%**

**Question 131 Answer: d, 10%**
*Explanation*: Dementia is the one of most common psychiatric comorbidities with a prevalence of 6%–10%.

**Question 132 Answer: c, 5%**

**Question 133 Answer: b, 2%**

**Question 134 Answer: c, 5%**
*Explanation*: Psychiatric comorbidity includes obsessive-compulsive disorder (2% of the patients, especially presenting with a need for excessive order or tidiness), depression, autism, bipolar disorder, psychosis and sleep apnoea. The average life expectancy of people with Down's syndrome is between 58 and 66 years. The most common cause of death is chest infection.

*Reference and Further Reading*: Collacott RA (1992). The effect of age and residential placement on adaptive behaviour of adults with Down's syndrome. *Br J Psychiatry*, 161: 675–679; Myers BA, Pueschel SM (1991). Psychiatric disorders in a population with Down syndrome. *J Nerv Ment Dis*, 179: 609–613; Puri BK, Treasaden I (eds) (2010). *Psychiatry: An Evidence-Based Text*. London: Hodder Arnold, pp. 467, 1082, 1087–1088.

## Theme: Genetics

**Question 135 Answer: b, 9%**

**Question 136 Answer: c, 13%**

**Question 137 Answer: a, 5%**
*Explanation*: The appropriate lifetime risks for the development of schizophrenia in the relatives of patients with schizophrenia are as documented:
Parents: 6%
All siblings: 10%
Siblings (when one parent has schizophrenia): 17%
Children: 13%
Children (when both parents have schizophrenia): 46%
Grandchildren: 4%
Uncles, aunts, nephews and nieces: 3%

*Further Reading*: Puri BK, Treasaden I (eds) (2010). *Psychiatry: An Evidence-Based Text*. London: Hodder Arnold, pp. 593–609.

## Theme: Psycho-pharmacology and neurology

**Question 138 Answer: e, QRS complex = 200 milliseconds, f, QTc = 500 milliseconds, r, Heart rate: 120 per minute**
*Explanation*: This patient suffers from tricyclic antidepressant overdose.

*Reference*: Olgun H, Yildirim ZK, Karacan M, Ceviz N (2009). Clinical, electrocardiographic, and laboratory findings in children with amitriptyline intoxication. *Pediatric Emergency Care*, 25: 170–173.

**Question 139 Answer: k, ST segment elevation with saddle, o, Diffuse T wave inversion, r, Heart rate: 120 per minute**
*Explanation*: This man suffers from clozapine-induced myocarditis.

*Reference*: Feldman AM, McNamara D (2000). Myocarditis. *New England. Journal of Medicine*, 343: 1388–1398.

**Question 140 Answer: k, ST segment elevation, p, Tall T waves, q, Q wave, r, Heart rate: 120 per minute**
*Explanation*: This man suffers from acute myocardial infarction caused by thyroxine treatment.

**Question 141 Answer: b, Biphasic P waves, i, R wave in $V_6$ = 30 mm, r, Heart rate: 120 per minute**
*Explanation*: This patient suffers from amphetamine-induced left ventricular hypertrophy.

*Reference*: Crean AM, Pohl JEF (2004). 'Ally McBeal heart?'– Drug induced cardiomyopathy in a young woman. *British Journal of Clinical Pharmacology*, 58: 558–559.

**Question 142 Answer: d, PR interval = 300 ms, s, Heart rate = 30 per minute**

*Explanation*: This patient suffers from acetylcholinesterase inhibitor-induced sinus bradycardia and first-degree AV block.

*Reference*: Rowland JP, Rigby J, Harper AC, Rowlan R (2007). Cardiovascular monitoring with acetylcholinesterase inhibitors: A clinical protocol. *Advances in Psychiatric Treatment*, 13: 178–184.

**Question 143 Answer: d, Huntington's disease**

*Explanation*: This is a progressive, inherited neurodegenerative disease that is characterized by autosomal dominant transmission and the emergence of abnormal involuntary movements and cognitive deterioration, with progression to dementia and death over 10–20 years.

**Question 144 Answer: i, Variant Creutzfeldt–Jakob disease**

*Explanation*: The hockey stick sign refers to bilateral symmetrical regions of hyperintensity in the pulvinar and the dorsomedial nuclei of the thalami.

*Reference*: Sánchez-Juan, P, Houben J, Hoff I, Jansen C, et al. (2007). The first case of variant Creutzfeldt–Jakob disease in the Netherlands. *Journal of Neurology*, 254: 958–960.

**Question 145 Answer: j, Wernicke's encephalopathy**

*Explanation*: This condition is caused by severe deficiency of thiamine (Vitamin B1), which is usually caused by alcohol abuse in the Western countries. Post-mortem examination of the brains of those dying of Wernicke's encephalopathy reveals petechial haemorrhages in the mammillary bodies, walls of the third ventricle (less common than in the mammillary bodies) and periaqueductal grey matter, as well as the floor of the fourth ventricle and inferior colliculi.

**Question 146 Answer: i, Variant Creutzfeldt–Jakob disease**
*Explanation*: Microscopy of brain material reveals vacuolar changes in grey matter, particularly in cerebral and cerebellar cortex, creating characteristic spongiform appearances.

## Theme: Neuroanatomy

**Question 147 Answer: a, Broca's area**
*Explanation*: Broca's area is the core of the frontal operculum on the dominant (usually left) side and consists mainly of areas 44 and 45. A lesion involving this area would lead to expressive (motor) aphasia.

**Question 148 Answer: d, Orbital cortex**
*Explanation*: Lesions of the orbital cortex on either side could lead to a form of acquired sociopathy.

**Question 149 Answer: Superior mesial region**
*Explanation*: A lesion of the left or right superior mesial region can lead to akinetic mutism.

**Question 150 Answer: e, Basal forebrain**
*Explanation*: Lesions of the basal forebrain (either side) could lead to amnesia and confabulation.

*Reference*: Puri BK, Hall A, Ho R (2014). *Revision Notes in Psychiatry*. London: CRC Press, p. 177.

## Theme: Neuropathology

**Question 151 Answer: a, Glioma**
*Explanation*: Glioma is the most common tumour. It is derived from the glial cells and their precursors and includes astrocytomas, oligodendrocytomas and ependymomas.

**Question 152 Answer: d, Pituitary adenomas**
*Explanation*: Null cell adenoma is one of the types of pituitary adenomas. The most common variant is the sparsely granulated PRL cell adenoma.

**Question 153 Answer: f, Haemangioblastomas**
*Explanation*: These are derived from blood vessels.

**Question 154 Answer: g, Medulloblastoma**
*Explanation*: These are cerebellar tumours which are embryonal in nature.

*Reference*: Puri BK, Hall A, Ho R (2014). *Revision Notes in Psychiatry*. London: CRC Press, p. 197.

## Theme: Advanced psychological process and treatment – group therapy

**Question 155 Answer: e, Continuous group therapy**
*Explanation*: In continuous group therapy, there is no definite end date of the group therapy. The therapy may last for years. Old members would leave, and new members could join.

**Question 156 Answer: a, Open-group therapy**
*Explanation*: In open-group therapy, replacement of group members is allowed for. This is in contrast to closed-group therapy, in which no replacement of group members is allowed for.

**Question 157 Answer: c, Heterogeneous group therapy**
*Explanation*: Heterogeneous group therapy allows for a mixture of clients with different backgrounds and conditions. This is in contrast to homogenous group

therapy, in which only members of the same gender, similar background and same conditions are included into the group.

*Reference*: Puri BK, Hall A, Ho R (2014). *Revision Notes in Psychiatry*. London: CRC Press, p. 344.

## Theme: Psychiatric epidemiology

**Question 158 Answer: f, Number needed to treat**
*Explanation*: The number needed to treat expresses the benefit for an active treatment over a placebo. It could be used in summarizing the results of a trial and in individualized medical decision making. It takes the value of nearest integer (or whole number) equal to or higher than.

**Question 159 Answer: g, Odds ratio**
*Explanation*: The odds ratio is the ratio of the odds that subjects in the disease group were exposed to the factor to the odds that subjects in the control group were exposed to the factor.

**Question 160 Answer: b, Attributable risk**
*Explanation*: This is the incidence of the disease in the group exposed to the risk factor of interest minus the incidence in the group not exposed to the risk factor.

**Question 161 Answer: d, Absolute risk reduction**
*Explanation*: The explanation is as per the preceding question.

**Question 162 Answer: a, Relative risk**
*Explanation*: Similarly in a cohort study, the relative risk is then the ratio of the probability of a positive outcome in the cohort group (exposed) to the probability of a positive outcome in the control group (not exposed).

*Reference*:  Puri BK, Hall A, Ho R (2014). *Revision Notes in Psychiatry*. London: CRC Press, p. 281.

## Theme: Genetics and morbid risks in first-degree relatives

**Question 163 Answer: b, 3.5%**
*Explanation*: The MR in first-degree relatives has been estimated to be approximately 3.5%.

**Question 164 Answer: f, 24.6%**
*Explanation*: In the second generation of Afro-Caribbean individuals, the morbid risk has been estimated to be around 24.6%.

**Question 165 Answer: c, 5%**
*Explanation*: The morbid risks of bipolar disorder amongst first-degree relatives has been estimated to be around 5%.

**Question 166 Answer: d, 10%**

*Explanation*: The morbid risks have been estimated to be around 10%.

**Question 167 Answer: g, 15%**

*Explanation*: The morbid risk in first-degree relatives has been estimated to be around 15%. This is estimated to be three times the risk for the general population.

**Question 168 Answer: a, 3%**

*Explanation*: The morbid risk has been estimated to be around 3%.

*Reference*: Puri BK, Hall A, Ho R (2014). *Revision Notes in Psychiatry*. London: CRC Press, p. 272.

## Theme: Neurochemistry of neuropeptides

**Question 169 Answer: a, CRF and c TRH**

*Explanation*: CRF concentration is increased in the CSF of depressed patients. After antidepressant treatment, there is a reduction in the CRF levels. It is also important to note that 25%–30% of euthyroid depressives have blunted TSH response to TRH challenge or abnormal T3/T4 levels.

**Question 170 Answer: a, CRF**

*Explanation*: CRH overactivity provokes the excessive release of NA in panic attacks as well as in alcohol withdrawal.

**Question 171 Answer: b, Somatostatin**

*Explanation*: This neuropeptide has an inhibitory effect on growth hormone release. It is reduced in Alzheimer's disease and the CSF concentration is also reduced in unipolar and bipolar depression.

**Question 172 Answer: d, CCK**

*Explanation*: CCK regulates the postprandial release of bile locally in the gut and controls the appetite in the CNS. It is involved in appetite and feeding as well as in the modulation of emotional behaviour.

**Question 173 Answer: e, VIP**

*Explanation*: The aforementioned is true with regards to VIP. It is found in the cerebral cortex, hypothalamus, amygdala, hippocampus, autonomic ganglia, and intestinal and respiratory tracts.

*Reference*: Puri BK, Hall A, Ho R (2014). *Revision Notes in Psychiatry*. London: CRC Press, p. 234.

## Theme: Neuropathology

**Question 174 Answer: b, Autism**

*Explanation*: Both neuropathological and structural neuroimaging studies have indicated that hypoplasia of the cerebellar vermis as well as hypoplasia of the cerebellar hemispheres occurs in individuals diagnosed with autism.

**Question 175 Answer: c, Parkinson's disease**
*Explanation*: The histological changes in idiopathic Parkinson's disease include neuronal loss, reactive astrocytosis and the presence of Lewy bodies in the substantia nigra.

**Question 176 Answer: d, Huntington's disease**
*Explanation*: In this condition, the typical changes are a small brain with reduced mass, along with marked atrophy of the corpus striatum and particularly that of the caudate nucleus. There is the associated dilatation of the lateral and the third ventricle.

*Reference*: Puri BK, Hall A, Ho R (2014). *Revision Notes in Psychiatry*. London: CRC Press, p. 200.

## Theme: Neurochemistry of serotonin

**Question 177 Answer: a, 5-HT1A**
*Explanation*: Buspirone exerts anxiolytic and antidepressant effects through the partial agonism of the 5-HT1A receptor. Aripiprazole is a 5-HT1A agonist.

**Question 178 Answer: b, 5-HT1B**
*Explanation*: It is an autoreceptor which is coupled with a G protein that inhibits the intracellular messenger. It reduces the 5-HT release and is implicated in Type II alcoholism.

**Question 179 Answer: g, 5-HT4**
*Explanation*: It is found in the brain stem, the substantia nigra, hippocampus as well as the frontal cortex. It is also present in the heart. The receptor does mediate cortisol secretion and contraction of the colon and the bladder.

**Question 180 Answer: h, 5-HT6**
*Explanation*: 5-HT6 is present in high levels in the olfactory tubercle, corpus striatum, the nucleus accumbens and hippocampus as well as in the cerebellum and the hippocampus. The receptor helps to regulate the release of neurotrophic factors. Antagonism may enhance the cognition.

**Question 181 Answer: i, 5-HT7**
*Explanation*: 5-HT7 is predominant in the thalamus and it is involved in the circadian rhythm.

*Reference*: Puri BK, Hall A, Ho R (2014). *Revision Notes in Psychiatry*. London: CRC Press, p. 230–231.

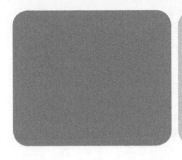

# MRCPSYCH PAPER A2 MOCK EXAMINATION 5: QUESTIONS

## GET THROUGH MRCPSYCH PAPER A2: MOCK EXAMINATION

Total number of questions: 175 (118 MCQs, 57 EMIs)
Total time provided: 180 minutes

**Question 1**
Which of the following statements about the structural brain abnormalities in schizophrenia is incorrect?
  a. There is a significant reduction in brain volume of the cerebral hemispheres, cerebral cortex and central grey matter.
  b. Ventricular enlargement has been found in post-mortem studies.
  c. Hippocampal formation was noted to be significantly smaller in the right and the left hemispheres.
  d. The reduction in hippocampal volume in male schizophrenics was smaller than that in female schizophrenics.
  e. Changes have been observed in the entorhinal cortex, which are indicative of disturbed development.

**Question 2**
Which of the following statement is incorrect with regards to the signalling that occurs at the synapse?
  a. Chemical synapse is the commoner type, in which a chemical neurotransmitter is stored in the presynaptic vesicles.
  b. Electrical synapse works much faster that the chemical synapse, due to the direct membrane to membrane connection via the gap junctions.
  c. Excitatory postsynaptic potentials could occur in the postsynaptic membrane, following the release of an excitatory neurotransmitter.
  d. Inhibitory postsynaptic potentials could occur following the release of an inhibitory neurotransmitter from the presynaptic neuron at the central inhibitory synapses.
  e. One EPSP is usually sufficient to initiate an action potential.

**Question 3**
Which of the following is not one of the structural changes seen on neuroimaging for patients with depression?
a. Ventricular enlargement
b. Sulcal widening
c. Hippocampus atrophy
d. Reduction in the size of the frontal lobe, cerebellum and basal ganglia
e. Asymmetry in temporal lobe

**Question 4**
Varenicline could be used for tobacco withdrawal syndrome, which develops usually if a person stops smoking after 3–10 weeks of tobacco consumption. The mechanism of action of varenicline is that
a. Alpha-4, beta-2 nicotinic partial agonist
b. Alpha-4, beta-2 nicotinic agonist
c. Alpha-4, beta-2 antagonist
d. Alpha-4 agonist
e. Alpha-4 partial agonist

**Question 5**
Bupropion is one of the other alternative medications that has been indicated for the treatment of tobacco withdrawal syndrome. Which one of the following statements about it is incorrect?
a. It is actually an antidepressant with noradrenergic activity that reduces the effect of nicotine withdrawal.
b. The starting dose is usually 150 mg per day.
c. The most common side effect is insomnia.
d. The major side effect and risk is the development of epilepsy.
e. Contraindications to treatment would include a past history of epilepsy, eating disorders, CNS tumour and bipolar disorder.

**Question 6**
Robertsonian translocations that occur in Down's syndrome usually involve chromosome 21 and which one of the following chromosomes?
a. Chromosome 1
b. Chromosome 14
c. Chromosome 15
d. Chromosome 18
e. Sex chromosome

**Question 7**
A 30-year-old female has a child diagnosed with Down's syndrome. She is concerned about having another child with Down's syndrome. Which one of the following maternal serum markers at 16 weeks of gestation is indicative of an increased likelihood of Down's syndrome?
a. Increased HCG, lowered alpha-fetoprotein, lowered unconjugated estriol
b. Increased HCG, increased alpha-fetoprotein, lowered unconjugated estriol

c. Increased HCG, alpha-fetoprotein, estriol
d. Decreased HCG, alpha-fetoprotein, estriol
e. Normal HCG, increased alpha-fetoprotein, estriol

## Question 8
In which of the following genetic conditions is the concept of anticipation best seen in?
a. Huntington's
b. Wilson's
c. Rett's syndrome
d. Niemann–Pick disease
e. Velocardiofacial syndrome

## Question 9
Based on neuroanatomy, which one of the following marks the division between the frontal and the parietal lobe?
a. Ventricular system
b. Medial longitudinal fissure
c. Lateral sulcus
d. Central sulcus
e. None of the above

## Question 10
In this particular form of amnesia, the clinical presentation is usually atypical and cannot be simply explained by ordinary forgetfulness. It is also commonly associated with 'la belle indifference' and has a highly unpredictable course. Which one of the following terminology best describes this particular form of amnesia?
a. Anterograde amnesia
b. Retrograde amnesia
c. Post-traumatic amnesia
d. Psychogenic amnesia
e. False memory

## Question 11
Which of the following medications should not be used in the treatment of an acute manic episode?
a. Risperidone
b. Quetiapine
c. Lithium carbonate
d. Lorazepam
e. Tricyclics

## Question 12
Based on the theories of genetic inheritance, male-to-male transmission is not possible for which of the following?
a. Autosomal dominant
b. Autosomal recessive
c. X-linked recessive

d. X-linked dominant
    e. Mitochondrial inheritance

## Question 13

Working through, enactment, containment of anxiety and resolution of conflicts are part of which modality of psychotherapy?
    a. Brief dynamic psychotherapy
    b. Cognitive behavioural therapy
    c. Cognitive analytic therapy
    d. Supportive therapy
    e. Interpersonal therapy

## Question 14

Which of the following statements about what Carl Jung has proposed as compared to Freud is incorrect?
    a. Jung discounted libido being confined to being sexual, but considered libido as being the unitary force out of every manifestation of psychic energy.
    b. Jung proposed the ideology of the collective unconscious.
    c. Jung's theory consists of causality and teleology only.
    d. Jung's theory views the contents of dreams within a framework in which archetypes may be projected onto others.
    e. Five important type of archetypes are identified in his theory.

## Question 15

Which of the following statements about mitochondrial inheritance is true?
    a. Mitochondrial DNA is essentially maternally inherited.
    b. There is the occurrence of anticipation amongst the generations.
    c. Mitochondrial inheritance leads to the effect of genomic imprinting.
    d. Mitochondrial inheritance leads to the effect of mosaicism.
    e. Mitochondrial inheritance leads to the effect of uniparental disomy.

## Question 16

The posterior part of the superior temporal gyrus forms which one of the following structures?
    a. Wernicke's area
    b. Broca's area
    c. Visual association area
    d. Somatosensory area
    e. Motor area

## Question 17

The neuroimaging scan showed that James has suffered an injury involving his dorsolateral prefrontal cortex. Which of the following is not one of the residual symptoms that he might have?
    a. Alexia without agraphia
    b. Utilization behaviour
    c. Motor Jacksonian fits

d. Aphasia

e. Anosmia

## Question 18

Which of the following correctly describes the mechanism of action of lofexidine, which is a substitute non-opiate usually given for opiate treatment?

a. Alpha-2 agonist

b. Opioid antagonist

c. GABA agonist and glutamate antagonist

d. Inhibition of ALDH2

e. Alpha-1 agonist

## Question 19

Concordance between monozygotic twins in an autosomal dominant disorder has been estimated to be

a. 10%

b. 25%

c. 50%

d. 75%

e. 100%

## Question 20

Cognitive analytic therapy is a combination of cognitive and analytic therapy. Which of the following terminology correctly describes the extreme pessimism about the future, even before a plan is started?

a. Traps

b. Dilemma

c. Snag

d. Mentalization

e. Automatic negative thoughts

## Question 21

Reframing and circular questioning are commonly used in which forms of the following therapies?

a. Systemic family therapy

b. Strategic family therapy

c. Eclectic family therapy

d. Psychodynamic therapy

e. None of the above

## Question 22

Research has found multiple genes to be associated with the onset of schizophrenia. In particular, the neuregulin gene has been implicated. On which of the following chromosome could the gene be located?

a. Chromosome 6

b. Chromosome 8

c. Chromosome 14

d. Chromosome 21
e. Chromosome 22

## Question 23
Based on classification by size, which of the following is the largest neuron?
a. Golgi type I
b. Golgi type II
c. Golgi type III
d. Amacrine type I
e. Amacrine type II

## Question 24
Which of the following statements about action potential is incorrect?
a. During an action potential, the membrane potential rapidly becomes positive, before returning to become negative.
b. An action potential is propagated by the depolarization spreading laterally to adjacent parts of the neuron.
c. The passage of an action potential along a neuron is an all or none phenomenon.
d. The greater the diameter of the un-myelinated fibre, the slower the rate of conduction.
e. For conduction in myelinated fibres, the action potential appears to jump from one node of Ranvier to the next.

## Question 25
A core trainee has been asked to assess James, who has suffered from an infarction involving the anterior cerebral artery. Which of the following psychiatric manifestations would be the most commonly seen for patients like James?
a. Auditory hallucinations
b. Visual hallucinations
c. Paranoid delusions
d. Formal thought disorder
e. Personality changes

## Question 26
Which of the following correctly describes the mechanism of action of ketamine, a commonly abused substance in the United Kingdom?
a. Competitive inhibition of the NMDA receptor complex
b. Inhibitory action on the GABA-A receptor
c. Blockage of the NMDA glutamate receptors
d. 5-HT antagonism
e. Dopamine antagonism

**Question 27**

The catechol-O-methyltransferase (COMT) gene has been implicated in the causation of schizophrenia as well as bipolar disorder. On which one of the following chromosomes could the gene be located?

a. Chromosome 6
b. Chromosome 8
c. Chromosome 14
d. Chromosome 21
e. Chromosome 22

**Question 28**

A child has chronic clinginess and ambivalence towards the mother. Which form of attachment type is this?

a. Secure attachment
b. Insecure attachment
c. Avoidant attachment
d. Separation anxiety
e. Dependent attachment

**Question 29**

Which of the following is not one of the objectives of cognitive behavioural therapy (CBT) when it is being used to treat individuals with depression?

a. Alleviation of symptoms by allowing the client to identify and challenge negative cognitions
b. Developing alternative and flexible schema
c. Helping them to rehearse new cognitive responses towards difficult situations
d. Helping them to rehearse new behaviour responses towards difficult situations
e. Helping them to improve self-understanding by developing capacity for self-reflection

**Question 30**

Which of the following statements about XYY syndrome is incorrect?

a. It tends to affect around 1 in 1000 male neonates.
b. An estimated 3% of patients in maximum security hospitals tend to have the XYY karyotype.
c. Individuals, especially females, with this genotype tend to have an increased rate of petty crime.
d. The mode of inheritance of this disorder is due to the primary nondisjunction of the Y chromosome.
e. Almost 10% of them have mosaic, which means that they have 46XY and 47 XYY chromosomes.

### Question 31
Connecting pathways of the limbic systems include all of the following, with the exception of
a. Anterior commissure
b. Cingulum
c. Dorsal longitudinal fissure
d. Lateral longitudinal fissure
e. Posterior commissure

### Question 32
Which of the following about the ultrastructural pathology of the deposits found in Alzheimer's dementia is correct?
a. Predominantly amyloid
b. Predominantly straight neurofilaments
c. Predominantly paired helical filaments
d. Predominantly unpaired helical filaments
e. Predominantly microtubule assembly protein

### Question 33
Which of the following statements about the CATIE (Clinical Antipsychotic Trials of Intervention Effectiveness) is incorrect?
a. The comparison drugs include olanzapine, quetiapine, risperidone, ziprasidone and perphenazine.
b. The sample size involved almost 150 subjects.
c. The trial demonstrated that the efficacy of first-generation antipsychotics was inferior to that of second-generation antipsychotics.
d. Olanzapine was considered to be the most effective in terms of the rates of discontinuation.
e. Olanzapine was associated with greater weight gain and an increase in the measure of glucose and lipid metabolism.

### Question 34
Which of the following terminologies correctly describes the process by which proteins are being generated from the original DNA template?
a. Mitosis
b. Meiosis I
c. Meiosis II
d. Transcription
e. Translation

### Question 35
Which of the following statements about psychological treatments for OCD is incorrect?
a. For initial treatment of OCD, exposure and response prevention (ERP) of up to 10 therapist hours per client is indicated.
b. For initial treatment of OCD, brief individual CBT using self-help materials and by telephone and group CBT should be offered.

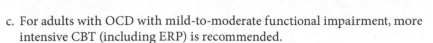

c. For adults with OCD with mild-to-moderate functional impairment, more intensive CBT (including ERP) is recommended.

d. For children and young people with OCD with mild functional impairments, CBT and ERP are first-line treatments.

e. For children and young people with OCD with moderate-to-severe functional impairment, CBT and ERP are not the first line of treatment.

## Question 36
Which of the following psychological therapies will be the most effective for an individual with excessive fears of contamination and recurrent compulsions of hand washing?
a. Brief psychodynamic psychotherapy
b. Supportive psychotherapy
c. Cognitive analytical therapy
d. Exposure and response prevention
e. Dialectical behaviour therapy

## Question 37
Patients with the karyotype XXY would have all of the following clinical features, with the exception of
a. Mild learning disability
b. Better verbal skills as compared to performance skills
c. Aggression and antisocial traits in adulthood
d. Normal sexual orientation
e. In-fertile

## Question 38
Which of the following antidepressants has the lowest approximate prevalence of sexual dysfunction?
a. Tricyclics
b. Monoamine oxidase (MAO)Is
c. SSRIs
d. Venlafaxine
e. Mirtazapine

## Question 39
The main types of neuroglia which are present in the CNS include all of the following, except
a. Astrocytes
b. Oligodendrocytes
c. Microglia
d. Ependyma
e. Satellite cells

## Question 40
Which of the following is not affected by age?
a. Speed of processing
b. Familiarity and novelty

c. Problem-solving
d. Creativity
e. Psychomotor speed

## Question 41

Which of the following statements about mania in patients who have suffered from cerebrovascular accident (CVA) is incorrect?
a. The incidence and prevalence of mania have been estimated to be around 0.5%–.1%.
b. CVA in the left hemisphere has a stronger association with mania.
c. Post-CVA mania is usually associated with cortical and subcortical lesions.
d. CVA in the thalamus is associated with mania.
e. Post-CVA mania usually occurs 3–9 months after stroke, and the first episode could either be mania or depression.

## Question 42

It has been known that variable expressivity could cause clinical features of autosomal dominant disorder to vary between affected individuals. Which terminology refers to whether a particular disorder would be manifested?
a. Transmission
b. Expressivity
c. Heritability
d. Inheritance
e. Penetrance

## Question 43

Which of the following modality of psychological therapy has been demonstrated to be of some benefit for patients with post-myocardial infarction depression?
a. Cognitive behavioural therapy
b. Cognitive analytical therapy
c. Supportive therapy
d. Psychodynamic therapy
e. Group therapy

## Question 44

Which of the following statements about structural family therapy, as previously proposed, is incorrect?
a. Families are viewed as systems that operate through subsystems.
b. Each subsystem would require adequate boundaries.
c. Family problems tend to arise when the boundaries are too tight, thus resulting in enmeshment.
d. Structural family therapy identifies the set of unspoken rules governing the hierarchy, sharing of responsibilities and boundaries.
e. Therapist might present the identified rules to the family in a paradoxical way to bring about changes.

## Question 45
Which of the following is not considered to be an external indicator for family-based therapy?
a. Addition of members to the family
b. Knowledge that a family member has been recently diagnosed with a particular terminal illness
c. Change in financial status within the family
d. Change in marital status within the family
e. Behaviour control problems

## Question 46
A 12-year-old obese boy has a learning disability and was referred to the learning disability service. His parents commented that he seemed to have excessive hunger drive and he will resort to excessive skin picking at times. Which of the following conditions is he most likely to have?
a. Prader–Willi syndrome
b. Angelman syndrome
c. William syndrome
d. DiGeorge syndrome
e. Smith–Magenis syndrome

## Question 47
Which of the following drugs is not considered to be established treatments for bipolar depression?
a. Lithium
b. Lithium and antidepressant
c. Lamotrigine
d. Quetiapine
e. Valproate

## Question 48
What is the known mechanism of action of memantine?
a. Inhibition of AChE
b. Inhibition of AChE and BChE
c. Modulation of nicotine receptor via upregulation
d. Modulation of nicotine receptor via down-regulation
e. Uncompetitive antagonist at the NMDA receptor

## Question 49
All of the following are known functions of astrocytes, with the exception of
a. Provision of structural support of neurons
b. Phagocytosis
c. Formation of the CNS neuroglial scar tissue
d. Contributing to the blood–brain barrier
e. CNS myelin sheath formation

## Question 50
The neurological condition of alexia without agraphia is usually caused by a lesion involving which areas of the cortex?
a. Left occipital lobe
b. Right occipital lobe
c. Right parietal lobe
d. Left parietal lobe
e. Temporal lobe

## Question 51
A lesion involving the left inferior frontal lobe as well as the insula would lead to which of the following type of apraxia?
a. Ideational apraxia
b. Ideo-motor apraxia
c. Orobuccal apraxia
d. Construction apraxia
e. Global apraxia

## Question 52
Which of the following statements about the CUTLASS (Cost Utility of the Latest Antipsychotic Drugs in Schizophrenia Study) is incorrect?
a. The study compared first-generation antipsychotics with second-generation antipsychotics.
b. The study included clozapine in the intervention.
c. The participants were randomly prescribed either first-generation antipsychotics or second-generation antipsychotics.
d. Patients in the first-generation antipsychotic arm showed a trend towards greater improvement in quality-of-life scale and symptom scales.
e. Overall, all the patients reported no clear preference for either first- or second-generation antipsychotics.

## Question 53
Which of the following antipsychotics has the greatest propensity to raise prolactin?
a. Risperidone
b. Olanzapine
c. Haloperidol
d. Quetiapine
e. Aripiprazole

## Question 54
Based on current research, which one of the following proteins is the most significant risk factor for late-onset Alzheimer's dementia?
a. PS1 gene on chromosome 14
b. PS2 gene on chromosome 1
c. Apolipoprotein E4

d. Apolipoprotein E2
e. Apolipoprotein E3

## Question 55
Interpretation and confrontation are techniques commonly used in which one of the following psychological therapies?
a. Brief dynamic psychotherapy
b. Cognitive behavioural therapy
c. Supportive therapy
d. Interpersonal therapy
e. Dialectical behaviour therapy

## Question 56
Approximately what percentage of patients with anorexia nervosa will continue to have no improvement in their weight, menstrual pattern and eating behaviour and might even die from the condition?
a. 5%
b. 10%
c. 15%
d. 20%
e. 30%

## Question 57
The presence of which of the following factors will help to reduce the risk of Alzheimer's dementia?
a. High level of education
b. Previous known psychiatric history with previous treatment
c. Known vascular risk factors, but under treatment
d. Moderate level of physical activity (less than three times a week)
e. Smoking

## Question 58
A child has a relatively short stature, but with relatively mild learning disability. In addition, there are some subtle defects in visuospatial perception. Which of the following genetic deficits could this be due to?
a. 45XO
b. 45XX
c. 46XXY
d. 46XY
e. 47XXY

## Question 59
A 6-year-old boy has the following clinical features: ventricular septal defect, hypocalcaemia and short stature. This is likely to be due to a microdeletion involving which one of the following chromosomes?
a. 7q
b. 14q

c. 17q
d. 21q
e. 22q

## Question 60
A 25-year-old male has been on lithium monotherapy has the following symptoms: convulsions, syncope and oliguria. Which one of the following treatments should be considered immediately?
a. Intravenous fluid replacement
b. Haemodialysis
c. Peritoneal dialysis
d. Chelation using charcoal
e. Immediate diuresis

## Question 61
Based on the neuroanatomical findings, the cerebellum is derived from which one of the following primitive structures?
a. Telencephalon
b. Diencephalon
c. Prosencephalon
d. Rhombencephalon
e. Myelencephalon

## Question 62
Nondominant temporal lobe damage would lead to significant impairments in terms of performance on this particular test
a. Rey–Osterrieth Test
b. Paired associate learning test
c. Synonym learning test
d. Object learning test
e. Rey Auditory Verbal Learning Test

## Question 63
Which of the following statements about the neurochemical 'acetylcholine' is incorrect?
a. It is synthesized from both acetyl-CoA and choline.
b. It is made usually in the cytoplasm of the cholinergic nerve terminals.
c. Choline is usually obtained from dietary sources.
d. The final step in the synthesis is usually catalysed by the enzyme choline acetyltransferase.
e. In Alzheimer's dementia, the activity of the enzyme is increased and this leads to a reduction in the synthesis of acetylcholine.

## Question 64
Pick's disease has an average age of onset of 45–65 years, with a female-to-male ratio of 2:1. Fifty per cent of patients who have this disorder are due to inheritance of which chromosome?
a. Chromosome 1
b. Chromosome 14
c. Chromosome 17
d. Chromosome 21
e. Chromosome 22

## Question 65
Having a history of deliberate self-harm is a long-term predictor of suicide. Approximately what percentage of patients eventually kill themselves in the year following their deliberate self-harm?
a. 0.5%
b. 1%
c. 1.5%
d. 2%
e. 3%

## Question 66
Based on the findings from the National Confidential Inquiry into Suicide, what is the estimated number of general population suicides that occur per year in England and Wales?
a. 1000
b. 2500
c. 3000
d. 4500
e. 6000

## Question 67
With regards to the genetic condition known as fragile X, individuals with full mutations usually have approximately how many repeats at the fragile X mental retardation gene?
a. 30
b. 50
c. 100
d. 150
e. 200

## Question 68
Paliperidone acts on which one of the following dopamine receptors?
a. Dopamine D1 receptor
b. Dopamine D2 receptor

c. Dopamine D2 receptor
    d. Dopamine D4 receptor
    e. All of the above

## Question 69
Which of the following statements correctly describe the mechanism of action of the common dementia medication known as rivastigmine?
    a. It is a partial inhibitor of AChE.
    b. It is a complete inhibitor of AChE.
    c. It is an inhibitor of both AChE and BChE.
    d. It is a partial inhibitor of BChE.
    e. It is a complete inhibitor of BChE.

## Question 70
Which of the following is not a type of apraxia?
    a. Ideational apraxia
    b. Ideomotor apraxia
    c. Orobuccal apraxia
    d. Construction apraxia
    e. Global apraxia

## Question 71
In this particular condition, an individual is unable to recognize the overall meaning of a picture, whereas the individual details are still being understood. Which terminology best describes the aforementioned?
    a. Prosopagnosia
    b. Achromatopsia
    c. Simultanagnosia
    d. Anosognosia
    e. Asterognosia

## Question 72
Hypertensive crisis might result when food rich in tyramine is eaten when a patient has been started on MAO-I. Such a reaction will not happen when which one of the following is consumed?
    a. Cream cheese
    b. Yeast extracts
    c. Alcohol
    d. Caviar
    e. Beer

## Question 73
Which of the following antidepressants is indicated for the treatment of patients with post-myocardial infarction depression?
    a. Fluoxetine
    b. Sertraline
    c. Fluvoxamine

d. Paroxetine
e. Citalopram

## Question 74
Damage to which area of the brain will result in conduction dysphasia?
a. Wernicke's area
b. Broca's area
c. Lesion of the arcuate fasciculus
d. Middle cerebral artery infarction
e. Anterior cerebral artery infarction

## Question 75
It is not uncommon that patients with Down's syndrome do present with early-onset cognitive impairment and even dementia. This is mediated by the action of which one of the following chromosomes?
a. Chromosome 1
b. Chromosome 14
c. Chromosome 17
d. Chromosome 21
e. Chromosome 22

## Question 76
Which of the following is a confounder that needs to be adjusted for when calculating either the standardized mortality rate or the standardized mortality ratio?
a. Age
b. Total number of live births
c. Total number of deaths
d. Socioeconomic status
e. Ethnicity

## Question 77
Based on recent epidemiological studies, roughly what percentage of homicide perpetrators have a diagnosis of schizophrenia?
a. 1%
b. 2%
c. 3%
d. 4%
e. 5%

## Question 78
Linkage studies have identified several genes to be responsible for the development of schizophrenia. The gene that affects synaptic plasticity and growth of neurons, which has also been implicated in the causation of schizophrenia, has been found to be located on which chromosome?
a. Chromosome 1
b. Chromosome 5

c. Chromosome 6
d. Chromosome 8
e. Chromosome 22

## Question 79

How does monamine oxidase help in the treatment of depression?
a. Via the inhibition of the reuptake of noradrenaline and serotonin
b. Increasing the availability of monoamines by inhibiting their metabolic degradation
c. Increasing the availability of serotonin
d. Via the release of catecholamines from the neurons
e. Via the depletion of central monoaminergic neuronal stores of catecholamines

## Question 80

Several neuroanatomical areas have been implicated in depression based on imaging findings. Which of the following associations is incorrect?
a. Amygdala: associated with memories of emotional reactions
b. Cerebellum: psychomotor retardation
c. Hippocampus: memories
d. Nucleus accumbens: negative anticipation
e. Prefrontal cortex: associated with impairment in executive functions

## Question 81

PTSD patients tend to have a heightened physiological state after the traumatic event. This is due to the effects of which one of the following neurochemicals?
a. Dopamine
b. Serotonin
c. Neuropeptide Y
d. Acetylcholine
e. Adrenaline

## Question 82

It has been known that antipsychotics such as risperidone have a higher affinity for the D2 receptors than for the D3 receptors. It is believed that approximately what percentage of the blockade of the D2 receptors is needed in order to achieve therapeutic response?
a. 15%
b. 30%
c. 45%
d. 65%
e. 75%

## Question 83

Based on local epidemiological data, the highest number of post-discharge suicide cases occurred on which of the following day post-discharge?
a. 1st day
b. 2nd day
c. 3rd day

d. 4th day

e. 5th day

## Question 84

Based on epidemiological studies, as compared to Afro-Caribbean probands, the risk of siblings of Caucasians to develop schizophrenia has been estimated to be around what percentage?

a. 1%

b. 2%

c. 4%

d. 6%

e. 8%

## Question 85

Which of the following countries has been known to have the world's highest suicide rates?

a. Estonia

b. London

c. Scotland

d. Wales

e. France

## Question 86

Which of the following statements about the epidemiology of offending in the United Kingdom is incorrect?

a. The peak age of offending is around 14 years in girls.

b. The peak age of offending is around 15 years in boys.

c. Half of all the indictable crimes are committed by people under the age of 21 years.

d. By the age of 30 years, nearly 30% of all the males in the United Kingdom have been convicted of an indictable offense.

e. The sex ratio of convicted males to females in the United Kingdom has been estimated to be around 5:1.

## Question 87

Based on epidemiological studies, which of the following statements about depressive disorder is incorrect?

a. Prevalence in the general population is around 5%.

b. 1 in 4 men and 1 in 10 women have been estimated to have depressive disorder in their lifetime.

c. The lifetime risk for first-degree relative is 20%.

d. In the United Kingdom, the lifetime prevalence of major depression with a seasonal pattern is 0.4%.

e. Male gender and older age are associated with seasonal pattern.

**Question 88**
All of the following are candidate genes that are associated with the development of schizophrenia, with the exception of
a. CAPON
b. DISC1
c. DTNBP2
d. NRGI
e. PRODH

**Question 89**
Which of the following statements about the sleep changes which occur in ageing is incorrect?
a. There is increased sleep latency or time to fall asleep.
b. There is increased frequency of awakenings at night.
c. There are increased episodes of fragmentation of REM sleep.
d. There is increased duration of slow-wave sleep.
e. There is decreased sleep efficiency.

**Question 90**
Which of the following statements about the gender differences in schizophrenia is incorrect?
a. There is an approximate equal male-to-female ratio.
b. The mortality rate in men with schizophrenia is half that of women with schizophrenia.
c. Men with schizophrenia are most associated with more structural brain abnormalities.
d. Women tend to show a bimodal peak of incidence in their late 20s and 50s.
e. None of the above.

**Question 91**
It has been known that antipsychotics may block the D2 receptors in the nigrostriatal pathway and this might result in the development of extra-pyramidal side effects (EPSE). EPSE usually emerges when approximately what percentage of the D2 receptors are blocked?
a. 10%
b. 20%
c. 40%
d. 60%
e. 80%

**Question 92**
Based on local epidemiological data, what percentage of suicide occurs on the ward?
a. 2%
b. 4%

c. 5%
d. 15%
e. 30%

## Question 93
Approximately what percentage of patients with prodromal psychosis, which has developed into full-fledged schizophrenia, will achieve stable remission within 1 year?
 a. 10%
 b. 20%
 c. 40%
 d. 60%
 e. 80%

## Question 94
For those with prodromal symptoms suggestive of psychosis, the conversation rate to schizophrenia has been estimated to be around
 a. 5%
 b. 10%
 c. 15%
 d. 30%
 e. 35%

## Question 95
Damage to which area of the brain will result in expressive dysphasia?
 a. Wernicke's area
 b. Broca's area
 c. Lesion of the arcuate fasciculus
 d. Middle cerebral artery infarction
 e. Anterior cerebral artery infarction

## Question 96
A therapist decides that it will be ideal for a patient who has been diagnosed with agoraphobia to have repeated exposure to crowd. This is based on which one of the following basic psychological concepts?
 a. Extinction
 b. Generalization
 c. Discrimination
 d. Incubation
 e. Stimulus preparedness

## Question 97
A 32-year-old female came to the outpatient clinic and requested to stop her therapy sessions. She mentioned that the therapist was critical, which reminded of how her father used to treat her. This experience is termed as
 a. Transference
 b. Countertransference

c. Acting out behaviour
d. Negative therapeutic reaction
e. Resistance

## Question 98
Based on previous research findings, which one of the following is not a psychosocial factor that will predispose an individual towards developing PTSD?
a. Male gender
b. Previous psychiatric history of hyperactivity
c. Previous psychiatric history of antisocial behaviour
d. Perceived life threat
e. Low socioeconomic status

## Question 99
Based on epidemiological studies, which of the following is true with regards to the percentage of individuals in the community who have severe learning disabilities?
a. 0.5%
b. 1.0%
c. 1.5%
d. 2.0%
e. 3.0%

## Question 100
A lesion in the arcuate fasciculus would result in impairments in the following, with the exception of
a. Fluency
b. Repetition
c. Comprehension
d. Naming
e. None of the above

## Question 101
Which of the following statements about the epidemiology of substance misuse is incorrect?
a. For adolescents and young adults in the United Kingdom, approximately 50% have taken illicit drugs at some point in time.
b. Around 20% have used illicit drugs in the previous month.
c. The peak age of substance misuse is 15 years.
d. The male-to-female ratio has been estimated to be 3:1.
e. For opiate misuse, the mortality is increased by 12 times and the suicide rate is increased by 10 times.

## Question 102
According to the model proposed by Brown and Harris in 1978, which of the following psychosocial factors will not predispose an individual towards depression?
a. Having three or more children
b. Having children who are younger than the age of 11

c. Unemployment
d. Lack of a confiding relationship
e. Bereavement

## Question 103
Habit reversal is a useful psychological intervention for which of the following conditions?
a. ADHD
b. Autistic disorder
c. School refusal
d. Conduct disorder
e. Tourette's syndrome

## Question 104
A damage to which area of the brain will result in receptive dysphasia?
a. Wernicke's area
b. Broca's area
c. Lesion of the arcuate fasciculus
d. Middle cerebral artery infarction
e. Anterior cerebral artery infarction

## Question 105
Which of the following statements about the epidemiology of insomnia is incorrect?
a. The estimated prevalence of the disorder is between 1% and 10% in the general population.
b. The estimated 1-year prevalence for adults could range to as high as 60%.
c. Prevalence is especially higher in the elderly population.
d. It has been estimated to affect around one fourth of the elderly population.
e. There is a predisposition for females to have the disorder as compared to males.

## Question 106
Based on existing epidemiological studies, what has been estimated to be the prevalence of schizophrenia amongst those with learning disabilities?
a. 0.5%
b. 1%
c. 1.5%
d. 2%
e. 3%

## Question 107
A 60-year-old male has recently suffered from a cerebrovascular event. Ever since the incident, he is unable to copy shapes or to discriminate between two versions of the same objects. This is most likely due to a lesion involving the
a. Frontal lobes
b. Right parietal lobe
c. Left parietal lobe
d. Occipital lobe
e. Temporal lobe

## Question 108

The autopsy report of a man who died of Creutzfeldt–Jakob disease shows spongiform change in his brain. Which of the following pathological findings is associated with the spongiform change?
a. Amyloid beta deposition in entorhinal cortex
b. Hirano bodies in hippocampal pyramidal cells
c. Hyaline eosinophilic bodies in neocortex
d. Neurofibrillary tangles in raphe nuclei
e. Vacuolation of the glial cells

## Question 109

Which of the following genes is associated with Pick's disease?
a. Amyloid precursor protein gene on chromosome 21
b. Apolipoprotein E gene on chromosome 19
c. Presenilin 1 gene on chromosome 14
d. Presenilin 2 gene on chromosome 1
e. Tau gene on chromosome 17

## Question 110

A 60-year-old man suffers from mild cognitive impairment and his son wants to find out the rate of conversion into dementia every year. Your answer is
a. 2%–5%
b. 10%–15%
c. 20%–25%
d. 30%–35%
e. 40%–45%

## Question 111

Buprenorphine acts as a partial agonist at which of the following receptors?
a. Beta opioid receptor
b. Delta opioid receptor
c. Mu opioid receptor
d. Kappa opioid receptor
e. Sigma opioid receptor

## Question 112

Deletion in which of the following genes is associated with ubiquitin-positive and tau-negative frontotemporal dementia (FTD)?
a. Epidermal growth factor gene
b. Latent-transforming growth factor beta-binding protein gene
c. Nerve growth factor gene
d. Neurotrophin gene
e. Progranulin gene

## Question 113

Which of the following statements correctly describes confounding bias?
a. This bias occurs in clinical trials when treatment is chosen by personnel involved without randomization.
b. This bias occurs when comparisons are made between groups of participants that differ with respect to determinants of outcome other than those under study.
c. This bias occurs when the methods of measurements are consistently dissimilar among groups of participants.
d. This bias occurs when participants in one group are more likely to remember past events than participants in another study group.
e. This bias occurs when studies based on the prevalence produce very different results when compared with studies based on incidence of a disease.

## Question 114

A 40-year-old woman suffers from depression and has taken tranylcypromine for 2 years. She presents to the Accident and Emergency Department with a blood pressure of 220/120 mmHg. A few hours ago, she went for a buffet dinner and consumed a large amount of mature cheese, red wine and smoked salmon. The Accident and Emergency Department consultant wants to find out from you the best medication to reduce her blood pressure. Your answer is
a. Lisinopril
b. Phentolamine
c. Propranolol
d. Nifedipine
e. Thiazide

## Question 115

A 4-year-old child is referred to you with delayed speech and language. He was initially suspected to suffer from autism. He has gaze aversion and social avoidance. His IQ is 60. He also has attention deficit. Physical examination shows enlarged testes, large ears, a long face and flat feet. Mental state examination reveals limited eye contact, perseveration of words, echolalia and hand flapping. The genetic mutation responsible for this disorder is
a. CAA repeats
b. CCC repeats
c. CAG repeats
d. CCG repeats
e. CGG repeats

## Question 116

A 75-year-old man seems to develop Alzheimer's disease. His daughter has read an article stating that a magnetic resonance imaging (MRI) scan can establish the diagnosis of early Alzheimer's disease. Which of the following MRI findings is associated with the diagnosis of early Alzheimer's disease?
a. Atrophy of frontal lobe
b. Atrophy of lateral parietal lobe

c. Atrophy of medial parietal lobe
d. Atrophy of lateral temporal lobe
e. Atrophy of medial temporal lobe

**Question 117**
Rivastigmine is a
a. Reversible acetylcholinesterase inhibitor
b. Pseudo-irreversible acetylcholinesterase inhibitor
c. Reversible butyrylcholinesterase inhibitor
d. Reversible acetylcholinesterase and butyrylcholinesterase inhibitor
e. Pseudo-irreversible acetylcholinesterase and butyrylcholinesterase inhibitor

**Question 118**
Which of the following risk factors causes the late onset (ages 12–14 years) of
delinquent behaviour in males?
a. Difficulty concentrating
b. Dishonesty
c. Hyperactivity
d. Neglect
e. Physical problems

# Extended Matching Items (EMIs)

### Theme: General adult psychiatry
**Options:**
a. Aggressive obsession
b. Contamination obsession
c. Symmetry obsession
d. Religious obsession
e. Somatic obsession
f. Sexual obsession
g. Checking compulsion
h. Cleaning compulsion
i. Counting compulsion
j. Hoarding obsession
k. Ordering compulsion
l. Repeating compulsion
m. Saving compulsion

**Lead in:** A 35-year-old man suffers from treatment refractory OCD. The core
trainee wants to find out more about OCD symptoms and the relationship with
treatment outcome. Each option might be used once, more than once or not at all.

**Question 119**
Name two symptoms associated with poor response to SSRIs. (Choose two
options.)

**Question 120**

Name two symptoms associated with poor response to CBT. (Choose two options.)

**Question 121**

Name the most common obsession. (Choose one option.)

**Question 122**

Name the most common compulsion. (Choose one option.)

## Theme: Advanced psychology

**Options:**
a. Altruism
b. Acting out
c. Anticipation
d. Denial
e. Displacement
f. Humour
g. Idealization
h. Identification
i. Intellectualization
j. Introjection
k. Isolation of affect
l. Projection
m. Projective identification
n. Rationalization
o. Reaction formation
p. Repression
q. Regression
r. Splitting
s. Sublimation
t. Suppression
u. Undoing
v. Asceticism

**Lead in:** A 25-year-old woman is admitted to the psychiatric ward with a history of emotionally unstable personality disorder, borderline type and alcohol dependence. She was physically abused by her parents as a child, and she mentions that she feels the hospital staff have become abusive to her like her parents used to. Select the most appropriate defence mechanisms for each of the following situations. Each option can be used once or more than once.

**Question 123**

The nurse asks the client if she can go through her things to ensure there are not any sharp objects that she could use to self-harm. The client becomes upset and feels like punching the nurse. Later when the client sees a psychotherapist she realizes that her desire to hit the nurse was related to her mother hitting her as a child. (Choose one option.)

**Question 124**
The client told the core trainee that she has thoughts of harming her partner and she has to tap on a table five times in order to dispel these thoughts. (Choose one option.)

**Question 125**
The core trainee inquires about her alcohol dependence, and the client informs her that she is not dependent on alcohol and that drinking is a way to ease the stress in her life. She feels that her drinking was within reason and gave an explanation for this. (Choose one option.)

**Question 126**
After speaking to the core trainee, she believes that the trainee is the best doctor whom she has ever seen. From now on, the patient only wants to see this core trainee as her doctor. (Choose two options.)

**Question 127**
The core trainee asks you to give some examples of primitive defence. (Choose seven options.)

**Question 128**
On the second day, the client worries that the consultant may give her a warning for hitting the nurse and behaving like a child on the ward. (Choose one option.)

**Question 129**
Her behaviour became uncontrollable and she almost set fire to part of the ward. The consultant has decided to send her to a secure hospital. She complains that no one cares about her. She was chased away by her parents and now by the consultant. This verifies her belief that hospital staff are as abusive as her parents. (Choose one option.)

## Theme: Advanced psychology
**Options:**
   a. Altruism
   b. Acting out
   c. Anticipation
   d. Denial
   e. Displacement
   f. Humour
   g. Idealization
   h. Identification
   i. Intellectualization
   j. Introjection
   k. Isolation of affect
   l. Projection
   m. Projective identification

n. Rationalization
o. Reaction formation
p. Repression
q. Regression
r. Splitting
s. Sublimation
t. Suppression
u. Undoing
v. Asceticism

**Lead in:** A 20-year-old man is referred by his GP for assessment for abnormal grief. His father was a businessman who died suddenly during an elective operation 4 weeks ago and his family intends to take legal action against the hospital seeking compensation, as they believe his death was preventable. Select the most appropriate defence mechanism for each of the following situations. Each option can be used once or more than once.

**Question 130**
The GP mentioned in his referral letter that the client has tried to separate himself from his emotions since his father died. (Choose one option.)

**Question 131**
During the interview, the client tells you that he has tried to block and expel grief from entering his mind. (Choose one option.)

**Question 132**
During the interviewing, the client refers to abstract philosophy to explain his current state. (Choose one option.)

**Question 133**
One month later, the client appears to take on the quality of his father by behaving like him. (Choose one option.)

**Question 134**
Two months later, the client informs you that he has internalized the hostility of his father to scold other staff in the business, as he feels sad for his father's sudden death. (Choose one option.)

**Question 135**
You speak to his mother who expresses sympathy to doctors, as they are always busy and medical errors seem to be inevitable. She wants to apologize to the doctors who looked after her husband, as she was rude to him. Two weeks later, the client informs you that his mother is proceeding with the legal case and hopes to get a huge amount of compensation from the hospital. What is the defence mechanism used by his mother? (Choose one option.)

## Theme: Neuroanatomy – occipital lobes lesions

**Options:**
a. Dorsal and adjourning parietal lesion
b. Bilateral dorsal lesions
c. Left ventral lesions
d. Right ventral lesions

**Lead in:** Please select the most appropriate options from the aforementioned for each of the following questions.

**Question 136**
A 52-year-old has been admitted to the neurology unit. On clinical examination, he has optic ataxia, simultanagnosia and ocular apraxia.

**Question 137**
A 32-year-old male has been having contralateral hemiachromatopsia and dyslexia.

**Question 138**
A 45-year-old male presents to the emergency department with new-onset asteropsis and impaired visual motion perception.

**Question 139**
A 45-year-old female presents to the emergency department with new-onset apperceptive visual agnosia.

## Theme: Neurophysiology

**Options:**
a. Adrenocorticotropic hormone (ACTH)
b. Follicle-stimulating hormone (FSH)
c. Luteinizing hormone (LH)
d. Melanocyte-stimulating hormone (MSH)
e. Prolactin
f. Growth hormone (GH)
g. Thyroid-stimulating hormone (TSH)
h. Antidiuretic hormone (ADH/AVP)
i. Oxytocin

**Lead in:** Please select the most appropriate options from the aforementioned for each of the following questions.

**Question 140**
This is a peptic hormone that is involved in the stimulation of the hepatic secretion of insulin-like growth factor 1.

**Question 141**
This is a single-chain peptide that has an action on lactation.

**Question 142**
In males, this hormone stimulates the seminiferous tubule Sertoli cells to promote the growth of spermatozoa.

**Question 143**
This hormone consists of two peptide chains, and the alpha chain is similar to that of FSH.

**Question 144**
This hormone has a natriuretic action for both males and females.

## Theme: Neurophysiology – EEG and effects of drugs

**Options:**
- a. Increased alpha activity
- b. Decreased alpha activity
- c. Increased beta activity
- d. Decreased beta activity
- e. Increased delta activity
- f. Decreased delta activity
- g. No significant changes

**Lead in:** Please select the most appropriate options from the aforementioned for each of the following questions pertaining to the effects of drugs on the EEG rhythm.

**Question 145**
The usage of anxiolytics would cause which TWO of the changes on the EEG?

**Question 146**
The usage of antidepressant would cause which ONE of the changes on the EEG?

**Question 147**
The usage of antipsychotic drugs would cause which TWO of the following changes on the EEG?

## Theme: Neurophysiology – sleep

**Options:**
- a. Increased complexity of dreams
- b. Decreased complexity of dreams
- c. Decreased recall of dreams
- d. Upwards ocular deviation
- e. Decreased cerebral blood flow
- f. Occasional myoclonic jerks
- g. Increased penile erection

**Lead in:** Based on your understanding of the sleep cycle, please select the appropriate options for each of the following questions.

**Question 148**
Select four options that are characteristic for non-rapid eye movement (NREM) sleep.

**Question 149**
Select three options that are characteristic of rapid eye movement (REM) sleep.

## Theme: Neurochemical and common disorders
**Options:**
  a. Decreased dopamine in mesocortical pathway
  b. Increased dopamine in mesocortical pathway
  c. Decreased dopamine in mesolimbic pathway
  d. Increased dopamine in mesolimbic pathway
  e. Increased dopamine in nigrostriatal pathway
  f. Decreased dopamine in nigrostriatal pathway
  g. Decreased CSF homovanillic acid (HVA) levels
  h. Increased CSF HVA levels

**Lead in:** There are disease processes that are caused by dysregulation of dopamine. Please select the appropriate options for each of the following questions.

**Question 150**
Select TWO of the aforementiond changes that are common in schizophrenia.

**Question 151**
Select ONE of the aforementioned changes that is common for OCD.

**Question 152**
Select TWO of the aforementioned changes that are common for bipolar disorder.

## Theme: Genetics (I)
**Options:**
  a. Chromosome 2
  b. Chromosome 4
  c. Chromosome 5
  d. Chromosome 13
  e. Chromosome 15
  f. Chromosome 18
  g. Chromosome 20
  h. Chromosome 22

**Lead in:** Please select the most appropriate options for each of the following questions.

**Question 153**
This chromosome is implicated in DiGeorge syndrome.

**Question 154**
This chromosome has been associated with autism.

**Question 155**
Patau's syndrome is due to abnormalities with this particular chromosome.

**Question 156**
Both of these genetic conditions (Angelman's and Prader–Willi) are due to abnormalities on this chromosome.

**Question 157**
Which of the chromosomes has been implicated in inherited CJD?

## Theme: Genetics (II)

**Options:**
a. Substitution mutation
b. Transition mutation
c. Transversion mutation
d. Silent mutation
e. Missense mutation
f. Nonsense mutation
g. Frameshift mutation

**Lead in:** Please select the appropriate mutations from the aforementioned list for each of the following case scenarios.

**Question 158**
This could potentially give rise to either silent or missense mutations.

**Question 159**
This refers to a mutation that causes a change from a purine to a pyrimidine.

**Question 160**
In this form of mutation, the mutation involves a change from a purine to a purine base.

**Question 161**
This results in the creation of a stop codon.

**Question 162**
This particular type of mutation results in a change in a reading frame, which might cause a loss-of-function mutation.

## Theme: Advanced psychological process and treatment

**Options:**
a. Supportive psychotherapy
b. Brief dynamic psychotherapy
c. Cognitive behavioural therapy
d. Dialectical behaviour therapy
e. Mentalization-based treatment

f. Cognitive analytic therapy
g. Interpersonal therapy
h. Family therapy

**Lead in:** Please select the most appropriate psychological therapy for each of the following scenarios.

**Question 163**
Presence of behavioural control problems within the family

**Question 164**
The common indications for this particular form of psychotherapy include dysthymia, depressive disorder and, in particular, bulimia nervosa.

**Question 165**
This particular form of therapy is suitable for borderline personality disorders. The core conceptualization of this form of therapy is that individuals are unable to interpret their actions or others' actions.

**Question 166**
This particular form of therapy involves dealing with faculty procedures such as traps, dilemma and snag.

**Question 167**
One part of this form of therapy is based on Mowrer's two-factor model.

**Question 168**
Some of the possible negative reactions during this process of psychological therapy include resistance, acting-out, acting-in and negative therapeutic reaction.

## Theme: Psychiatric epidemiology (I)

| Test Result | Positive | Negative |
|---|---|---|
| Positive | a | b |
| Negative | c | d |

**Options:**
a. Positive predictive value
b. Negative predictive value
c. Screen prevalence
d. Disease prevalence
e. Test accuracy

**Lead in:** Making use of the aforementioned table, please select the most appropriate options for each of the following questions.

**Question 169**
This is computed by the following formula (a/a+b).

**Question 170**
This is computed by the following formula (d/c+d).

**Question 171**
This is computed by the following formula (a+b/a+b+c+d).

## Theme: Psychiatric epidemiology (II)

**Options:**
  a. Crude mortality rate
  b. Age-specific mortality rate
  c. Proportionate mortality
  d. Case fatality rate
  e. Child mortality rate
  f. Infant mortality rate
  g. Postnatal mortality rate
  h. Neonatal mortality rate
  i. Stillbirth
  j. Perinatal mortality rate

**Lead in:** Please select the most appropriate options for each of the following questions.

**Question 172**
This is based on the number of deaths in the first 28 days over the total number of live births in a 1-year period.

**Question 173**
This is computed based on the number of deaths in the first 28 days over the total number of live births in one year.

**Question 174**
This takes into consideration the mortality due to a condition within a specified time period.

**Question 174**
This is computed based on the number of deaths and the mid-year population.

# GET THROUGH MRCPSYCH PAPER A2: MOCK EXAMINATION

**Question 1 Answer: d, The reduction in hippocampal volume in male schizophrenics was smaller than that in females.**
*Explanation*: As compared to controls, in the schizophrenic group, the hippocampal formation was significantly smaller in the right as compared to the left hemisphere. The reduction in hippocampal volume in male schizophrenics was greater than that in females.

*Reference*: Puri BK, Hall A, Ho R (2014). *Revision Notes in Psychiatry*. London: CRC Press, p. 198.

**Question 2 Answer: e, One EPSP is usually sufficient to initiate an action potential.**
*Explanation*: This is incorrect. Summation (temporal or spatial) can occur to allow the degree of depolarization to reach the critical threshold.

*Reference*: Puri BK, Hall A, Ho R (2014). *Revision Notes in Psychiatry*. London: CRC Press, p. 210.

**Question 3 Answer: e, Asymmetry in temporal lobe**
*Explanation*: Asymmetry in temporal lobe is commonly observed in patients with bipolar disorder and not observed on neuroimaging in patients with depressive disorder.

*Reference*: Puri BK, Hall A, Ho R (2014). *Revision Notes in Psychiatry*. London: CRC Press, p. 388.

**Question 4 Answer: a, Alpha-4, beta-2 nicotinic partial agonist**
*Explanation*: The tobacco withdrawal syndrome usually develops when a person stops smoking after 3–10 weeks of tobacco consumption. The onset may be within an hour after the last cigarette. The aforementioned medication has high affinity to the alpha-4 beta-2 nicotine Ach receptors and helps to prevent the withdrawal syndrome.

*Reference*: Puri BK, Hall A, Ho R (2014). *Revision Notes in Psychiatry*. London: CRC Press, p. 545.

### Question 5 Answer: c, The most common side effect is insomnia.
*Explanation*: Based on existing research, the most common side effect is headache that occurs in around 30% of patients, followed closely by insomnia and then rash.

*Reference*: Puri BK, Hall A, Ho R (2014). *Revision Notes in Psychiatry*. London: CRC Press, p. 545.

### Question 6 Answer: b, Chromosome 14
*Explanation*: Robertsonian translocations are caused by the fusion of chromosome 14 and chromosome 21. The extra chromosome is usually of maternal origin and this happens in around 90% of the cases.

*Reference*: Puri BK, Hall A, Ho R (2014). *Revision Notes in Psychiatry*. London: CRC Press, p. 665.

### Question 7 Answer: a, Increased HCG, lowered alpha-fetoprotein, lowered unconjugated estriol
*Explanation*: The aforementioned combination of maternal serum markers present at 16 weeks is indicative of the likelihood of the development of Down's syndrome.

*Reference*: Puri BK, Hall A, Ho R (2014). *Revision Notes in Psychiatry*. London: CRC Press, p. 665.

### Question 8 Answer: a, Huntington's
*Explanation*: The concept of anticipation refers to the occurrence of an autonomic dominant disorder at earlier ages of onset and with greater severity in the succeeding generations. Huntington's disease is caused by the expansions of unstable triplet repeat sequences.

*Reference*: Puri BK, Hall A, Ho R (2014). *Revision Notes in Psychiatry*. London: CRC Press, p. 271.

### Question 9 Answer: d, Central sulcus
*Explanation*: The central sulcus marks the division between the frontal and the parietal lobes.

*Reference*: Puri BK, Hall A, Ho R (2014). *Revision Notes in Psychiatry*. London: CRC Press, p. 175.

### Question 10 Answer: d, Psychogenic amnesia
*Explanation*: Psychogenic amnesia is part of the dissociative disorder consisting of a sudden inability to recall important personal data. The amnesia may be

localized or generalized. The amnesia may be selective or continuous. It is true that the clinical presentation is usually atypical and cannot be explained by ordinary forgetfulness. Psychogenic amnesia is associated with la belle indifference (lack of concern) and a highly unpredictable course.

*Reference*: Puri BK, Hall A, Ho R (2014). *Revision Notes in Psychiatry*. London: CRC Press, p. 104.

### Question 11 Answer: e, Tricyclics
*Explanation*: The treatment of acute mania is usually with antipsychotics, such as (a) and (b). Lithium carbonate could be used in the prophylaxis, or could also be used in the treatment of acute mania episodes. Neuroleptics are usually preferred as the first-line drug of choice, though. Short-term benzodiazepines could also be used to help control behaviour difficulties or agitation. It is essential to ensure that medications such as antidepressants are stopped, as they could precipitate the manic episode.

*Reference*: Puri BK, Hall A, Ho R (2014). *Revision Notes in Psychiatry*. London: CRC Press, p. 394.

### Question 12 Answer: c, X-linked recessive
*Explanation*: For X-linked recessive disorder, male-to-male transmission would not take place. Males are far more likely to be affected with X-linked recessive disorder, and females are more likely to be carriers.

*Reference*: Puri BK, Hall A, Ho R (2014). *Revision Notes in Psychiatry*. London: CRC Press, p. 267.

### Question 13 Answer: a, Brief dynamic therapy
*Explanation*: These are part of brief dynamic therapy. In brief dynamic therapy, it is important to establish a therapeutic alliance, and then set goals and allow free association by the client. There is a need to focus on internal conflicts and interpretation of transference. Confrontation, working through and enactment can be used. Eventually, it is hoped that there will be resolution of conflicts and the client would be able to link the past, present and the transference.

*Reference*: Puri BK, Hall A, Ho R (2014). *Revision Notes in Psychiatry*. London: CRC Press, p. 331.

### Question 14 Answer: c, Jung's theory consists of causality and teleology only
*Explanation*: His theory also includes synchronicity, which offers an explanation in terms of causation at the boundary of the physical world with the psychical world.

*Reference*: Puri BK, Hall A, Ho R (2014). *Revision Notes in Psychiatry*. London: CRC Press, p. 133.

**Question 15 Answer: a, Mitochondrial DNA is essentially maternally inherited.**
*Explanation*: The aforementioned is true. Mitochondrial inheritance may explain some cases of disorders that affect both males and females but that are transmitted through females and not through males.

*Reference*: Puri BK, Hall A, Ho R (2014). *Revision Notes in Psychiatry*. London: CRC Press, p. 269.

**Question 16 Answer: a, Wernicke's area**
*Explanation*: The posterior part of the superior temporal gyrus, area 22, forms on the left, the Wernicke's area. It has been noted that lesions involved with this particular area could lead to a resultant receptive aphasia.

*Reference*: Puri BK, Hall A, Ho R (2014). *Revision Notes in Psychiatry*. London: CRC Press, p. 178.

**Question 17 Answer: a, Alexia without agraphia**
*Explanation*: All of the aforementioned options are the residual symptoms caused by frontal lobe lesions, with the exception of alexia without agraphia. Alexia without agraphia occurs when there is an occlusion of the left posterior cerebral artery which leads to an infarction of the medial aspect of the left occipital lobe and the splenium of the corpus callosum.

*Reference*: Puri BK, Hall A, Ho R (2014). *Revision Notes in Psychiatry*. London: CRC Press, p. 110.

**Question 18 Answer: a, Alpha-2 agonist**
*Explanation*: It acts primarily as an alpha-2 agonist, which acts centrally to reduce the sympathetic tone and hence will lead to a reduction in the blood pressure. The indication for use are for detoxification within a short period of time and for dependence in young people.

*Reference*: Puri BK, Hall A, Ho R (2014). *Revision Notes in Psychiatry*. London: CRC Press, p. 531.

**Question 19 Answer: e, 100%**
*Explanation*: Autosomal dominant disorders result from the presence of an abnormal dominant allele, thus causing the individual to manifest the abnormal phenotypic trait. Males and females are affected, and male-to-male transmission can take place.

*Reference*: Puri BK, Hall A, Ho R (2014). *Revision Notes in Psychiatry*. London: CRC Press, p. 266.

**Question 20 Answer: c, Snag**
*Explanation*: Snag refers to the extreme pessimism about the future, which would halt a plan before it even starts. Traps refer to the repetitive cycles of behaviour

and their consequences become perpetuation. Dilemma refers to false choices or unduly narrowed options.

*Reference*: Puri BK, Hall A, Ho R (2014). *Revision Notes in Psychiatry*. London: CRC Press, p. 339.

### Question 21 Answer: a, Systemic family therapy
*Explanation*: Systemic family therapy uses the aforementioned techniques. Reframing occurs when an individual's problem is being framed as a family problem. Circular questioning is used to examine perspective of each family member on interfamily member relationship. Circular questioning aims at discovering and clarifying conflicting views. Hypothesis could be formed from conflicting views and the therapist can propose further changes.

*Reference*: Puri BK, Hall A, Ho R (2014). *Revision Notes in Psychiatry*. London: CRC Press, p. 344.

### Question 22 Answer: b, Chromosome 8
*Explanation*: The gene responsible is located on chromosome 8.

*Reference*: Puri BK, Hall A, Ho R (2014). *Revision Notes in Psychiatry*. London: CRC Press, p. 260.

### Question 23 Answer: a, Golgi type I
*Explanation*: Golgi type I would be the largest neuron due to it having a relatively long axon.

*Reference*: Puri BK, Hall A, Ho R (2014). *Revision Notes in Psychiatry*. London: CRC Press, p. 176.

### Question 24 Answer: d, The greater the diameter of the unmyelinated fibre, the slower the rates of conduction
*Explanation*: This is incorrect. The greater the diameter of the fibre, the faster is the rate of transmission.

*Reference*: Puri BK, Hall A, Ho R (2014). *Revision Notes in Psychiatry*. London: CRC Press, p. 209.

### Question 25 Answer: e, Personality changes
*Explanation*: An insult to the frontal lobe is likely to result in personality changes. It is important to note that left frontal lobe damage would result in non-fluent speech as well as depression. Involvement of the right frontal lobe would result in disinhibition and antisocial behaviour.

*Reference*: Puri BK, Hall A, Ho R (2014). *Revision Notes in Psychiatry*. London: CRC Press, p. 110.

**Question 26 Answer: a, Competitive inhibition of the NMDA receptor complex**
*Explanation*: Ketamine is considered to be the shorter-acting derivative of PCP. The action of ketamine is mediated via competitive inhibition from the NMDA receptor complex. Use of ketamine will lead to cramps, fatigue, depression and irritability. It may also lead to violent reactions such as flashbacks and harm to others.

*Reference*: Puri BK, Hall A, Ho R (2014). *Revision Notes in Psychiatry*. London: CRC Press, p. 543.

**Question 27 Answer: e, Chromosome 22**
*Explanation*: The COMT gene that is responsible for the causation of both schizophrenia and bipolar disorder is located on chromosome 22.

*Reference*: Puri BK, Hall A, Ho R (2014). *Revision Notes in Psychiatry*. London: CRC Press, p. 260.

**Question 28 Answer: b, Insecure attachment**
*Explanation*: In insecure attachment, there is chronic clinginess and ambivalence towards the mother. Clinically, this is very relevant, as it could lead to childhood emotional disorders (such as school refusal) as well as disorders in childhood and adulthood.

*Reference*: Puri BK, Hall A, Ho R (2014). *Revision Notes in Psychiatry*. London: CRC Press, p. 64.

**Question 29 Answer: e, Helping them to improve self-understanding by developing capacity for self-reflection**
*Explanation*: The objectives of CBT for depression are as aforementioned, with the exception of (e). That is an objective of brief dynamic psychotherapy.

*Reference*: Puri BK, Hall A, Ho R (2014). *Revision Notes in Psychiatry*. London: CRC Press, p. 334.

**Question 30 Answer: c, Individuals, especially females, with this genotype tend to have an increased rate of petty crime.**
*Explanation*: It has been shown that males with this particular genotype tend to have an increased rate of petty crime instead. This could be a result of the resultant impulsiveness.

*Reference*: Puri BK, Hall A, Ho R (2014). *Revision Notes in Psychiatry*. London: CRC Press, p. 664.

**Question 31 Answer: e, Posterior commissure**
*Explanation*: All of the aforementioned represent connecting pathways of the limbic system, with the exception of (e).

*Reference*: Puri BK, Hall A, Ho R (2014). *Revision Notes in Psychiatry*. London: CRC Press, p. 182.

### Question 32 Answer: a, Predominantly amyloid
*Explanation*: The plaques that are found contain mainly a core of amyloid. This consists of 8-nm extracellular filaments made up mainly of amyloid beta peptide. This has been derived from the membrane-bound beta amyloid precursor protein.

*Reference*: Puri BK, Hall A, Ho R (2014). *Revision Notes in Psychiatry*. London: CRC Press, p. 195.

### Question 33 Answer: c, The trial demonstrated that the efficacy of first-generation antipsychotic was inferior to that of second-generation antipsychotics.
*Explanation*: The trial showed similar efficacy for first-generation and second-generation antipsychotics.

*Reference*: Puri BK, Hall A, Ho R (2014). *Revision Notes in Psychiatry*. London: CRC Press, p. 249.

### Question 34 Answer: e, Translation
*Explanation*: It is known that following transcription, splicing and nuclear transport, translation is the process in gene expression whereby the mRNA acts as a template allowing the genetic code to be deciphered to allow the formation of a peptide chain.

*Reference*: Puri BK, Hall A, Ho R (2014). *Revision Notes in Psychiatry*. London: CRC Press, p. 261.

### Question 35 Answer: e, For children and young people with OCD with moderate-to-severe functional impairment, CBT and ERP are not the first line of treatment.
*Explanation*: CBT and ERP are indicated to be the first line of treatment for children and young people even if they have moderate-to-severe functional impairments.

*Reference*: Puri BK, Hall A, Ho R (2014). *Revision Notes in Psychiatry*. London: CRC Press, p. 414.

### Question 36 Answer: d, Exposure and response prevention
*Explanation*: Based on the NICE guidelines, exposure and response prevention (up to 10 therapist hours per client) is indicated for the initial treatment of OCD.

*Reference*: Puri BK, Hall A, Ho R (2014). *Revision Notes in Psychiatry*. London: CRC Press, p. 414.

### Question 37 Answer: b, Better verbal skills as compared to performance skills
*Explanation*: It has been noted that those with the aforementioned karyotype would have difficulties in acquiring verbal skills, along with a mild level of intellectual disability.

*Reference*: Puri BK, Hall A, Ho R (2014). *Revision Notes in Psychiatry*. London: CRC Press, p. 663.

### Question 38 Answer: e, Mirtazapine
*Explanation*: Among all the options, it has the lowest prevalence of sexual dysfunction, estimated to be at 25%. It does cause decreased libido and delayed orgasm. Erectile dysfunction and absence of orgasm are less common.

*Reference*: Puri BK, Hall A, Ho R (2014). *Revision Notes in Psychiatry*. London: CRC Press, p. 414.

### Question 39 Answer: e, Satellite cells
*Explanation*: These are the main types of neuroglia which are present in the peripheral nervous system instead of the central nervous system.

*Reference*: Puri BK, Hall A, Ho R (2014). *Revision Notes in Psychiatry*. London: CRC Press, p. 176.

### Question 40 Answer: b, Familiarity and novelty
*Explanation*: Option (b) is not influenced by age changes. Tasks that have been learnt over a lifetime relying on overlearned abilities are actually the most resistant to age-related changes. This is also known as crystallized intelligence. It is of importance to note that tasks that require the less practised processing of new information are most sensitive to age-related decline, or also known as fluid intelligence.

*Reference*: Puri BK, Hall A, Ho R (2014). *Revision Notes in Psychiatry*. London: CRC Press, p. 679.

### Question 41 Answer: b, CVA in the left hemisphere has a stronger association with mania.
*Explanation*: It has been shown that CVA in the right hemisphere has a stronger association with mania in comparison to CVA in the left hemisphere.

*Reference*: Puri BK, Hall A, Ho R (2014). *Revision Notes in Psychiatry*. London: CRC Press, p. 494.

### Question 42 Answer: e, Penetrance
*Explanation*: Penetrance refers to the percentage of individuals who would express a particular phenotype. Variable expressivity, in association with penetrance might at times give the impression that a particular disorder has skipped a generation.

*Reference*: Puri BK, Hall A, Ho R (2014). *Revision Notes in Psychiatry*. London: CRC Press, p. 268.

### Question 43 Answer: a, Cognitive behavioural therapy
*Explanation*: Based on the ENRICHD (Enhancing Recovery in Coronary Heart Disease Study), there was noted to be substantial improvement in the severity of

depression 6 months after the commencement of CBT. However, these beneficial effects have seemed to have diminished after 30 months.

*Reference*: Puri BK, Hall A, Ho R (2014). *Revision Notes in Psychiatry*. London: CRC Press, p. 469.

**Question 44 Answer: c, Family problems tend to arise when the boundaries are too tight, thus resulting in enmeshment.**
*Explanation*: When the boundaries are too tight, this would result in disengagement. When the boundaries are too loose, it will result in enmeshment.

*Reference*: Puri BK, Hall A, Ho R (2014). *Revision Notes in Psychiatry*. London: CRC Press, p. 341.

**Question 45 Answer: e, Behaviour control problems**
*Explanation*: Behaviour control problems are considered to be internal indicators for family-based therapy. When there are behaviour control problems within the family, it is pertinent to engage the family to deliver the behaviour therapy within the context of the home environment.

*Reference*: Puri BK, Hall A, Ho R (2014). *Revision Notes in Psychiatry*. London: CRC Press, p. 341.

**Question 46 Answer: a, Prader–Willi syndrome**
*Explanation*: The clinical presentation is characteristic for Prader–Willi syndrome. This is an autosomal dominant disorder that is commonly due to the deletion of chromosome of the paternal origin.

*Reference*: Puri BK, Hall A, Ho R (2014). *Revision Notes in Psychiatry*. London: CRC Press, p. 673.

**Question 47 Answer: e, Valproate**
*Explanation*: The aforementioned options are considered to be established treatments for bipolar depression, with the exception of valproate. There is limited evidence of using valproate. It will probably protect against a depressive relapse but the current research database is small.

*Reference*: Puri BK, Hall A, Ho R (2014). *Revision Notes in Psychiatry*. London: CRC Press, p. 414.

**Question 48 Answer: e, Uncompetitive antagonist at the NMDA receptor**
*Explanation*: Memantine is a low-affinity voltage-dependent uncompetitive antagonist at the NMDA receptor. It might be neuro-protective and disease modifying.

*Reference*: Puri BK, Hall A, Ho R (2014). *Revision Notes in Psychiatry*. London: CRC Press, p. 694.

**Question 49 Answer: e, CNS myelin sheath formation**
*Explanation*: CNS myelin sheath formation is a function of the oligo-dendrocytes and not a function of the astrocytes.

*Reference*: Puri BK, Hall A, Ho R (2014). *Revision Notes in Psychiatry*. London: CRC Press, p. 176.

**Question 50 Answer: a, Left occipital lobe**
*Explanation*: This is usually due to an occlusion of the left posterior cerebral artery, which leads to infarction of the medial aspect of the left occipital lobe and the splenium of the corpus callosum.

*Reference*: Puri BK, Hall A, Ho R (2014). *Revision Notes in Psychiatry*. London: CRC Press, p. 108.

**Question 51 Answer: c, Orobuccal apraxia**
*Explanation*: An insult to the left inferior frontal lobe and insula would lead to orobuccal apraxia. The patient will have difficulty in preforming learned, skilled movements of the face, lips, tongue, check, larynx and pharynx on command.

*Reference*: Puri BK, Hall A, Ho R (2014). *Revision Notes in Psychiatry*. London: CRC Press, p. 109.

**Question 52 Answer: b, The study included clozapine in the intervention.**
*Explanation*: (b) is incorrect. In the study, second-generation antipsychotics were included, but with the exception of clozapine.

*Reference*: Puri BK, Hall A, Ho R (2014). *Revision Notes in Psychiatry*. London: CRC Press, p. 249.

**Question 53 Answer: a, Risperidone**
*Explanation*: Antipsychotics decrease dopaminergic transmission, which in itself can decrease libido but may also increase prolactin levels via negative feedback. The overall propensity of an antipsychotic to cause sexual dysfunction is much similar to its propensity to raise prolactin: risperidone > haloperidol > olanzapine > quetiapine > aripiprazole.

*Reference*: Puri BK, Hall A, Ho R (2014). *Revision Notes in Psychiatry*. London: CRC Press, p. 414.

**Question 54 Answer: c, Apolipoprotein E4**
*Explanation*: It is believed that late-onset AD is an autosomal dominant trait with age-dependent expression and low penetrance, resulting in apparent sporadic causes (to add explanation).

*Reference*: Puri BK, Hall A, Ho R (2014). *Revision Notes in Psychiatry*. London: CRC Press, p. 694.

**Question 55 Answer: a, Brief dynamic psychotherapy**
*Explanation*: Interpretation of transference and confrontation, which is an attempt to make the client face the issues that are close to consciousness but are repressed or denied by the client, is an aspect of brief dynamic psychotherapy.

*Reference*: Puri BK, Hall A, Ho R (2014). *Revision Notes in Psychiatry*. London: CRC Press, p. 331.

**Question 56 Answer: d, 20%**
*Explanation*: Approximately 20% of patients with anorexia nervosa will have poor outcome with no improvement and will eventually result in death.

*Reference*: Puri BK, Hall A, Ho R (2014). *Revision Notes in Psychiatry*. London: CRC Press, p. 294.

**Question 57 Answer: a, High level of education**
*Explanation*: Protective factors that would reduce the risk of development of Alzheimer's dementia include the following: bilingualism, cognitive engagement and late retirement, fish intake (more than once a week), high level of education (longer than 15 years), high level of physical activities (more than three times a week) and the use of NSAIDs and statin.

*Reference*: Puri BK, Hall A, Ho R (2014). *Revision Notes in Psychiatry*. London: CRC Press, p. 690.

**Question 58 Answer: a, 45XO**
*Explanation*: The clinical features are suggestive of Turner's syndrome. This is usually due to nondisjunction of the paternal XY that results in sexual chromosomal monosomy; 50% of the patients will have a karyotype consisting of 45XO or 46XX.

*Reference*: Puri BK, Hall A, Ho R (2014). *Revision Notes in Psychiatry*. London: CRC Press, p. 662.

**Question 59 Answer: e, 22q**
*Explanation*: The clinical features are congruent with DiGeorge syndrome. This involves a microdeletion in the chromosome 22q11.2.

*Reference*: Puri BK, Hall A, Ho R (2014). *Revision Notes in Psychiatry*. London: CRC Press, p. 677.

**Question 60 Answer: b, Haemodialysis**
*Explanation*: He is having signs and symptoms of a severe overdose of lithium, with the expected lithium plasma level of more than 2mM. Immediate haemodialysis should be commenced.

*Reference*: Puri BK, Hall A, Ho R (2014). *Revision Notes in Psychiatry*. London: CRC Press, p. 252.

### Question 61 Answer: d, Rhombencephalon

*Explanation*: The cerebellum is derived from the aforementioned structure. The oral part of the medulla oblongata as well as the cerebellum is also derived from the aforementioned structure.

*Reference*: Puri BK, Hall A, Ho R (2014). *Revision Notes in Psychiatry*. London: CRC Press, p. 176.

### Question 62 Answer: a, Rey–Osterrieth Test

*Explanation*: This is a visual memory test in which the subject is presented with a complex design. The subject is asked to copy the design and then, 40 minutes later, without previous notification that this will occur, is then asked to draw the same design from memory. It is noted that nondominant temporal lobe damage will lead to impaired performance on this test. Dominant temporal lobe damage would lead to verbal memory difficulties.

*Reference*: Puri BK, Hall A, Ho R (2014). *Revision Notes in Psychiatry*. London: CRC Press, p. 95.

### Question 63 Answer: e, In Alzheimer's dementia, the activity of the enzyme is increased and this leads to a reduction in the synthesis of acetylcholine.

*Explanation*: This is incorrect. The activity of the enzyme is reduced, and hence there is a reduction in the synthesis of the acetylcholine.

*Reference*: Puri BK, Hall A, Ho R (2014). *Revision Notes in Psychiatry*. London: CRC Press, p. 220.

### Question 64 Answer: c, Chromosome 17

*Explanation*: 50% of patients with this disorder are caused by autosomal dominant inheritance of tau gene on chromosome 17. This will result in abnormal insoluble tau isoforms being accumulated in the neurons and also in the glia.

*Reference*: Puri BK, Hall A, Ho R (2014). *Revision Notes in Psychiatry*. London: CRC Press, p. 697.

### Question 65 Answer: b, 1%

*Explanation*: Approximately 1% of patients eventually kill themselves in the year following their deliberate self-harm.

*Reference*: Puri BK, Hall A, Ho R (2014). *Revision Notes in Psychiatry*. London: CRC Press, p. 287.

**Question 66 Answer: d, 4500**

*Explanation*: The estimated number of general population suicides that occur per year in England and Wales has been estimated to be between 4500 and 5000.

*Reference*: Puri BK, Hall A, Ho R (2014). *Revision Notes in Psychiatry*. London: CRC Press, p. 286.

**Question 67 Answer: e, 200**

*Explanation*: The normal number of repeats has been estimated to be 30. For carriers, they usually will have between 55 to 200 repeats. Full mutation usually involves having more than 200 repeats, which leads to hypermethylation at the gene.

*Reference*: Puri BK, Hall A, Ho R (2014). *Revision Notes in Psychiatry*. London: CRC Press, p. 661.

**Question 68 Answer: b, Dopamine D2 receptors**

*Explanation*: It has its action on the dopamine D2 receptors. All clinically effective antipsychotic drugs occupy a substantial proportion of the D2 receptors in the brain. This is usually between 70% and 80% at normal doses of the antipsychotics.

*Reference*: Puri BK, Hall A, Ho R (2014). *Revision Notes in Psychiatry*. London: CRC Press, p. 359.

**Question 69 Answer: c, It is an inhibitor of both AChE and BChE**

*Explanation*: AChEIs are largely broadly similar in their mechanism of action, and they are chosen usually based on their costs, their side effect profiles and patients' preferences. Rivastigmine is commonly used for AD as well as DLB and dementia related to Parkinson's disease. It inhibits both the enzymes. It does not modulate the nicotine receptor.

*Reference*: Puri BK, Hall A, Ho R (2014). *Revision Notes in Psychiatry*. London: CRC Press, p. 693.

**Question 70 Answer: e, Global apraxia**

*Explanation*: Apraxia refers to an inability in performing purposive volitional acts, which does not result from paresis, incoordination, sensory loss or involuntary movements. Global apraxia is not one of the commonly known forms of apraxia.

*Reference*: Puri BK, Hall A, Ho R (2014). *Revision Notes in Psychiatry*. London: CRC Press, p. 108.

**Question 71 Answer: c, Simultanagnosia**

*Explanation*: This is the correct terminology for the aforementioned deficits. This is usually associated with a lesion in the anterior part of the occipital lobe.

*Reference*: Puri BK, Hall A, Ho R (2014). *Revision Notes in Psychiatry*. London: CRC Press, p. 107.

## Question 72 Answer: a, Cream cheese
*Explanation*: Cheese, with the exception of cottage cheese and cream cheese, does cause the typical reaction when consumed.

*Reference*: Puri BK, Hall A, Ho R (2014). *Revision Notes in Psychiatry*. London: CRC Press, p. 255.

## Question 73 Answer: b, Sertraline
*Explanation*: Based on the Sertraline Antidepressant Heart Attack Randomized Trial (SADHART), the study has found that sertraline is a safe treatment for depression immediately after myocardial infarction. It is notable that the effects of sertraline were greater in the patients with severe and recurrent depression.

*Reference*: Puri BK, Hall A, Ho R (2014). *Revision Notes in Psychiatry*. London: CRC Press, p. 468.

## Question 74 Answer: c, Lesion of the arcuate fasciculus
*Explanation*: Damage to the aforementioned region will result in conduction dysphasia in which the person is unable to repeat what is said by another. Of importance, comprehension and verbal fluency do remain intact.

*Reference*: Puri BK, Hall A, Ho R (2014). *Revision Notes in Psychiatry*. London: CRC Press, p. 105.

## Question 75 Answer: d, Chromosome 21
*Explanation*: Individuals with Down's syndrome are at a high risk for developing Alzheimer's dementia. Over the age of 40, there is a high incidence of neurofibrillary tangles and plaques with an increase in P300 latency. This is largely due to a defect at 21q21.1 that leads to the overexpression of genes that encode for amyloid precursor protein.

*Reference*: Puri BK, Hall A, Ho R (2014). *Revision Notes in Psychiatry*. London: CRC Press, p. 661.

## Question 76 Answer: a, Age
*Explanation*: The most important confounder that needs to be adjusted for is the age. The standardized mortality rate is the mortality rate adjusted to compensate for a confounder. The standardized mortality ratio is the ratio of the observed standardized mortality rate derived from the population being studied to the expected standardized mortality rate derived from a comparable standard population.

*Reference*: Puri BK, Hall A, Ho R (2014). *Revision Notes in Psychiatry*. London: CRC Press, p. 277.

## Question 77 Answer: e, 5%
*Explanation*: According to recent epidemiological studies, roughly 5% of homicide perpetrators have a diagnosis of schizophrenia. This percentage is much lower than the comorbidity of alcohol and drug misuse.

*Reference*: Puri BK, Hall A, Ho R (2014). *Revision Notes in Psychiatry*. London: CRC Press, p. 282.

## Question 78 Answer: d, Chromosome 8
*Explanation*: The gene that is being referred to here is neuregulin and it is located on chromosome 8p12. It has been implicated in the aetiology of schizophrenia.

*Reference*: Puri BK, Hall A, Ho R (2014). *Revision Notes in Psychiatry*. London: CRC Press, p. 357.

## Question 79 Answer: b, Increasing the availability of monoamines by inhibiting their metabolic degradation
*Explanation*: Monoamine oxidase inhibitors increase the availability of monoamines by inhibiting their metabolic degradation by monoamine oxidase.

*Reference*: Puri BK, Hall A, Ho R (2014). *Revision Notes in Psychiatry*. London: CRC Press, p. 386.

## Question 80 Answer: d, Nucleus accumbens: negative anticipation
*Explanation*: Based on neuroanatomy and imaging findings, the nucleus accumbens is associated with lack of motivation. The anterior cingulate cortex is associated with negative anticipation or poor judgement.

*Reference*: Puri BK, Hall A, Ho R (2014). *Revision Notes in Psychiatry*. London: CRC Press, p. 390.

## Question 81 Answer: a, Dopamine
*Explanation*: The heightened physiological state specific to PTSD is mediated by noradrenergic and also the dopaminergic neurotransmitter systems, as well as the HPA axis.

*Reference*: Puri BK, Hall A, Ho R (2014). *Revision Notes in Psychiatry*. London: CRC Press, p. 427.

## Question 82 Answer: e, 75%
*Explanation*: It has been proven that approximately 75% blockade of the D2 receptors is required for there to be therapeutic response.

*Reference*: Puri BK, Hall A, Ho R (2014). *Revision Notes in Psychiatry*. London: CRC Press, p. 224.

**Question 83 Answer: a, 1st Day**
*Explanation*: Post-discharge suicide is the most frequent in the first 2 weeks after leaving the hospital. The highest number usually occurred on the first day after leaving the hospital.

*Reference*: Puri BK, Hall A, Ho R (2014). *Revision Notes in Psychiatry*. London: CRC Press, p. 288.

**Question 84 Answer: b, 2%**
*Explanation*: In the UK, the risk of siblings of the Afro-Caribbean probands to develop schizophrenia has been estimated to be around 16%. In contrast, the risk of siblings of the Caucasian to develop schizophrenia has been estimated to be around 2%.

*Reference*: Puri BK, Hall A, Ho R (2014). *Revision Notes in Psychiatry*. London: CRC Press, p. 281.

**Question 85 Answer: a, Estonia**
*Explanation*: Lithuania, Estonia and Latvia are the countries that have been known to have the highest rate of suicide in the world.

*Reference*: Puri BK, Hall A, Ho R (2014). *Revision Notes in Psychiatry*. London: CRC Press, p. 286.

**Question 86 Answer: b, The peak age of offending is around 15 years in boys**
*Explanation*: All of the aforementioned statements are true, with the exception of (b). The peak age of offending is around 17–18 years in boys.

*Reference*: Puri BK, Hall A, Ho R (2014). *Revision Notes in Psychiatry*. London: CRC Press, p. 719.

**Question 87 Answer: b, One in four men and one in 10 women have been estimated to have depressive disorder in their lifetime.**
*Explanation*: Based on epidemiological studies, it has been estimated that one in four women and one in 10 men will have depressive disorder in their lifetime.

*Reference*: Puri BK, Hall A, Ho R (2014). *Revision Notes in Psychiatry*. London: CRC Press, p. 285.

**Question 88 Answer: c, DTBNP2**
*Explanation*: It should be DTBNP1 (dystrobrevin-binding protein 1).

*Reference*: Puri BK, Hall A, Ho R (2014). *Revision Notes in Psychiatry*. London: CRC Press, p. 357.

**Question 89 Answer: d, There is increased duration of slow-wave sleep.**
*Explanation*: With ageing, there is decreased duration of slow-wave sleep, sleep efficacy as well as the total sleep time.

*Reference*: Puri BK, Hall A, Ho R (2014). *Revision Notes in Psychiatry*. London: CRC Press, p. 679.

**Question 90 Answer: b, The mortality rate in men with schizophrenia is half that of women with schizophrenia.**
*Explanation*: Based on current literature, the mortality rate in men with schizophrenia has been estimated to be twice that of women with the similar condition.

*Reference*: Puri BK, Hall A, Ho R (2014). *Revision Notes in Psychiatry*. London: CRC Press, p. 281.

**Question 91 Answer: e, 80%**
*Explanation*: EPSE emerge when around 80% of the D2 receptors in the nigrostriatal pathway are blocked.

*Reference*: Puri BK, Hall A, Ho R (2014). *Revision Notes in Psychiatry*. London: CRC Press, p. 224.

**Question 92 Answer: e, 30%**
*Explanation*: 30% of suicide occurs on the ward, with the most common method being hanging.

*Reference*: Puri BK, Hall A, Ho R (2014). *Revision Notes in Psychiatry*. London: CRC Press, p. 288.

**Question 93 Answer: e, 80%**
*Explanation*: Approximately 80% of patients are able to achieve stable remission within 1 year.

*Reference*: Puri BK, Hall A, Ho R (2014). *Revision Notes in Psychiatry*. London: CRC Press, p. 369.

**Question 94 Answer: e, 35%**
*Explanation*: The conversion rate to schizophrenia has been estimated to be around 35% for those who are prodromal.

*Reference*: Puri BK, Hall A, Ho R (2014). *Revision Notes in Psychiatry*. London: CRC Press, p. 369.

**Question 95 Answer: b, Broca's area**
*Explanation*: Damage to the Broca's area will result in the loss of rhythm, intonation and grammatical aspects of speech. Comprehension is still normal, and the patient is

aware that his or her speech is difficult for others to follow, thus resulting in marked distress and frustration.

*Reference*: Puri BK, Hall A, Ho R (2014). *Revision Notes in Psychiatry*. London: CRC Press, p. 105.

### Question 96 Answer: a, Extinction

*Explanation*: This is based on the concept of extinction. Extinction refers to the gradual disappearance of a conditioned response when the conditioned stimulus has been repeatedly presented without the unconditioned stimulus.

*Reference*: Puri BK, Hall A, Ho R (2014). *Revision Notes in Psychiatry*. London: CRC Press, p. 26.

### Question 97 Answer: a, Transference

*Explanation*: This is an example of transference. Transference is an unconscious process in which the patient transfers to the therapist feelings, emotions and attitudes that were experienced previously.

*Reference*: Puri BK, Hall A, Ho R (2014). *Revision Notes in Psychiatry*. London: CRC Press, p. 132.

### Question 98 Answer: a, Male gender

*Explanation*: Based on previous research, all of the aforementioned are predisposing psychosocial factors. However, females tend to be more affected than males.

*Reference*: Puri BK, Hall A, Ho R (2014). *Revision Notes in Psychiatry*. London: CRC Press, p. 427.

### Question 99 Answer: e, 3.0%

*Explanation*: The definition for severe mental retardation will include those whose IQ range is between 20 and 34. This affects around 3% of those who have learning disability.

*Reference*: Puri BK, Hall A, Ho R (2014). *Revision Notes in Psychiatry*. London: CRC Press, p. 659.

### Question 100 Answer: b, Repetition

*Explanation*: It is the region of the brain that is responsible for transmission of information between the Wernicke's area and the Broca's area. A lesion involving that area would cause repetition to be impaired, but with preserved functioning in terms of fluency, comprehension and naming.

*Reference*: Puri BK, Hall A, Ho R (2014). *Revision Notes in Psychiatry*. London: CRC Press, p. 105.

**Question 101 Answer: c, The peak age of substance misuse is 15 years**
*Explanation*: The peak age of substance misuse is 15 years based on existing epidemiological studies.

*Reference*: Puri BK, Hall A, Ho R (2014). *Revision Notes in Psychiatry*. London: CRC Press, p. 298.

**Question 102 Answer: e, Bereavement**
*Explanation*: Bereavement is not one of the predisposing factors that would predispose an individual to depressive disorder.

*Reference*: Puri BK, Hall A, Ho R (2014). *Revision Notes in Psychiatry*. London: CRC Press, p. 284.

**Question 103 Answer: e, Tourette's syndrome**
*Explanation*: Habit reversal is an effective technique for Tourette's syndrome. It involves performing simultaneous incompatible movements to reduce the unwanted movements.

*Reference*: Puri BK, Hall A, Ho R (2014). *Revision Notes in Psychiatry*. London: CRC Press, p. 637.

**Question 104 Answer: a, Wernicke's area**
*Explanation*: It is important to note that damage to the Wernicke's area would disrupt the ability to comprehend language, either written or spoken. The patient also is unaware that his or her dysphasic speech is difficult for others to comprehend

*Reference*: Puri BK, Hall A, Ho R (2014). *Revision Notes in Psychiatry*. London: CRC Press, p. 105.

**Question 105 Answer: b, The estimated 1-year prevalence for adults could range to as high as 60%.**
*Explanation*: The estimated 1-year prevalence in adults usually range between 15 and 40%.

*Reference*: Puri BK, Hall A, Ho R (2014). *Revision Notes in Psychiatry*. London: CRC Press, p. 609.

**Question 106 Answer: e, 3%**
*Explanation*: The prevalence of people with learning disabilities who also have schizophrenia has been estimated to be around 3%. This is much higher than the average prevalence in the general population. It has been noted that the prevalence of schizophrenia is inversely related to the intelligence quotient (IQ). More importantly, a diagnosis of schizophrenia cannot be made if the IQ is considered to be less than 45.

*Reference*: Puri BK, Hall A, Ho R (2014). *Revision Notes in Psychiatry*. London: CRC Press, p. 670.

### Question 107 Answer: b, Right parietal lobe

*Explanation*: It is essential to note that visuospatial elements are being perceived together into complete perceptions in the right parietal lobe. A lesion at the level of the right parietal lobe would result in apperceptive agnosia. Hence, the individual would not be able to copy shapes or discriminate between two versions of the same objects. In addition, he is not able to name the object when he or she sees it or touches it.

*Reference*: Puri BK, Hall A, Ho R (2014). *Revision Notes in Psychiatry*. London: CRC Press, p. 106.

### Question 108 Answer: e, Vacuolation of the glial cells

*Explanation*: Microscopy of the brain materials reveals vacuolar changes in the grey matter particularly in cerebral and cerebellar cortex, creating characteristic spongiform changes.

*Further Reading*: Puri BK, Treasaden I (eds) (2010). *Psychiatry: An Evidence-Based Text*. London: Hodder Arnold, pp. 571–573, 1101.

### Question 109 Answer: e, *Tau* gene on chromosome 17

*Explanation*: 50% of cases are caused by autosomal dominant inheritance of the tau gene on chromosome 17. This results in abnormal insoluble tau isoforms which accumulate in the neurons and the glia.

*Further Reading*: Puri BK, Treasaden I (eds) (2010). *Psychiatry: An Evidence-Based Text*. London: Hodder Arnold, pp. 95, 438, 463, 1107.

### Question 110 Answer: b, 10%–15%

*Explanation*: The conversion rate to dementia has been estimated to be around 10% per year.

*Reference and Further Reading*: Petersen RC, Doody R, Kurz A, et al. (2001). Current concepts in mild cognitive impairment. *Archives of Neurology*, 58: 1985–1992; Puri BK, Treasaden I (eds) (2010). *Psychiatry: An Evidence-Based Text*. London: Hodder Arnold, pp. 524, 1103.

### Question 111 Answer: c, Mu opioid receptor

*Explanation*: It is known to be a partial mu opioid agonist.

*Reference and Further Reading*: Ho RCM, Chen KY, Broekman B, Mak A (2009). Buprenorphine prescription, misuse and service provision: A global perspective. *Advances in Psychiatric Treatment*, 15: 354–363; Puri BK, Treasaden I (eds) (2010). *Psychiatry: An Evidence-Based Text*. London: Hodder Arnold, pp. 717, 1037, 1039–1040.

**Question 112 Answer: e, *Progranulin* gene**
*Explanation*: Progranulin is a growth factor protein and its genetic locus deletion is associated with frontotemporal dementia.

*Reference and Further Reading*: Gijselinck I, van der Zee J, Engelborghs S (2008). Progranulin locus deletion in frontotemporal dementia. *Human Mutation*, 29: 53–58; Puri BK, Treasaden I (eds) (2010). *Psychiatry: An Evidence-Based Text*. London: Hodder Arnold, pp. 507, 1107.

**Question 113 Answer: b, This bias occurs when comparisons are made between groups of participants that differ with respect to determinants of outcome other than those understudy.**
*Explanation*:
  Option (a) refers to selection bias.
  Option (c) refers to measurement bias.
  Option (d) refers to recall bias.
  Option (e) refers to Neyman bias.

*Further Reading*: Puri BK, Treasaden I (eds) (2010). *Psychiatry: An Evidence-Based Text*. London: Hodder Arnold, pp. 43, 72, 74, 75, 86.

**Question 114 Answer: b, Phentolamine**
*Explanation*: This lady suffers from hypertensive crisis owing to consumption of food containing high levels of tyramine.

*Further Reading*: Puri BK, Treasaden I (eds) (2010). *Psychiatry: An Evidence-Based Text*. London: Hodder Arnold, pp. 425, 426, 708, 907.

**Question 115 Answer: e, CGG repeats**
*Explanation*: This child suffers from fragile X syndrome.

*Further Reading*: Puri BK, Treasaden I (eds) (2010). *Psychiatry: An Evidence-Based Text*. London: Hodder Arnold, pp. 1082, 1088, 1091.

**Question 116 Answer: e, Atrophy of medial temporal lobe**

*Reference and Further Reading*: Duara R, Loewenstein DA, Potter E, et al. (2008). Medial temporal lobe atrophy on MRI scans and the diagnosis of Alzheimer disease. *Neurology*, 71: 1986–1992; Puri BK, Treasaden I (eds) (2010). Psychiatry: An Evidence-Based Text. London: Hodder Arnold, pp. 1103–1104.

**Question 117 Answer: e, Pseudo-irreversible acetylcholinesterase and butyryl-cholinesterase inhibitor**
*Explanation*:
  Option (d) refers to tacrine.
  Option (a) refers to donepezil and galantamine.

*Further Reading*: Puri BK,Treasaden I (eds) (2010). *Psychiatry: An Evidence-Based Text*. London: Hodder Arnold, pp. 906, 1104, 1106.

**Question 118 Answer: a, Difficulty concentrating**
*Explanation*: Options (b) to (e) are risk factors for early-onset (ages 6–11 years) delinquent behaviour.

*Reference and Further Reading*: Office of the Surgeon General. 2001. *Youth Violence: A Report of the Surgeon General*. Washington, DC: U.S. Department of Health and Human Services, Office of the Secretary, Office of Public Health and Science, Office of the Surgeon General .Retrieved from: www.surgeongeneral.gov/library/youthviolence; Puri BK,Treasaden I (eds) (2010). *Psychiatry: An Evidence-Based Text*. London: Hodder Arnold, pp. 1156–1157.

# Extended Matching Items (EMIs)

**Question 119 Answer: j, Hoarding obsession, m, Saving compulsion**

**Question 120 Answer: g, Checking compulsion, j, Hoarding obsession**

**Question 121 Answer: b, Contamination obsession (45%)**

**Question 122 Answer: g, Checking compulsion (63%)**
*Explanation*: The most common obsessions (in descending order) are fear of contamination, doubting, fear of illness, germs or bodily fear, symmetry and sexual or aggressive thoughts. The most common compulsions are checking, washing and counting.

*References:* Rufer M, Fricke S, Moritz S, Kloss M, Hand I (2006). Symptom dimensions in obsessive-compulsive disorder: Prediction of cognitive-behavior therapy outcome. *Acta Psychiatric Scandinavia*, 113: 440–446; Mataix-Cols D, Wooderson S, Lawerence N, Brammer MJ, Speckens A, Phillips ML (2004). Distinct neural correlates of washing, checking and hoarding symptom dimensions in obsessive-compulsive disorder. *Archives of General Psychiatry*, 61: 564–576; Saxena S, Maidment KM, Vapnik , et al. (2002). Obsessive-compulsive hoarding: Symptom severity and response to multimodal treatment. *Journal of Clinical Psychiatry*, 63: 21–27.

**Question 123 Answer: b, Acting out**
*Explanation*: Acting out is enacting an unconscious wish or fantasy impulsively as a way of avoiding painful affect.

*Reference*: Puri BK,Treasaden I (eds) (2010). *Psychiatry: An Evidence-Based Text*. London: Hodder Arnold, pp. 940, 948–949.

**Question 124 Answer: u, Undoing**

*Explanation*: Undoing is an attempt to negate sexual, aggressive or shameful implications from a previous comment or behaviour by elaborating, clarifying or doing the opposite.

**Question 125 Answer: n, Rationalization**

*Explanation*: Rationalization refers to the justification of unacceptable attitudes, beliefs or behaviours and making them tolerable to oneself.

**Question 126 Answer: g, Idealization, r, Splitting**

*Explanation*: Idealization refers to the attribution of perfect or near-perfect qualities to others as a way of avoiding anxiety or negative feelings.

Splitting is compartmentalizing experiences of self and others such that integration is not possible.

**Question 127 Answer: b, Acting out, d, Denial, g, Idealization, l, Projection, m, Projective identification, q, Regression, r, Splitting**

*Explanation*: Melanie Klein described projection and splitting but not denial.

**Question 128 Answer: q, Regression**

*Explanation*: Regression refers to an earlier phase or functioning to avoid the conflicts and tensions associated with current situation.

**Question 129 Answer: m, Projective identification**

*Explanation*: Projective identification has two phases: (1) the client first projected an internal object (i.e. uncaring parents in this case) to the consultant; (2) then, pressure is placed on the consultant to take on characteristics of the uncaring parents.

*Reference*: Puri BK,Treasaden I (eds) (2010). *Psychiatry: An Evidence-Based Text*. London: Hodder Arnold, pp. 949–950, 979.

## Theme: Advanced psychology

**Question 130 Answer: k, Isolation of affect**

*Explanation*: Isolation of affect refers to the separation of an idea from its associated affect to avoid emotional turmoil.

**Question 131 Answer: t, Suppression**

*Explanation*: Suppression refers to conscious effort not to attend to the certain state, feeling or impulse. On the other hand, repression refers to blockage or expulsion of unacceptable ideas or impulses in the inner states from entering the consciousness.

**Question 132 Answer: i, Intellectualization**

*Explanation*: Intellectualization refers to the excessive use of abstract ideation to avoid difficult feelings.

**Question 133 Answer: h, Identification**
*Explanation*: Identification refers to internalization of the qualities of another person by behaving like that person.

**Question 134 Answer: j, Introjection**
*Explanation*: Introjection means internalizing aspects of a significant person as a way of dealing with the loss of that person.

**Question 135 Answer: o, Reaction formation**
*Explanation*: Reaction formation refers to the transformation of an unacceptable wish or impulse into its opposite.

## Theme: Neuroanatomy – occipital lobes lesions

**Question 136 Answer: a, Dorsal and adjourning parietal lesion**
*Explanation*: The clinical features are representative of the Balint's syndrome. This is usually due to lesions of the dorsal region and the adjoining parietal regions.

**Question 137 Answer: c, Left ventral lesions**
*Explanation*: Lesions of the left ventral region (inferior to the calcarine fissure) could lead to contralateral (right) acquired (central) hemiachromatopsia and acquired dyslexia.

**Question 138 Answer: b, Bilateral dorsal lesions**
*Explanation*: A bilateral occipital dorsal lesion could lead to the aforementioned clinical features.

**Question 139 Answer: d, Right ventral lesions**
*Explanation*: Lesions of the right ventral region could lead to contralateral (left) acquired hemiachromatopsia and apperceptive visual agnosia.

*Reference*: Puri BK, Hall A, Ho R (2014). *Revision Notes in Psychiatry*. London: CRC Press, p. 216.

## Theme: Neurophysiology

**Question 140 Answer: f, GH**
*Explanation*: GH is a peptide hormone that stimulates the hepatic secretion of IGF-1. In turn, binding of IGF-1 to widespread IGF-binding proteins leads to stimulation of anabolism.

**Question 141 Answer: e, Prolactin**
*Explanation*: Prolactin is a single-chain peptide hormone that acts on the mammary glands to stimulate the secretion of milk (normally during lactation). It also inhibits the activity of the testes and the ovaries.

**Question 142 Answer: b, FSH**
*Explanation*: This hormone, in males, also stimulates the release of inhibin A and inhibin B.

**Question 143 Answer: c, LH**
*Explanation*: LH consists of two peptide chains; the alpha chain is the same as that of the FSH. LH also stimulates the gonads (ovaries and testes).

**Question 144 Answer: i, Oxytocin**
*Explanation*: This hormone is a nonapeptide that stimulates the contraction of the uterine myometrium during parturition. In addition, it also stimulates the ejection of milk from the mammary glands during lactation.

*Reference*: Puri BK, Hall A, Ho R (2014). *Revision Notes in Psychiatry*. London: CRC Press, pp. 211–212.

## Theme: Neurophysiology – EEG and effects of drugs
**Question 145 Answer: c, Increased beta activity and b, decreased alpha activity**
*Explanation*: They tend to cause an increase in the beta activity and a corresponding decrease in the alpha activity (sometimes).

**Question 146 Answer: e, Increased delta activity**
*Explanation*: Antidepressants tend to cause an increase in delta activity.

**Question 147 Answer: d, Decreased beta activity and e, increased delta activity**
*Explanation*: Antipsychotic drugs could cause a decrease in beta activity as well as an increased in low-frequency delta activity and/or theta activity.

*Reference*: Puri BK, Hall A, Ho R (2014). *Revision Notes in Psychiatry*. London: CRC Press, p. 217.

## Theme: Neurophysiology – sleep
**Question 148 Answer: b, Decreased complexity of dreams, c, decreased recall of dreams, d, upwards ocular deviation, and e, decreased cerebral blood flow**
*Explanation*: The characteristic features of NREM sleep include decreased recall of dreaming, decreased complexity of dreams, increased parasympathetic tone, upward ocular deviation with few or no movements, abolition of tendon reflexes, decreased heart rate, decreased systolic blood pressure, decreased respiratory rate and decreased cerebral blood flow. The penis is not usually erect as well.

**Question 149 Answer: a, Increased complexity of dreams, f, occasional myoclonic jerks, and g, increased penile erection**
*Explanation*: The characteristic features include increased recall of dreaming, increased complexity of dreams, increased sympathetic activity, transient runs of conjugate ocular movements, maximal loss of muscle tone, increased heart rate, increased systolic blood pressure, increased respiratory rate and increased cerebral blood flow. There will also be penile erection or increased vaginal blood flow. In rat brains, increased protein synthesis is noted.

*Reference*: Puri BK, Hall A, Ho R (2014). *Revision Notes in Psychiatry*. London: CRC Press, p. 216.

## Theme: Neurochemical and common disorders

**Question 150 Answer: a, Decreased dopamine in mesocortical pathway, and d, increased dopamine in mesolimbic pathway**

*Explanation*: In schizophrenia, there is a reduction in the dopamine in the mesocortical pathway and this causes anergy and loss of drive (predominantly the negative symptoms). The dopamine hypothesis proposes that increased levels of DA or DA receptors could cause schizophrenia. Galactorrhoea is seen in antipsychotic treatment as a result of the blockade of DA receptors.

**Question 151 Answer: e, Increased dopamine in the nigrostriatal pathway**

*Explanation*: In this condition (OCD), there is noted to be an increase in dopamine in the nigrostriatal pathway. This is, in turn, responsible for the development of compulsive behaviour.

**Question 152 Answer: e, Increased dopamine in the nigrostriatal pathway, and h, increased CSF HVA levels**

*Explanation*: The increased dopamine would cause an increased in sensory stimuli and movement. There is also, in turn, an increase in the CSF HVA levels in manic patients.

*Reference*: Puri BK, Hall A, Ho R (2014). *Revision Notes in Psychiatry*. London: CRC Press, p. 223.

## Theme: Genetics (I)

**Question 153 Answer: h, Chromosome 22**

*Explanation*: Chromosome 22 is associated with DiGeorge syndrome. In addition, it also codes for the COMT gene, which is implicated in schizophrenia and bipolar disorder.

**Question 154 Answer: a, Chromosome 2**

*Explanation*: Chromosome 2q and Chromosome 7 have been implicated in autism.

**Question 155 Answer: d, Chromosome 13**

*Explanation*: There has been an association between Wilson's disease and this particular chromosome as well.

**Question 156 Answer: e, Chromosome 15**

*Explanation*: Angelman's syndrome is due to a maternal chromosome 15 microdeletion, whereas Prader–Willi syndrome is due to a paternal chromosome 15 microdeletion.

**Question 157 Answer: g, Chromosome 20**

*Explanation*: Chromosome 20 has been implicated in inherited CJD.

*Reference*: Puri BK, Hall A, Ho R (2014). *Revision Notes in Psychiatry*. London: CRC Press, p. 260.

## Theme: Genetics (II)

**Question 158 Answer: a, Substitution mutations**
*Explanation*: Substitution mutations could result in silent, missense or nonsense mutations.

**Question 159 Answer: c, Transversion mutation**
*Explanation*: A tranversion mutation causes a change from a purine to a pyrimidine or a pyrimidine to a purine.

**Question 160 Answer: b, Transition mutation**
*Explanation*: In a transition mutation, the change is usually from a purine to a purine or a pyrimidine to a pyrimidine.

**Question 161 Answer: f, Nonsense mutation**
*Explanation*: A nonsense mutation would result in the creation of a stop codon, thus resulting in the premature termination of a protein that is being synthesized.

**Question 162 Answer: g, Frameshift mutation**
*Explanation*: If the number of nucleotides deleted or inserted in an exon involves multiples of three, then the sequence of codons or the reading frame is preserved. If it does not, the reading frame will be disrupted and this would result in a frameshift mutation with a truncated protein product.

*Reference*: Puri BK, Hall A, Ho R (2014). *Revision Notes in Psychiatry*. London: CRC Press, p. 263.

## Theme: Advanced psychological process and treatment

**Question 163 Answer: h, Family therapy**
*Explanation*: Behavioural control problems such as conduct disorder in a child are an internal indication for family-based therapy. Family therapy helps to engage the family to deliver behaviour therapy in a home environment.

**Question 164 Answer: g, Interpersonal therapy**
*Explanation*: Research has indicated that interpersonal therapy for depressive disorder is equally effective as CBT. In addition, it is also indicated for eating disorder such as bulimia nervosa. Dysthymia disorder is another indication. Other issues that would render such a therapy useful include interpersonal disputes, role transition, grief as well as dealing with loss.

**Question 165 Answer: e, Mentalization-based treatment**
*Explanation*: Mentalization refers to psychological minded and empathy. It is developed in people who have responsive parents providing secure attachment in childhood. Patients with BPD have impaired mentalization. As a result, they are not able to interpret their actions or others' actions based on intentional mental states such as beliefs, feelings and preferences. Impaired mentalization is associated with affect dysregulation and incoherent sense of self.

**Question 166 Answer: f, Cognitive analytic therapy**
*Explanation*: Traps refers to repetitive cycles of behaviour and their consequences that become perpetuation. Dilemma refers to false choices or unduly narrowed options. Snag refers to extreme pessimism about the future and halts a plan before it even starts.

**Question 167 Answer: c, Cognitive behavioural therapy**
*Explanation*: The theory states that the fear of a specific stimulus is acquired through classical conditioning and the client tries to reduce fear by avoiding the conditioned stimulus through operant conditioning. The cognitive component is based on Beck's cognitive model of depression that includes the effect of early experiences, core beliefs, underlying assumptions, cognitive distortions, automatic thoughts and the negative cognitive triad.

**Question 168 Answer: b, Brief dynamic psychotherapy**
*Explanation*: In resistance, the client is ambivalent about getting help and may even oppose attempts from the therapist who offers help. Resistance may manifest in the form of silence, avoidance or absences. In acting out, it refers to the poor containment of strong feelings triggered by the therapy. In acting in, it refers to the exploration of the therapist's personal and private information by the client or presenting a symbolic gift to the therapist. Negative therapeutic reaction refers to the sudden and unexpected deterioration or regression in apparent progression during therapy.

*Reference*: Puri BK, Hall A, Ho R (2014). *Revision Notes in Psychiatry*. London: CRC Press, pp. 331–336.

## Theme: Psychiatric epidemiology (I)

**Question 169 Answer: a, Positive predictive value**
*Explanation*: The predictive value of a positive test result is the proportion of the positive result that is truly positive.

**Question 170 Answer: b, Negative predictive value**
*Explanation*: This refers to the proportion of the negative results that is truly negative.

**Question 171 Answer: c, Screen prevalence**
*Explanation*: This is known as screen prevalence or also as disease prevalence and test accuracy.

*Reference*: Puri BK, Hall A, Ho R (2014). *Revision Notes in Psychiatry*. London: CRC Press, p. 278.

## Theme: Psychiatric epidemiology (II)

**Question 172 Answer: h, Neonatal mortality rate**
*Explanation*: The estimated neonatal mortality rate is 3.4/1000 in the United Kingdom.

**Question 173 Answer: g, Postnatal mortality rate**

*Explanation*: The aforementioned definition is that of the postnatal mortality rate.

**Question 174 Answer: d, Case fatality rate**

*Explanation*: It should be noted that the typical reference period for this is usually within a specified time period.

**Question 175 Answer: a, Crude mortality rate**

*Explanation*: The crude mortality rate refers to the number of deaths over the midyear population.

*Reference*: Puri BK, Hall A, Ho R (2014). *Revision Notes in Psychiatry*. London: CRC Press, p. 280.

# INDEX